SYNOPSIS OF
CLINICAL PULMONARY
DISEASE

SYNOPSIS OF
CLINICAL PULMONARY DISEASE

Edited by

ROGER S. MITCHELL, M.D.

Professor of Medicine Emeritus; formerly Director,
Webb-Waring Lung Institute; Head, Division of Pulmonary Sciences; and
Chief of Staff, Veterans Administration Medical Center,
University of Colorado Health Sciences Center,
Denver, Colorado

THOMAS L. PETTY, M.D.

Professor of Medicine and Anesthesia and
Head, Division of Pulmonary Sciences,
University of Colorado Health Sciences Center,
Denver, Colorado

THIRD EDITION

with **89** *illustrations*

The C. V. Mosby Company

ST. LOUIS • TORONTO • LONDON   1982

MOSBY

A TRADITION OF PUBLISHING EXCELLENCE

Editor: John E. Lotz
Manuscript editor: Ann Calandro
Design: Susan Trail
Production: Ginny Douglas

THIRD EDITION

The C.V. Mosby Company
11830 Westline Industrial Drive, St. Louis, Missouri 63141

Library of Congress Cataloging in Publication Data

Main entry under title:

Synopsis of clinical pulmonary disease.

  Bibliography: p.
  Includes index.
  1. Lungs—Diseases. I. Mitchell, Roger S.
II. Petty, Thomas L. [DNLM: 1. Lung diseases.
WF 600 S993]
RC756.S94   1982   616.2′4   81-14154
ISBN 0-8016-3474-1   AACR2

AC/D/D 9 8 7 6 5 4 3 2 1   01/B/056

CONTRIBUTORS

DARRYL D. BINDSCHADLER, M.D.

Associate Clinical Professor of Medicine,
University of Colorado Health Sciences Center,
Denver, Colorado; now of Cheyenne, Wyoming

REUBEN M. CHERNIACK, M.D.

Chairman, Department of Medicine,
National Jewish Hospital; Professor and
Vice-Chairman, Department of Medicine,
University of Colorado Health Sciences Center,
Denver, Colorado

PAUL T. DAVIDSON, M.D.

Assistant Professor of Medicine,
National Jewish Hospital,
University of Colorado Health Sciences Center,
Denver, Colorado

ROBERT B. DREISIN, M.D.

Assistant Professor of Medicine,
National Jewish Hospital,
University of Colorado Health Sciences Center,
Denver, Colorado

JAMES H. ELLIS, Jr., M.D.

Associate Clinical Professor of Medicine and
Chief, Pulmonary Department,
Rose Medical Center,
University of Colorado Health Sciences Center,
Denver, Colorado

ENRIQUE FERNANDEZ, M.D.

Assistant Professor of Medicine,
National Jewish Hospital,
University of Colorado Health Sciences Center,
Denver, Colorado

JAMES T. GOOD, Jr., M.D.

Assistant Professor of Medicine,
Denver General Hospital,
University of Colorado Health Sciences Center,
Denver, Colorado

FREDERICK N. HANSON, M.D.

Senior Fellow in Pulmonary Medicine,
Cardiovascular-Pulmonary Research
Laboratory, University of
Colorado Health Sciences Center,
Denver, Colorado

RUTH N. HARADA, M.D.

Assistant Professor of Medicine,
Webb-Waring Lung Institute,
University of Colorado Health Sciences Center,
Denver, Colorado

DAVID W. HUDGEL, M.D.

Assistant Professor of Medicine,
National Jewish Hospital,
University of Colorado Health Sciences Center,
Denver, Colorado

THOMAS M. HYERS, M.D.

Assistant Professor of Medicine,
Veterans Administration Medical Center,
University of Colorado Health Sciences Center,
Denver, Colorado

MICHAEL D. ISEMAN, M.D.

Associate Professor of Medicine and
Associate Director, Pulmonary Medicine
Service, Denver General Hospital,
University of Colorado Health Sciences Center,
Denver, Colorado

TALMADGE E. KING, Jr., M.D.

Assistant Professor of Medicine,
Veterans Administration Medical Center,
University of Colorado Health Sciences Center,
Denver, Colorado

ROGER S. MITCHELL, M.D.

Professor of Medicine Emeritus; formerly
Director, Webb-Waring Lung Institute;
Head, Division of Pulmonary Sciences; and
Chief of Staff, Veterans Administration
Medical Center, University of Colorado
Health Sciences Center,
Denver, Colorado

THOMAS A. NEFF, M.D.

Associate Professor of Medicine and Chief,
Pulmonary Service, Denver General Hospital,
University of Colorado Health Sciences Center,
Denver, Colorado

THOMAS L. PETTY, M.D.

Professor of Medicine and Anesthesia and
Head, Division of Pulmonary Sciences,
University of Colorado Health Sciences Center,
Denver, Colorado

JOHN E. REPINE, M.D.

Associate Professor of Medicine and Assistant
Director, Webb-Waring Lung Institute,
University of Colorado Health Sciences Center,
Denver, Colorado

LAWRENCE H. REPSHER, M.D.

Associate Clinical Professor of Medicine,
Lutheran Medical Center, University of
Colorado Health Sciences Center,
Denver, Colorado

STEVEN A. SAHN, M.D.

Associate Professor of Medicine,
University Hospital, University of
Colorado Health Sciences Center,
Denver, Colorado

JOHN A. SBARBARO, M.D.

Associate Professor of Medicine and Deputy
Director, Department of Health and Hospitals,
University of Colorado Health Sciences Center,
Denver, Colorado

MARVIN I. SCHWARZ, M.D.

Associate Professor of Medicine and
Chief, Pulmonary Medicine,
Veterans Administration Medical Center,
University of Colorado Health Sciences Center,
Denver, Colorado

CHARLES SCOGGIN, M.D.

Associate Professor of Medicine,
University Hospital, University of
Colorado Health Sciences Center,
Denver, Colorado

MICHAEL SHASBY, M.D.

Assistant Professor of Medicine,
University of Virginia School of Medicine,
Charlottesville, Virginia

RICHARD H. SIMON, M.D.

Senior Fellow in Pulmonary Medicine,
University Hospital, University of
Colorado Health Sciences Center,
Denver, Colorado

CHARLES W. VAN WAY III, M.D.

Associate Professor of Surgery and Chief,
Surgical Service, Denver General Hospital,
University of Colorado Health Sciences Center,
Denver, Colorado

H. DENNIS WAITE, M.D.

Assistant Clinical Professor of Medicine,
Rose Medical Center,
University of Colorado Health Sciences Center,
Denver, Colorado

FOREWORD

Pulmonary medicine has come a long way in the past 20 years. It seems incredible that 23 years ago as a senior medical student I chose an elective in pulmonary medicine with Dr. Mitchell. Very clearly, as I look back, this was the major force that kindled my interest in the fascinating field of pulmonary medicine. Since that time many medical students have sought elective training in pulmonary medicine at the University of Colorado Health Sciences Center. Currently over 50% of our graduating class and many students from other medical schools choose our elective in the senior year. Hopefully they all become "turned on" to the delights of the practice and science of pulmonary disease.

Thus, members of the Division of Pulmonary Sciences have been particularly dedicated to the task of revising chapters from the first two editions of this synopsis, or writing new chapters, with the hope that collectively we may be able to spark the imagination of many more undergraduate physicians, house officers, and colleagues in the allied health professions who will be tomorrow's servants for patients with diseases of the respiratory system.

I personally thank my former chief for his continued efforts in medical education in our field, particularly for the effort of this synopsis and all it means.

Thomas L. Petty

PREFACE

The first edition of this introduction to the intricacies of chest medicine, published in 1974, was sufficiently successful to prompt a second edition. This third edition is the result of a request from the publisher. In response to suggestions, the present volume goes into more detail, adds many illustrations, including both chest films and tabular material, and updates and expands the bibliographies.

As before, the intended audience for this book includes both undergraduate and postgraduate medical students and practitioners other than the pulmonary specialist.

All of the contributors have been members of the faculty of the University of Colorado Health Sciences Center, and all but one, a surgeon, are members of the Division of Pulmonary Sciences, Department of Medicine, to which all proceeds derived from the sale of this volume will again be donated.

I am very pleased to have my friend and colleague, Thomas L. Petty, join me in editing this third edition.

Roger S. Mitchell

CONTENTS

SYNOPSIS OF
CLINICAL PULMONARY
DISEASE

Chapter 1

LUNG STRUCTURE AS RELATED TO FUNCTION

Ruth N. Harada *and* **John E. Repine**

Human beings can live for weeks without food and days without water, but they cannot survive for more than a few minutes without oxygen. A continuous external supply of oxygen is essential for survival because no significant amount of oxygen is stored in the body.

RESPIRATORY SYSTEM FUNCTION

The major function of the respiratory system—the lungs—is to procure oxygen from the external environment and to eliminate carbon dioxide at rates required by tissue metabolism. The overall success of the lungs depends on a patent airway system, intact pulmonary parenchyma (including the vascular bed), adequate cardiac output, normal neuromuscular function, and intact central nervous system (CNS) ventilatory control. Other less obvious but equally important respiratory tract functions include the ability to generate airflow for speech, to act as a mechanical and immunologic sieve for noxious gases or inert and infectious particles in the environment, to degrade drugs and endogenous chemical substances, and to synthesize and secrete numerous proteins and lipids.

RESPIRATORY SYSTEM STRUCTURE

The respiratory tract consists of two basic parts: the *conducting airways* and the *respiratory unit* (Fig. 1-1). The conducting airways are passageways through which inspired air from the external environment reaches the alveoli; conversely, expired air from the alveoli is removed to the atmosphere. The upper airways consist of the nose, pharynx, and larynx; they warm and humidify air as well as remove aerosol particles. The *tracheobronchial tree*

1

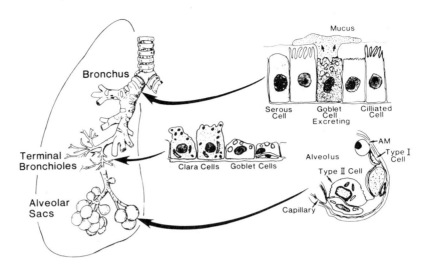

FIG. 1-1. Schematic gross and microscopic lung anatomy.

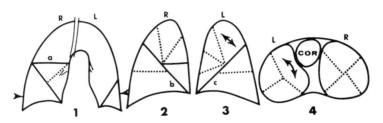

FIG. 1-2. Schematic lung segmental anatomy.

branches irregularly and provides increasing surface area at each branching. The 16 segmental bronchi arising at the tracheobronchial tree's third branching are conduits for anatomic segments of the lungs (Fig. 1-2). The walls of the airways—that is, the *trachea* and the *bronchi*—contain incomplete, cartilaginous, support rings that are lined with pseudostratified, ciliated, columnar epithelium interspersed with *goblet cells* and *mucous glands*.

The respiratory unit consists of the terminal bronchiole, respiratory bronchiole, alveolar ducts, and the alveoli. The alveolar ducts and alveoli are the functional area of gas exchange. The bronchiolar walls consist mainly of a few ciliated cells and many nonciliated cells called Clara cells. The alveoli are composed of two types of epithelial cells. Type I pneumocytes are simple squamous cells that form a thin layer over most of the alveolar wall and seem anatomically specialized to provide a slender barrier for gaseous diffusion.

Type II cells (granular pneumocytes) are metabolically active and elaborate surfactant, a lipoprotein that lines and stabilizes the inherently unstable alveolar surface. In addition, alveolar macrophages are normally found adherent to alveolar walls and are a major defense against inhaled particles and microorganisms.

MECHANICS OF RESPIRATION

Gas transfer between the external atmosphere and the internal gas phase of lung alveoli is accomplished through a "bellows" mechanism (i.e., the alternate expansion and contraction of a hollow chamber in communication with the atmosphere). In humans the *thoracic cage* is a hollow chamber able to expand in volume by contraction of the intercostal muscles, the diaphragm, and, to a lesser extent, the scalene and abdominal muscles. During expansion of the thoracic cage, intrapleural pressures become subatmospheric, causing air to enter the lung. In contrast, during expiration the intrapleural pressure becomes greater than the atmospheric pressure, and air leaves the lung. Expiration results from the intrinsic elastic recoil of the lung and the contraction and relaxation of various respiratory muscles. After fresh air enters the alveoli it is brought into contact with a thin membrane consisting of alveolar and capillary endothelial cells. At this location, a passive diffusion of oxygen and carbon dioxide takes place.

Factors that determine the rate of gas diffusion through the pulmonary membrane are as follows: (1) the greater the pressure difference across the membrane, the greater the rate of gas exchange, (2) the greater the area of pulmonary membrane (normal adults have an estimated 90 m² effective gas exchange surface), the greater the amount of diffusion, and (3) the thinner the pulmonary membrane, the greater the diffusion rate. Finally, note that the diffusion coefficient of a gas determines the amount of a given gas that dissolves in the membrane. This is important, since carbon dioxide is approximately 20 times more soluble than oxygen.

CONTROL OF BREATHING

The respiratory control system regulates a complex series of activities. It must maintain a rhythmic breathing pattern as well as adjust minute ventilation through changes in tidal volume and respiratory rate to meet the demands for gas exchange in the lung. This system must also adjust the breathing pattern during speech, change in posture, swallowing, and other activities.

Anatomically the respiratory centers have not been precisely defined, but they are believed to consist of neurons scattered throughout the cerebral cortex, pons, and medulla. Cerebral control is probably responsible for voluntary acts of breathing such as hyperventilation and breath holding. The involuntary breathing centers consist of neurons in the pons and medulla. The medullary oscillatory pattern is modulated by neural inputs from the cortex and pons and from peripheral and central chemoreceptors. Peripheral chemoreceptors are located at the bifurcation of the common carotid artery (carotid body), in proximity to the aortic arch (aortic body), and centrally in proximity to the medulla. Stimulation of these receptors increases the rate and depth of breathing. The most potent stimulus to chemoreceptors is hypoxemia (Pa_{O_2} less than 60 mm Hg). Hypercarbia, acidosis, decreased cardiac output, and hyperthermia also stimulate the chemoreceptors and thereby increase ventilation.

VENTILATION-PERFUSION RELATIONSHIPS

The job of pulmonary gas exchange is to bring air and blood into juxtaposition on either side of a thin diffusion membrane so that oxygen and carbon dioxide transfer can occur. Even in healthy people, however, neither all the "fresh" inspired air nor all the "stale" systemic venous blood reaches the effective exchange membrane. In disease states this inefficiency of ventilation, perfusion, or both may be greatly magnified.

The relationship of alveolar ventilation ($\dot{V}A$) to pulmonary capillary blood flow ($\dot{Q}c$) is called the ventilation-perfusion ratio (V/Q). Each gas exchange unit has its own V/Q ratio, and the sum of these ratios is the overall V/Q ratio of the lungs. V/Q abnormalities can arise as follows:

1. Inspired air can remain in the conducting airways; indeed, some of it normally does. This anatomic dead space consists of trachea, bronchi, and bronchioles and is approximately 150 cc, or one third of every tidal breath.
2. Inspired air can reach nonperfused alveoli.
3. Systemic venous blood can pass through anatomic channels that bypass alveoli.
4. Systemic venous blood can reach nonventilated alveoli.

Conditions 1 and 2 are *anatomic* and *physiologic dead space*, or *wasted*, ventilation. Conditions 3 and 4 are *anatomic* and *physiologic shunts*. Wasted ventilation implies adequate ventilation with decreased or absent perfusion; a shunt implies adequate blood flow with absent or decreased ventilation. A V/Q disturbance is the most common cause of hypoxemia in the absence of hypoxia or circulatory impairment.

PULMONARY VASCULATURE

The pulmonary circulation is unlike the systemic circulation because (1) the entire cardiac output passes through the lungs and (2) pulmonary circulation replenishes blood with oxygen rather than delivering oxygen to tissues. Another unique characteristic of the pulmonary circulation is the expansile nature of the pulmonary vasculature; venous pressure and vascular resistance are only one tenth that of the systemic circulation. A fivefold increase in pulmonary blood flow is associated with only a minimal increase in pulmonary arterial pressure. In experimental animal models 75% of the pulmonary vascular bed must be occluded before pulmonary hypertension develops. The presence of pulmonary hypertension therefore implies the existence of widespread vascular disease.

Hypoxia and acidosis can cause generalized or localized pulmonary arteriolar constriction. Poorly aerated areas of the lung develop hypoxemia and acidosis, which in turn lead to pulmonary vasoconstriction and decreased blood flow.

LUNG ACTIVITIES
Metabolic functions

Although the metabolic activities that occur in the lung are not unique, the lung is unique in that it filters the body's entire blood volume before blood enters the systemic circulation. It has recently been established that the lung has an important pharmacokinetic function: the cells and enzyme systems of the pulmonary vascular bed change the biologic activity of a variety of substances presented to them. Thus the pulmonary circulation is well suited to monitor and control levels of circulating hormones and biologically active substances and, consequently, to modify their effects on the arterial circulation. Just as the respiratory function adds oxygen and removes carbon dioxide from the lung, so the metabolic function adds angiotensin II, histamine, and prostaglandins and removes 5-hydroxytryptamine, bradykinin, and noradrenaline from the systemic circulation. Thus the lung has pharmacokinetic functions of uptake, storage, and enzymatic degradation as well as "endocrine" functions. Various stimuli have been shown to release vasoactive substances from the lung, including histamine, serotonin, vasoactive prostaglandins, and still-unidentified vasoactive lung peptides.

Immune functions

The respiratory tract exposes a total surface area of approximately 90 m² to approximately 10,000 L of ambient air every day. Ambient inspired air not only contains the oxygen vital to survival; it contains noxious gases and a multitude of particulates that the lungs must exclude to maintain good health.

The upper respiratory tract removes most noxious gases and particles, including potential pathogens. Small inhaled particles less than 5 μm may be deposited distal to ciliated epithelial portions of the tracheobronchial tree and enter the alveolar spaces. The mechanism of removal of many noxious gases and particulates in the upper respiratory tract is the *mucociliary escalator*. Most of the noxious gases and large particles are absorbed in the mucous lining of the upper airways and tracheobronchial tree; they are eventually coughed up or swallowed through rhythmic and unidirectional beating of the cilia.

When a particle or gas enters the alveolar spaces, a different clearance apparatus takes over. In the alveolus, the resident phagocytic cell—the alveolar macrophage—and immunoglobulins and enzymes inactivate and remove particles by way of the mucociliary escalator or through lymphatic channels. When local defenses fail, chemical mediators from the inflamed part of the lung can recruit polymorphonuclear leukocytes and other cellular and humoral factors from the blood. Interestingly, recent evidence indicates that many of these mechanisms that usually protect the lung against infection may, under such circumstances as cigarette smoking, environmental exposure, or allergy, mediate lung damage.

· · ·

In summary, the lung mediates not only gas exchange, but also regulates numerous immunologic and biochemical functions. Abnormalities in the lung's various structures and/or functions and how they contribute to various lung disorders will be described in subsequent chapters.

LUNG SEGMENTAL ANATOMY (Fig. 1-2)

In view 1 the horizontal fissure *(a)* separates the right upper lobe from the right middle lobe, the dotted line separates the two segments of the right middle lobe (medial and lateral), and the two diagonal lines near the base mark the lateral and inferior margins of the right middle lobe and the left upper lobe, respectively.

In view 2, a lateral view of the right lung, the long (diagonal) fissure *(b)* separates the right lower lobe from the right upper and middle lobes. The dotted lines in the right upper lobe demarcate its three segments (anterior, apical, and posterior); the dotted line in the right lower lobe identifies the superior segment of the right lower lobe.

In view 3, a lateral view of the left lung, the long (diagonal) fissure *(c)* separates the left upper lobe from the left lower lobe; the dotted lines show the left upper lobe segments (apical posterior [the fusion indicated by the double arrow], anterior, superior lingular, and inferior lingular); and the superior segment of the left lower lobe is again identified.

In view 4, a horizontal section at the level noted by the two markers in view 1, the basal segments of both lower lobes are identified—on the right are the medial, lateral, anterior, and posterior basal, and on the left the anteromedial basal fusion is again identified by a double arrow.

Segmental anomalies are not uncommon.

Atelectasis of the right middle lobe may be seen on the lateral projection as an angulated linear shadow; atelectasis of the upper and lower lobes may be seen on the posteroanterior projection as linear shadows, except when held laterally by dense pleural adhesions.

SUGGESTED READINGS

Bakhle, Y.S., and Vane, J.R., editors: Metabolic functions of the lung, New York City, 1977, Marcel Dekker, Inc.

Bates, D.V., Macklem, P.T., and Christie, R.V.: Respiratory function in disease: an introduction to the integrated study of the lung, ed. 2, Philadelphia, 1971, W.B. Saunders Co.

Bouhuys, A.: Breathing: physiology, environment and lung disease, New York City, 1974, Grune & Stratton, Inc.

Brain, J.D., Proctor, D.I., and Reid, L.M., editors: Respiratory defense mechanisms, New York City, 1977, Marcel Dekker, Inc.

Crystal, R.G., editor: The biochemical basis of pulmonary function, New York City, 1976, Marcel Dekker, Inc.

Davies, D.G., and Barnes, C.D., editors: Regulation of ventilation and gas exchange, New York City, 1978, Academic Press, Inc.

Fishman, A.P.: Pulmonary disease and disorders, New York City, 1980, McGraw-Hill Book Co.

Grodins, F.S., and Yamashiro, S.M.: Respiratory function of the lung and its control, New York City, 1978, Macmillan Publishing Co., Inc.

Junod, A.F., and deHaller, R., editors: Lung metabolism, New York City, 1975, Academic Press, Inc.

Kirkpatrick, C.H., and Reynolds, H.F., editors: Immunologic and infectious reactions in the lung, New York City, 1976, Marcel Dekker, Inc.

Murray, J.F.: The normal lung, Philadelphia, 1976, W.B. Saunders Co.

Chapter 2

HISTORY AND PHYSICAL EXAMINATION IN PATIENTS WITH PULMONARY PROBLEMS

Roger S. Mitchell

History

In taking the medical history of a patient with pulmonary problems, the physician should note the primary symptoms of pulmonary disease and also any symptoms arising from other organ systems that may bear on pulmonary disorders. These primary symptoms are cough, expectoration, dyspnea, hemoptysis, wheezing, and chest pain. Key points in the patient's past medical history include smoking, allergies, and occupational exposure to potential disease-producing environments.

Perhaps the most neglected pulmonary symptom is *cough*. An acute change in cough pattern is quite obvious to the patient, family, and physician; however, determination of the chronic cough pattern requires special attention. Too often, a chronic cough is taken for granted by both physician and patient. "Doesn't everyone cough upon arising in the morning?" Many smokers do; but when they do, it is the common early warning sign of a potentially serious disease: chronic bronchitis. The crucial point is that *chronic cough is not normal.* The physician should inquire carefully into the patient's cough pattern, including frequency, severity, character, and associated sputum production.

Coughing is a normal response to the inhalation of foreign material such as dust particles, irritant gases, and nasal mucus; it may be caused by an upper respiratory problem unrelated to the pulmonary parenchyma, such as an upper respiratory infection. However, chronic daily cough suggests pulmonary disease.

Some smokers do not cough because they have not smoked long enough, they do not inhale, or they have an inherently efficient tracheobronchial clearance mechanism. The point the physician should stress is that daily

8

cough or cough equivalent such as throat clearing is abnormal, especially when it is *productive*.

The amount, viscosity, color, and odor of *sputum* are very important features, and the physician should observe the sputum during the history taking.

The presence and degree of *dyspnea*—exertional, noneffort dependent, or episodic—should be carefully determined. This should include inquiry into exercise tolerance, for example, the distance the patient can walk or how many steps the patient can climb without having to stop for breath, whether the dysnpea is worsening, and its relation to body position (orthopnea). True *paroxysmal nocturnal dyspnea* is classically a sudden awakening from sleep with an overwhelming sensation of air hunger that simply demands the erect or slightly forward position. It may be accompanied or followed by wheezing ("cardiac asthma") and cough productive of blood-stained froth; this kind of attack is clearly an episode of acute left ventricular failure. On the other hand, patients with chronic obstructive pulmonary disease (COPD) frequently have intense dyspnea at night, usually preceded by a bout of coughing that sitting up generally relieves somewhat.

Hemoptysis is a direct and meaningful symptom of lung disease. However, blood from the mouth does not necessarily come from the lungs. When it does, it is usually accompanied by cough and sometimes by chest rattling; furthermore, true hemoptysis is apt to recur over a period of days. Other sources of blood in the mouth include the nose, pharynx, and gums; these sources usually can be ruled out by careful nose and throat examination. Hematemesis is usually detectable by being accompanied by vomiting.

Wheezing or noisy breathing is a common symptom of pulmonary disease. Even healthy persons can produce a wheeze by a forced expiration; however, to be significant, the wheezing should be involuntary. Sometimes wheezing is lateralized and even made worse or stopped by lateral recumbency, an observation suggesting the presence of a malignant bronchial narrowing or foreign body. The *stridor* of upper airway obstruction is predominant on both inspiration and expiration and is not easily confused with wheezing.

Chest pain must be reviewed in detail: quality of pain; location; radiation; duration; frequency; and relationship to food intake, swallowing, exertion, rest, position, and, most important, inspiration or cough. Pain made worse by inspiration, cough, or both is usually pleural in origin.

A history of *recurrent pneumonia*, especially in the same location (lung, lobe, or segment), suggests localized bronchial obstruction, bronchiectasis, or some form of reduced host defenses to infection.

Other patient symptoms on which the physician should concentrate are fever, chills, chilly sensations, sweating, night sweats, easy fatigability, loss of weight, anorexia, malaise, bone and joint pain (possibly osteoarthropathy), hoarseness, and dysphagia. The physician should also inquire about and attempt to obtain for review any previous chest radiographs. Details of current and past *medications* may also help in elucidating an obscure situation.

In patients with a history of *tuberculosis*, the details of sputum bacteriology, drug susceptibility tests, chemotherapy regimens, tuberculin reactivity, and surgical procedures are essential; inquiries must be sent to prior physicians and hospitals.

The patient's *occupational history* may be vital in the diagnosis of obscure pulmonary pathology. It should include the precise duration, nature of work, and location of exposure to industrial fumes and dusts as hard rock, coal, asbestos, uranium, talc, cotton and wool processing, moldy hay, silage, and animals, especially birds. *Geographic exposure* also has a distinct bearing on the possibility of certain diseases, especially parasitic and fungus diseases.

The patient's *smoking history* is of extreme importance in evaluating a pulmonary problem. Questions asked should include the following: age at starting; cigar, pipe, cigarette—hand made versus "tailor" made; quantity smoked, including variations over the years and length of cigarette smoked; habit of inhalation; attempts at stopping, including length of time, reason, and effects, if any, especially on cough and expectoration. The physician should also query the patient concerning possible use of oily nose drops, allergies, and drug sensitivities.

Physical examination

The physical examination should begin and continue during the history taking. The patient should be sitting in a chair and in a good light. Depth, frequency, and noisiness of breathing should be noted. Does the patient flare the alae nasi on inspiration? Does the patient use accessory muscles of respiration? The physician should listen for cough and loose sputum. He should look at the sputum if raised and attempt to persuade the patient to expectorate sputum into a tissue or cup for inspection; this is especially necessary for patients who do not like to expectorate, but, rather, tend to swallow sputum. What is the patient's skin color—cyanotic, plethoric, pallid?

Once the actual examination begins, the physician should look for signs of recent or chronic weight loss, Horner's syndrome, palpably enlarged lymph nodes (especially in the neck and axillae), and subcutaneous masses over the chest. In patients with suggestive symptoms, the physician should look for unilateral laryngeal paralysis through indirect laryngoscopy.

Clubbing of fingers or toes, especially when mild, is easily overlooked. Early clubbing may simply be a loss of the normal indentation at the nail-skin junction, softening at the base of the nail, or both.

In examining the heart the physician should pay particular attention to evidence of pulmonary hypertension, congestive right heart failure, or both. Evidence would include abnormal rhythms, right ventricular lift, S_3 (especially when the loudness of this sound varies with respiration) and S_4 gallop, sound and timing of pulmonary closure, distention or pulsation of neck veins, estimated venous pressure, liver enlargement or tenderness, and dependent edema.

Inspection of the chest wall should include evaluation of rib motion and diaphragmatic excursion. The anterior ribs normally rise and move laterally with inspiration. Hemidiaphragmatic movement can be measured by percussion at full inspiration and then at full expiration at each lung base. Overall diaphragmatic function can be assessed grossly by simply watching the rise of the patient's abdominal wall with inspiration and fall with expiration during spontaneous quiet breathing. Hoover's sign—indrawing rather than flaring of the anterior rib margins with inspiration—is a reliable sign of lung hyperinflation and is caused by horizontal rather than downward contraction of the diaphragm.

Percussion over normal lung has a *resonant* quality; this can be modified by the density of the overlying tissue (muscle, fat). The reflected sound of percussion over consolidated or compressed lung will be dampened, and the note will sound *dull* (short and nonmusical); an example is the sound and feel of percussion over the heart. The vibrations generated by percussion over fluid are completely dampened, that is, *flat;* percussing over the shoulder or thigh provides an example. In percussion over air (pneumothorax) the vibrations are enhanced and prolonged, that is, *hyperresonant* or *tympanitic,* as over the normal empty stomach. The *feeling* of percussion may be even more informative than the *sound.*

Tactile *fremitus* is the transmission of the spoken voice (low frequency vibrations), for example, "99," from the larynx and through the airways, the lungs, the pleurae, and the chest wall. It is influenced by the same considerations that modify the transmission of breath sounds, as discussed below.

Normal so-called *vesicular breath sounds* are the sounds of air moving into and out of the trachea and major bronchi, transmitted through the overlying lung and chest wall. If the lung is consolidated as in lobar pneumonia, the resultant *bronchial breath sounds* are similar to those heard directly over the trachea. A key point to distinguish bronchial from vesicular breath sounds (heard over all areas of the chest wall except the sternum and midscapular region) is the relative loudness of inspiration and expiration. Vesicular sounds are soft and short during expiration, whereas bronchial breath sounds are louder and more prolonged on expiration. (They become equal both in length and intensity to inspiration.) If the pleural space is filled with fluid, air, or a thick peel (so-called pleural thickening), the transmission of

TABLE 2-1. Chest physical findings

	Normal	Consolidation	Fluid*	Pneumothorax†	Fibrothorax	Cavity	Major atelectasis	Emphysema
Inspection and palpation	Good and equal rib and diaphragm movement	Slight restriction of motion	Slightly enlarged and restricted	Slightly enlarged and restricted	Small and very restricted		Slightly small and restricted	Enlarged and restricted bilaterally
Percussion	Resonant	Dull	Flat	Tympany	Dull or resonant		± slight dullness	Hyperresonant
Fremitus	Present	Increased	Absent	Absent	Present or reduced		Normal or reduced	Normal or reduced
Breath sounds	Vesicular	Bronchial	Absent‡	Absent	Reduced to absent	Amphoric	± reduced	Suppressed, with prolonged expiratory phase
Adventitious sounds	None	Rales often present	Friction rub early	None	None	"Consonating" rales	Rales ±	Occasional rhonchi; often fine rales late in inspiration

| Other | "Bronchophony" is normal spoken voice | "Egophony" (E to A) and whispered pectoriloquy | Contralateral Grocco's triangle; mediastinal shift away | Mediastinal shift away | Mediastinal shift toward | Coin sign | Tracheal and mediastinal shift toward | Hoover's sign; high clavicles; muscular wasting |

*A large amount, recently formed.

†A large pneumothorax, with almost total lung collapse and no adhesions.

‡Except for rim of consolidation findings at upper margin of large effusion.

NOTES

1. These findings pertain to the fully developed situations only and, except for the normal and emphysema, to the side or area involved. Lesser degrees of any one of them will frequently cause the signs to be normal or nearly normal.
2. In examining the recumbent patient unable to sit up, listen to both sides in the superior and dependent positions; the normal dependent lung ventilates slightly more than the upper one.
3. Normal dullness can be elicited over the heart, normal flatness over the shoulder, normal tympany over the stomach, typical bronchial breathing over the trachea.
4. The normal diaphragmatic excursion with a full breath is approximately two posterior interspaces.
5. Litten's sign is a ripple of contraction seen on the lower lateral anterior chest wall, caused by diaphragm descent.
6. Hoover's sign is an indrawing rather than flaring of the lower anterior ribs, caused by the low position of the diaphragm in emphysema.
7. Transmission of fremitus and breath sounds requires an open bronchus.
8. "Consonating" implies a hollow or resonating quality.

breath sounds is diminished by passing through these layers of varying density, and they sound softer or may be absent. When diffuse airways obstruction is present, breath sounds are softer and more difficult to hear and the duration of expiration is prolonged to a variable degree; with increasing severity of airways obstruction, the breath sounds may become virtually inaudible. Breath sounds have been said to have a *cavernous* or *amphoric* quality over a cavity, but this is only true when the cavity is quite large and surrounded by consolidated lung.

Rales, rhonchi, and *wheezes* are abnormal and are defined as *adventitious sounds.* These noises may be generated from a variety of mechanisms; they usually indicate abnormal fluid in airways, constriction of airways, or both. The character of these sounds is influenced by the *size of the tube*—the smaller the tube, the finer and more high pitched the sound, and by the *nature of the moisture*—the thinner and more fluid the moisture, the drier the sound. A musical quality to the sound seems to be generated by airway spasm and very sticky mucus. The term *rale* is usually applied to the short bursts of sounds; *wheeze,* to the coarsest and loudest sounds; and *rhonchi,* to those in between.

A *friction rub* is usually a low-pitched, repeatedly interrupted sound like leather surfaces creaking together. It is often repeated in the same phase of respiration (both inspiration and expiration) when purely pleural in origin, with the heart beat when pericardial based, or at both times when arising from both pleura and pericardium.

Table 2-1 outlines the physical findings in different pathologic conditions.

Chapter 3

RECENT TECHNICAL IMPROVEMENTS IN THE DIAGNOSIS OF PULMONARY DISEASE

James H. Ellis, Jr.

FLEXIBLE FIBEROPTIC BRONCHOSCOPY

In 1968 Ikeda described the flexible bronchofiberscope for the early diagnosis of peripherally located endobronchial neoplasms.[1] A fiberoptic bundle consists of several thousand closely packed glass fibers, about 10 μm in diameter, allowing transmission of light and a clear image around curves. An excellent selection of fiberoptic bronchoscopes is available with a variety of flexing angles, diameters, and size of aspiration channels. A 35 mm still camera or a 16 mm motion picture camera can be used to photograph laryngeal, tracheal, or endobronchial lesions or tracheobronchial dynamics.[2-4] Brushes and biopsy forceps can be passed through the aspiration channel[5-9] with or without fluoroscopic guidance, thus providing the most effective and widely applicable technique in diagnosing pulmonary diseases.[10,11]

Flexible fiberoptic bronchoscopy (FFB) is performed with a variety of individually selected premedications, topical anesthetics, and introduction techniques.[12-15] Careful cardiac screening and monitoring can reduce the majority of serious complications. Oxygen may be administered during the procedure by a nasal or mouth cannula, mask, or by way of the aspiration or oxygen channel of the bronchoscope. If special adaptors are used, patients with endotracheal tubes or tracheostomies, with or without assisted mechanical ventilation, can safely undergo fiberoptic bronchoscopy.

The advantages of fiberoptic bronchoscopy over conventional (rigid, straight-tube) bronchoscopy are (1) greater range of direct visibility,[16] (2) little patient discomfort, (3) safety even in very ill patients receiving assisted ventilation, and (4) the fact that it can be performed virtually anywhere (surgical suite, emergency room, bedside), although appropriate precautions must be followed. FFB is the procedure of choice in patients with cervical spine disease or those unable to tolerate hyperextension of the neck. At present it is not widely applicable in pediatric medicine because of the relative size of the airway and the bronchoscope, although special fiberoptic bronchoscopes are now available. It has not proved very useful for particulate matter aspiration.

The applications of fiberoptic bronchoscopy demonstrate its versatility.[17-21] It is useful in evaluating laryngeal obstructions, lesions, or paralysis; careful laryngeal examination is an essential part of the majority of procedures. It has proved helpful in performing difficult oral-tracheal intubations as well as in the evaluation of tracheal tube position and tracheal damage in intubated patients. Over half the procedures are used in the diagnosis of bronchogenic carcinomas and the evaluation of hemoptysis. Lung abscesses are approached from both a diagnostic and a therapeutic standpoint. Bronchoscopy is used to obtain specimens to ascertain the bacteriology of the lower tract and to perform tracheobronchial toilet in carefully selected patients. The removal of foreign bodies, previously an absolute indication for conventional bronchoscopy, is now possible by using a variety of grasping forceps and retrieval baskets. Pleural biopsy and pleuroscopy may be performed, usually after two negative needle pleural biopsies, in the evaluation of exudative pleural effusions.[22,23] Selective bronchography can be performed in conjunction with fiberoptic bronchoscopy and is routinely employed by certain endoscopists.[1,2] Research applications are increasing.

The indications for fiberoptic bronchoscopy in the intensive care unit are primarily therapeutic (radiographic atelectasis, retained secretions, difficult tracheal intubations) and occasionally diagnostic (hemoptysis, tracheal mucosa evaluation, collection of secretions, burn evaluation, slowly resolving infiltrates, diffuse lung disease, stridor, unexplained hypoxemia, lung abscess, and possible bronchial fracture). Bronchoscopy for atelectasis results in clinical and radiographic improvement in approximately 80% of patients when aggressive noninvasive techniques for retained secretions have failed.[24]

Transbronchial lung biopsy and *bronchial brushing* by way of the fiberoptic bronchoscope are adaptations of techniques developed by Andersen[25] and Fennessy.[20] Transbronchial lung biopsy with the flexible fiberoptic bronchoscope and the standard biopsy forceps that accompany this instrument have been used with[11] and without[26] fluoroscopic guidance with good results and few complications—fewer complications, in fact, than percutaneous lung biopsy techniques or thoracotomy. The technique is applicable in both stable and acutely ill patients and in both diffuse and localized lung diseases.[26-28] Bronchial brushing is performed during the same procedure.[11,29]

Transbronchial lung biopsy with the flexible fiberoptic bronchoscope has been useful in the evaluation of opportunistic infections.[30]

Complications of FFB relate largely to excessive premedication or topical anesthesia and consist principally of laryngospasm, bronchospasm (especially in asthmatic patients), pneumothorax, hemorrhage, and hypoxemia.[31-36] The complication rates remain very low, and deaths are rare.

PERCUTANEOUS NEEDLE BIOPSY OF THE LUNG

Percutaneous needle biopsy with or without fluoroscopic guidance has become an increasingly useful method in the diagnosis of diffuse or peripherally localized pulmonary lesions, thus obviating the need for thoracotomy in many cases. Contraindications to these procedures are abnormal coagulation studies, emphysematous blebs or bullae in the biopsy area, evidence of pulmonary hypertension, central or obviously vascular lesions, pulmonary function impairment of a degree indicating inability to tolerate significant pneumothorax, or inability to cooperate. Similar considerations are made before transbronchial lung biopsy.

Three current techniques are widely used: aspiration, cutting, and drill biopsy. In one series, aspiration needle biopsy gave positive cytologic or bacteriologic results in over 70% of cases with a complication rate of 23% (consisting of 14% simple pneumothorax, 5% pneumothorax requiring treatment, 3% hemoptysis, and 1% hemothorax) without fatality.[37] However, rare fatalities have occurred,[36] and the complications of cutting needle and drill biopsy techniques are much greater.

The value of any lung biopsy technique depends upon the operator's skill, diagnostic yield, and procedural risks. A careful selection of patients and procedures is imperative. The skills and experience of many physicians allow them to employ the fiberoptic bronchoscope with transbronchial lung biopsy and bronchial brushing, but all physicians must remain objective and versatile in order to serve patients most effectively.

REFERENCES

1. Ikeda, S., Yanai, N., and Ishikawa, S.: Flexible bronchofiberscope, Keio J. Med. **17:**1, 1968.
2. Ikeda, S.: Flexible bronchofiberscope, Ann. Otol. Rhinol. Laryngol. **79:**916, 1970.
3. Sackner, M.A., Wanner, A., and Landa, J.: Applications of bronchofiberoscopy, Chest **62:**70 (Suppl), 1972.
4. Rath, G.S., Schaff, J.T., and Snider, G.L.: Flexible fiberoptic bronchoscopy: techniques and review of 100 bronchoscopies, Chest **63:**689, 1973.
5. Fry, W.A., and Manalo-Estrella, P.: Bronchial brushing, Surg. Gynecol. Obstet. **130:**67, 1970.
6. Forrest, J.V.: Bronchial brush biopsy in lung cavities, Radiology **106:**69, 1973.
7. Zavala, D.C., Rossi, N.P., Bedeu, G.N., et al.: Bronchial brush biopsy: a valuable diagnostic technique in the presurgical evaluation of indeterminate lung densities, Ann. Thorac. Surg. **13:**519, 1972.

8. Bean, W.J., Graham, W.L., Jordan, B., et al.: Diagnosis of lung cancer by the transbronchial brush biopsy technique, J.A.M.A. **206**:1070, 1968.

9. Repsher, L.H., Schröter, G., and Hammond, W.S.: Diagnosis of *Pneumocystis carinii* pneumonitis by means of endobronchial brush biopsy, N. Engl. J. Med. **287**:340, 1972.

10. Levin, D.C., Wicks, A.B., Ellis, J.H., et al.: Transbronchial lung biopsy via the fiberoptic bronchoscope, Am. Rev. Respir. Dis. **110**:4, 1974.

11. Ellis, J.H.: Transbronchial lung biopsy via the fiberoptic bronchoscope: experience with 107 consecutive cases and comparison with bronchial brushing, Chest **68**:524, 1975.

12. Smiddy, J.F., Ruth, W.E., Kerby, G.R., et al.: Flexible fiberoptic bronchoscope, Ann. Intern. Med. **75**:971, 1971.

13. Smiddy, J.F., Ruth, W.E., and Kerby, G.R.: A new technique of bronchial visualization with fiberoptics, J. Kans. Med. Soc. **72**:441, 1971.

14. Renz, L.E., Smiddy, J.W., Rauscher, C.R., et al.: Bronchoscopy in respiratory failure, J.A.M.A. **219**:619, 1972.

15. Sackner, M.A., and Landa, J.F.: Bronchofiberoscopy: to intubate or not to intubate, Chest **63**:302, 1973.

16. Kovnat, D.M., Shankar-Ratch, G.S., Anderson, W.M., et al.: Maximal extent of visualization of bronchial tree by flexible fiberoptic bronchoscopy, Am. Rev. Respir. Dis. **110**:88, 1974.

17. Smiddy, J.F., and Elliott, R.C.: The evaluation of hemoptysis with fiberoptic bronchoscopy, Chest **64**:158, 1973.

18. Tucker, G.F., Olsen, A.M., Andrews, A.H., et al.: The flexible fiberscope in bronchoscopic perspective, Chest **64**:149, 1973.

19. King, E.G.: Expanding diagnostic and therapeutic horizons—fiberoptic bronchoscopy, Chest **63**:301, 1973.

20. Fennessy, J.J.: Bronchial brushing, Ann. Otol. Rhinol. Laryngol. **79**:924, 1970.

21. Zavala, D.C.: Diagnostic fiberoptic bronchoscopy: techniques and results of biopsy in 600 patients, Chest **68**:12, 1975.

22. Gwin, E., Pierce, G., Boggan, M., et al.: Pleuroscopy and pleural biopsy with the flexible fiberoptic bronchoscope, Chest **67**:527, 1975.

23. Senno, A., Moallem, S., Quijano, E.R., et al.: Thoracoscopy with the fiberoptic bronchoscope: a simple method in diagnosing pleuropulmonary diseases, J. Thorac. Cardiovasc. Surg. **67**:606, 1974.

24. Mahajan, V., Calron, P., and Huber, G.: The value of fiberoptic bronchoscopy in the management of pulmonary collapse, Chest **73**:817, 1978.

25. Andersen, H.A.: Lung biopsy via the bronchoscope, Ann. Otol. Rhinol. Laryngol. **79**:933, 1970.

26. Scheinhorn, D.J., Joyner, L.R., and Whitcomb, M.E.: Transbronchial forceps lung biopsy through the fiberoptic bronchoscope in *Pneumocystis carinii* pneumonia, Chest **66**:294, 1974.

27. Hanson, R.R., Zavala, D.C., Rhodes, M.L., et al.: Transbronchial biopsy via flexible fiberoptic bronchoscope: results in 164 patients, Am. Rev. Respir. Dis. **114**:67, 1976.

28. Koerner, S.K., Sakowitz, A.J., Appelman, R.I., et al.: Transbronchial lung biopsy for the diagnosis of sarcoidosis, N. Engl. J. Med. **293**:268, 1975.

29. Zavala, D.C., Richardson, R.H., Mukerjee, P.K., et al.: Use of the bronchofiberscope for bronchial brush biopsy: diagnostic results and comparison with other brushing techniques, Chest **63**:889, 1973.

30. Ellis, J.H.: Diagnosis of opportunistic infections using the flexible fiberoptic bronchoscope, Chest **735**:7135 (Suppl), 1978.

31. Pierson, D.J., Iseman, M.D., Sutton, F.D., et al.: Arterial blood gas changes in fiberoptic bronchoscopy during mechanical ventilation, Chest **66**:495, 1974.

32. Albertini, R.E., Harrell, J.H., II, and Moser, K.M.: Management of arterial hypoxemia induced by fiberoptic bronchoscopy, Chest **67**:134, 1975.

33. Dubrawsky, C., Awe, R.J., Jenkins, D.E., et al.: The effect of bronchofiberscopic examination on oxygenation status, Chest **67**:137, 1975.

34. Credle, W.F., Smiddy, J.F., Elliot, R.C., et al.: Complications of fiberoptic bronchoscopy, Am. Rev. Respir. Dis. **109**:67, 1974.
35. Suratt, P.M., Smiddy, J.F., Grubert, B., et al.: Deaths and complications associated with fiberoptic bronchoscopy, Chest **69**:747, 1976.
36. Sahn, S., and Scoggin, C.: Fiberoptic bronchoscopy in bronchial asthma: a word of caution, Chest **69**:39, 1976.
37. Dick, R., Heard, B.E., Hinson, K.F.W., et al.: Aspiration needle biopsy of thoracic lesions: an assessment of 227 biopsies, Br. J. Dis. Chest **68**:86, 1974.
38. Brandt, P.D., Blank, N., and Castellino, R.A.: Needle diagnosis of pneumonitis, J.A.M.A. **220**:1578, 1972.
39. Neff, T.A.: Appropriate alternatives to open thoracotomy for diagnosis of pulmonary lesions (editorial), Ann. Thorac. Surg. **13**:625, 1972.
40. Neff, T.A.: Percutaneous trephine biopsy of the lung, Chest **61**:18, 1972.
41. McCartney, R.L.: Hemorrhage following percutaneous lung biopsy, Radiology **112**:305, 1974.

Chapter 4

PULMONARY FUNCTION TESTING

Reuben M. Cherniack

Just as no physical examination is complete without determination of the patient's systolic and diastolic blood pressure, determination of his or her forced vital capacity maneuver (FVC), and forced expiratory volume in 1 second (FEV_1) is an integral component of clinical assessment. Advances in medical knowledge and management of hypertension have come about largely as a result of repeated measurement, over many years, of patients' blood pressure. If similar information about spirometry were available, physicians' understanding of chronic airflow limitation or interstitial lung disease would increase considerably. In all patients with respiratory symptomatology, this simple assessment, along with the history and the chest radiograph, allows the attending physician to gain an impression of the disease process present and the resultant physiologic disturbances. From repeated determinations of the FEV_1 and FVC, the physician can evaluate the progress of the disease process and assess the effect of therapeutic regimens.

Whether or not a spirometric abnormality has been demonstrated, many patients with chronic respiratory symptoms should be referred to a laboratory for further studies. The extent of further necessary evaluation will vary among patients, but as a minimum, lung volume and airflow characteristics and gas exchange and acid-base balance, both at rest and during exercise, should be determined.

Before discussing the tests performed in a pulmonary function laboratory and their interpretations, it is important to stress that no measurement or calculation is meaningful (and consequently no interpretation justified) unless the equipment used has been carefully calibrated and the variability and reproducibility of the test has been validated in each particular laboratory. For each test a set of the expected values must be derived from healthy individuals. Careful evaluation of the patient's and the technician's performance, in even the simplest test, must be ensured. In addition, the equipment must be quality controlled. Accuracy of measurement of volume and time by a spirometer, flow rate by a flow meter, and gas concentration by a gas analyzer is essential. When sensing devices are used simultaneously (such as in determination of thoracic gas volume or flow resistance), one must ensure an adequate frequency response of the various instruments and absence of a phase lag between the electronic responses.

VENTILATORY FUNCTION

Respiratory symptoms usually arise as a result of alterations of the elastic or flow-resistive properties of the lungs or chest wall, or both. In practice, one usually uses measurements of the total lung capacity (TLC) and its compartments to assess the elastic properties of the lungs and chest wall and of the airflow rate during a forced expiratory vital capacity as a reflection of flow resistance. However, valid interpretation of measurements of the mechanical properties of the lungs, whether determined directly, or indirectly from simple spirometry, requires knowledge of the absolute lung volumes at which these parameters were determined. Clearly, the advent of the body plethysmograph has greatly improved physicians' ability to assess the respiratory system's elastic or flow-resistive properties.

Elastic properties

The maximum volume of air in the lungs at TLC is determined by the balance of forces between the respiratory muscles and the elastic properties of the respiratory system. The absolute values of the subdivisions or compartments of TLC depend upon the patient's age, sex, and size, but their proportion of TLC is fairly constant. The functional residual capacity (FRC) is about 40% of TLC; the residual volume (RV), about 25%.

The finding of a lower than expected TLC generally indicates either a restrictive disorder or respiratory muscle weakness. Similarly, a lower than expected vital capacity (VC) may indicate a reduced compliance of the lungs (as in pulmonary fibrosis or congestion) or the chest wall (as in obesity or kyphoscoliosis). However, as depicted in Fig. 4-1, the VC may also be lower than expected in patients suffering from an obstructive disorder. In a restrictive disorder the low VC is associated with a reduced TLC and RV. On the other hand, in an obstructive disorder due to either increased flow resistance (as in asthma or bronchitis) or loss of lung elastic recoil (as in emphysema), or both, the low VC is associated with an increased RV and TLC.

The FRC is determined by using a gas dilution principle or a physical method based on Boyle's law. Although the dilution techniques also provide additional information about the distribution of ventilation, the physical

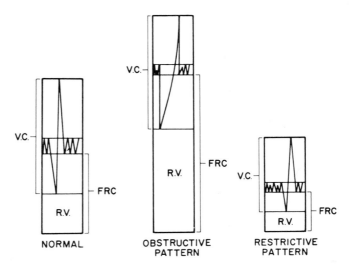

FIG. 4-1. Total lung capacity and its subdivisions in a healthy individual, a patient with obstructive lung disease, and a patient with restrictive lung disease.

method, employing a body plethysmograph, is quicker, easier, and particularly useful because the airway resistance (Raw) can also be determined.

The principle behind calculation of lung volume in the body plethysmograph is simple: pressure in the airways is determined while the subject makes inspiratory and expiratory efforts at a rate of approximately 120 breaths/min against a closed shutter. During the panting maneuver the air in the patient's chest is alternately compressed (airway pressure becomes positive) and decompressed (airway pressure becomes negative). The pressure of the gas in the airtight plethysmograph also changes, but in the opposite direction. The relationship between changes in pressure measured at the mouth ($\triangle P$), which are equal to alveolar pressure, and changes in thoracic gas volume ($\triangle V$), which are reflected by the changes in plethysmograph pressure, is observed continuously on an oscilloscope, and the slope ($\triangle P/\triangle V$) is determined.

Since the airway pressure (P_1) at the onset of the test is 970 cm water (atmospheric pressure minus water vapor pressure), the original volume of gas (V$_{TG}$) in the lungs is calculated from the change in lung volume ($\triangle V$) and airway pressure ($\triangle P$) during panting:

$$P_1 V_{TG} = P_2 V_2$$
$$P_1 V_{TG} = (P_1 + \triangle P)(V_{TG} + \triangle V)$$

Rearranging the equation:

$$V_{TG} = -P_1 \times \frac{\Delta V}{\Delta P}$$

Disregarding the sign and substituting the slope ($\Delta P/\Delta V$):

$$V_{TG} = \frac{970}{\Delta P/\Delta V}$$

Note that the determination of the TLC first involves measurement of the FRC; then a maximal inspiration (i.e., inspiratory capacity) is determined. Similarly, RV is determined by having the patient expire maximally from FRC (i.e., expiratory reserve volume [ERV] is determined), and this volume is subtracted from FRC. Clearly, these determinations will be influenced by patient effort, and the TLC may be lower than expected, the RV higher than expected, or both if the patient's respiratory muscle strength is reduced or if the patient is uncooperative. In some cases these results may be misinterpreted to indicate a mixed defect, in which a similar picture is seen. In general, a reduction in all lung compartments indicates a restrictive defect; an increase in all compartments indicates an obstructive disorder.

Other methods for measuring TLC are the helium dilution and nitrogen washout. Because these methods fail to include the gas content of bullae, the extent of any bullae present can be estimated by subtracting the TLC as measured by these methods from the TLC as measured by body plethysmography. The TLC can also be fairly reliably estimated by radiographic measurement.

Flow-resistive properties

In many laboratories Raw is estimated in a body plethysmograph by determination of the relationship of airway pressure (P_{AW}) and airflow ($\dot{V}$) during panting. Determination of total gas volume in the lungs involves measurement of the ratio between changes in mouth pressure (which are identical to P_{AW}) and plethysmograph pressure (P_P) during panting against a closed shutter. By determining the slope of the relationship between pressure and flow ($\dot{V}/P_P$) while the patient pants without obstruction, it is possible to calculate Raw from the ratio of $\dot{V}/P_P$ and P_{AW}/P_P:

$$Raw = \frac{P_{AW}/P_P}{\dot{V}/P_P} \text{ in cm } H_2O/1/sec$$

Ninety percent of the normal Raw determined by this technique is in the major airways. The fact that the measurement is made at the same time that lung volume is determined is particularly important, since the diameter of the bronchi and Raw depend on lung volume. To correct for the effect of lung volume, conductance (reciprocal of resistance) is calculated; it is expressed per unit lung volume, which is called *specific conductance.*

Considerable important information about the respiratory system's flow-resistive properties can be derived from analysis of the FVC. The amount of air expired during the first second (FEV$_1$), or the mean rate of change of volume during the middle half of the FVC (FEF$_{25-75}$),* is used most frequently.

Determination of the flow-volume relationship during the forced expiratory maneuver and assessment of the maximal expiratory flow rate ($\dot{V}_{max}$) at particular lung volumes is particularly useful not only in estimating flow limitation, but also in assessing the quality of the maneuver.

Since the FVC maneuver requires total patient effort, the finding of low flow rates or other parameters that are indexes of flow resistance may reflect patient effort rather than flow limitation. For this reason it is recommended that the FVC duration be at least 6 seconds and that a spirogram record of volume over time should always be obtained. When no spirogram record is available, observation of the flow-volume loop may help the physician assess the extent of patient cooperation. Fig. 4-2 illustrates the effect of reduced effort on the flow-volume relationship achieved during the FVC maneuver. As contrasted with the loop seen during maximal effort (Fig. 4-2, *A*), two types of loop may suggest poor effort. Fig. 4-2, *B* and *C* demonstrate two types of curves that may be seen when patient effort is less than maximum. In Fig. 4-2, *B* the patient does not try as hard initially but continues to blow as long as possible so that FVC is the same as in *A.* Fig. 4-2, *C* shows the flow-volume curve when the patient's initial effort was maximal; in this case the patient stopped expiring before residual volume was reached, and the flow rate cut off suddenly. Review of the flow-volume relationship during the FVC maneuver is therefore often used to determine the test's reliability; the values are considered reliable if the peak flows are reproducible in at least two curves and if abrupt cessation of flow is not evident at the end of the loop.

Provided maximum effort is ensured, the finding of an FEV$_1$, FEF$_{25-75}$, or $\dot{V}_{max}$ that is less than expected for a given age, height, and sex suggests the presence of expiratory airflow limitation. However, just as flow resistance varies with lung volume, Fig. 4-2 demonstrates that $\dot{V}_{max}$ during the FVC is also related to lung volume, being greatest at high lung volumes and falling as lung volume diminishes. Clearly, interpretation of expiratory flow rates or other parameters derived from the FVC must include the extent of patient effort and the lung volume at which the flow rates were achieved. An in-

---

*Formerly called maximal midexpiratory flow.

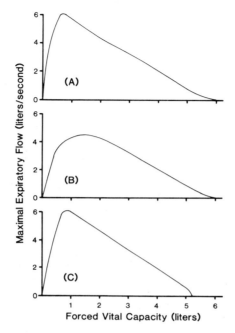

FIG. 4-2. Flow-volume relationship during a forced vital capacity maneuver in a healthy subject when maximal effort was exerted, **A,** when the initial effort was less than maximal, **B,** and when, despite maximal vital effort, the patient stopped expiring prematurely, **C.**

creased Raw can be inferred only if the airflow rate is different from that expected at an equivalent lung volume.

When absolute lung volume is not known, the FEV_1/FVC ratio is frequently used to determine whether expiratory airflow limitation is present. This ratio is usually within normal limits (i.e., greater than 70%) in patients suffering solely from restrictive disorders, but it is markedly reduced when there is obstruction to airflow. However, anything that will affect the patient's ability to expire fully, such as muscular weakness, pain, dyspnea, or lack of total effort (as in Fig. 4-2, *C*) may lead to a lower than possible FVC; as a result, the FEV_1/FVC ratio may appear greater than it actually is, and the presence of flow-limitation may be missed.

PATTERNS OF IMPAIRED VENTILATORY FUNCTION
Restrictive pulmonary disease

In restrictive pulmonary disease, lung volume is reduced, and the FEV_1, FEF_{25-75} and $\dot{V}_{max}$ are frequently lower than predicted values. As is seen in Fig.

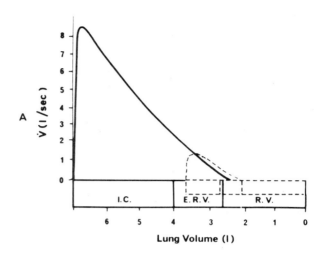

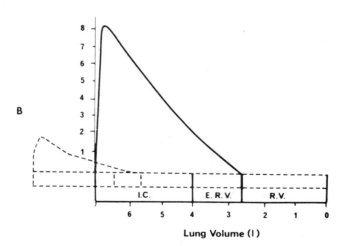

FIG. 4-3. The relationship between lung volume and $\dot{V}_{max}$ (---) in a patient with restrictive lung disease, **A**, and COPD, **B**. The solid lines represent predicted lung volumes and flow rates in a healthy individual of equivalent age, height, and sex.

TABLE 4-1. Patterns of ventilatory function

Parameter	Obstructive pattern	Restrictive pattern
VC	↓ ↔	↓
RV	↑	↓
FRC	↑	↓
TLC	↑ ↔	↓
FEV$_1$	↓	↓ ↔
FEF$_{25-75}$	↓	↓ ↔

4-3 and Table 4-1, the flow rates are low not because of an increase in flow resistance, but rather because they are being achieved at a low lung volume. In fact, the low expiratory flow rates may actually be higher than would be expected at any particular lung volume in such patients because the driving pressure (lung elastic retractive force) is increased (i.e., compliance is low). As a corollary, it is clear that if $\dot{V}_{max}$ is not higher than expected at a particular lung volume in a patient suffering from a restrictive disorder, then Raw is likely increased. As indicated earlier, the FEV$_1$/FVC ratio may be useful, but it is frequently normal in this condition.

In some cases it may be difficult to determine whether the finding of a low TLC and its compartments indicates a reduction in chest wall or lung compliance. If this question arises, it is possible to differentiate the mechanism underlying the altered lung volume by evaluating the shape of the curve relating the static transpulmonary pressure to the absolute lung volume (pressure-volume relationship) over the range of the expiratory vital capacity. As Fig. 4-4 shows, the pressure-volume curve is shifted downward (lung volume is less) and to the right (pressure is greater at any lung volume) and the slope of the curve at around FRC (compliance) is decreased in the patient with pulmonary fibrosis. If the low lung volume is due solely to a disorder of the chest wall, the slope of the curve will be normal.

Obstructive pulmonary disease

In obstructive pulmonary disease, TLC and its compartments are usually increased, and FEV$_1$, FEF$_{25-75}$, and $\dot{V}_{max}$ are reduced. Fig. 4-3 indicates that expiratory flow rates at a particular lung volume are lower than expected, indicating the presence of flow limitation. As in the case of a restrictive disorder, assessment of the lung's pressure-volume characteristics will help the physician differentiate whether an elevated lung volume and low expiratory flow rate are associated with an increase in Raw (as in asthma or bronchitis) or a loss of lung elastic recoil (as in emphysema). As Fig. 4-4

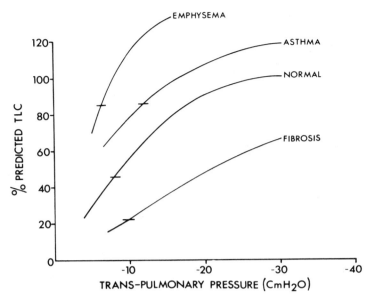

FIG. 4-4. Pressure-volume relationships of the lung in a healthy individual and in patients suffering from lung diseases. Note that the curve is shifted downward and slope is reduced in pulmonary fibrosis; it is shifted upward in both emphysema and asthma, but slope is increased in emphysema and unaltered in asthma.

indicates, the curve is shifted upward (lung volume is greater) and to the left (pressure is lower at any lung volume) in both emphysema and asthma. However, in emphysema the slope of the curve at FRC is increased, while in asthma or bronchitis the slope is normal.

BRONCHIAL REACTIVITY

When an obstructive pattern of abnormality is demonstrated, the physician should determine the pattern's potential reversibility by repeating the FVC maneuver after the patient has inhaled an adequate dose of nebulized bronchodilator. Improvement in parameters that reflect Raw indicates the presence of bronchial hyperreactivity and the benefit of bronchodilator therapy. However, it is important to point out that the converse may not be true, and a lack of change in flow rate does not necessarily imply failure to improve; any change in lung volume must be taken into account before reporting a lack of improvement following bronchodilator.

Fig. 4-5 illustrates two examples in which a beneficial effect of bronchodilator therapy may be missed. In one patient, FVC was unchanged after

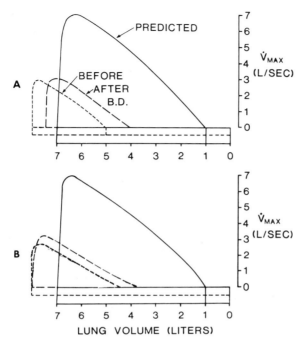

FIG. 4-5. The effect of nebulized bronchodilator on the flow-volume relationship in two patients with expiratory flow limitation. In **A,** TLC and RV fell after bronchodilator; FVC was unchanged so that FEF$_{25\text{-}75}$ was unchanged. In **B,** TLC was the same but FVC increased after bronchodilator; since FEF$_{25\text{-}75}$ was calculated over a larger volume, it was again unchanged. In both instances $\dot{V}_{max}$ at isovolume increased considerably. See text for explanation of symbols.

bronchodilator, but both TLC and RV fell. The postbronchodilator FEF$_{25\text{-}75}$ and $\dot{V}_{max50}$ were the same as before bronchodilator, but the flow rates were clearly greater at any particular lung volume (i.e., at isovolume). In the second patient, TLC was unchanged following bronchodilator but RV fell (i.e., VC increased). In this patient, the calculated FEF$_{25\text{-}75}$ and $\dot{V}_{max50}$ were also unchanged following bronchodilator because these parameters were calculated at a lower lung volume after bronchodilator. In both patients a hasty conclusion would suggest lack of benefit from nebulized bronchodilator. However, when the expiratory flow rates after use of aerosol are compared with those before bronchodilator at an equivalent lung volume (isovolume), patient improvement following inhaled bronchodilator is obvious.

In some patients the presence (or absence) of increased bronchial reactivity may be difficult to ascertain. In such individuals a reduction in FEV$_1$ or

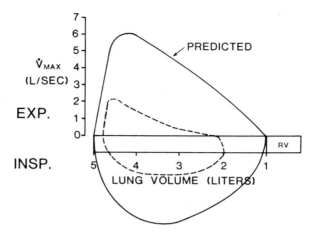

FIG. 4-6. Flow-volume relationship during inspiration and expiration in a patient with upper airways obstruction(---). Notice that compared with predicted values (——) the flow rates are reduced considerably during inspiration as well as expiration.

$\dot{V}_{max}$ in response to inhaled methacholine or histamine or following exercise indicates airway hyperreactivity. On the other hand, it must be recognized that airway hyperreactivity develops even in healthy individuals following an acute upper respiratory infection. Conversely, as with bronchodilator therapy, the physician should interpret hyperreactivity (or its absence) only after considering changes in lung volume also. The changes following bronchial challenge may be opposite to those shown in Fig. 4-5, and an increase in lung volume and an alteration of isovolume flow rates may be missed.

Maximal inspiratory flow measurements can also be useful if maximal patient effort is ensured, particularly when upper airway obstruction is suspected. Fig. 4-6 illustrates that when upper airway obstruction is present, inspiratory airflow is limited in addition to the reduction in $\dot{V}_{max}$.

GAS EXCHANGE

The assessment of arterial Pa_{O_2}, Pa_{CO_2}, and acid-base balance, both at rest and during exercise, is frequently informative in subjects with chronic respiratory symptoms. If expired gas is collected simultaneously with arterial blood, the respiratory quotient (R), alveolar oxygen tension (PA_{O_2}), alveolar-arterial oxygen tension gradient ($P[A-a]_{O_2}$), and the dead space-tidal volume ratio (V_D/V_T) can be determined. In particular, it is important to follow $P(A-a)_{O_2}$ when assessing a patient's progress or deterioration.

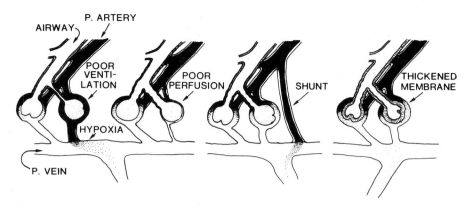

FIG. 4-7. Arterial hypoxemia (low P_{ao_2}) and an increased alveoloarterial P_{o_2} gradient ($P[_{A}-a]_{o_2}$) may result from mismatching of ventilation and perfusion, right-to-left shunt (true venous admixture), a diffusion defect, or a combination of these disturbances. In pure alveolar hypoventilation the $P(_{A}-a)_{o_2}$ remains within the normal range.

Even if expired air is not collected, the $P(_{A}-a)_{o_2}$ can be determined by assuming that R was 0.8 if the patient was breathing room air and 1.0 if he or she was breathing oxygen; a simplified alveolar air equation is used to calculate the P_{Ao_2}:

$$P_{AO_2} = P_{I}O_2 - \frac{Pa_{CO_2}}{R}$$

Then, on room air:

$$P_{AO_2} = P_{I}O_2 - (Pa_{CO_2} \times 1.25)$$

And:

$$P(_{A}-a)_{o_2} = P_{I}O_2 - (Pa_{CO_2} \times 1.25) - Pa_{o_2}$$

Even in healthy persons, the $P(_{A}-a)_{o_2}$ is about 10 to 15 mm Hg because of ventilation/perfusion mismatch ($\dot{V}/\dot{Q}$), and some mixing of venous blood with arterialized blood in the thebesian and bronchial veins. An increase in $P(_{A}-a)_{o_2}$ occurs when there is an increase in $\dot{V}/\dot{Q}$ mismatch, true venous admixture, a diffusion defect (Fig. 4-7), or a combination of these disturbances. In all these conditions, as well as in alveolar hypoventilation, the Pa_{o_2} will be less than normal. In the case of alveolar hypoventilation, however, oxygen equilibrates between the alveoli and the pulmonary capillary blood, making the $P(_{A}-a)_{o_2}$ within normal limits.

An elevation of Pa_{CO_2} occurs when the alveolar ventilation ($\dot{V}_A$) is inadequate relative to carbon dioxide production ($\dot{V}_{CO_2}$):

$$Pa_{CO_2} = \dot{V}_{CO_2}/\dot{V}_A \times 0.863$$

Thus, the $Paco_2$ will be elevated (and the Pao_2 will be low) when the work of breathing or total body metabolism is disproportionately high for a given $\dot{V}_A$ or the $\dot{V}_A$ falls without a concomitant reduction in carbon dioxide production. The former situation occurs particularly in COPD; the latter situation will develop when the minute ventilation falls or an excessive proportion of the minute ventilation is wasted (dead space–like ventilation). As indicated above, in uncomplicated alveolar hypoventilation the high $Paco_2$ and the low Pao_2 will be accompanied by a normal $P(A\text{-}a)o_2$. Conversely, the finding of an elevated $P(A\text{-}a)o_2$ in the presence of hypoxemia and hypercapnia indicates that the hypoxemia cannot be explained entirely by alveolar hypoventilation and that one or more of the other physiologic disturbances must be present.

$\dot{V}/\dot{Q}$ mismatch in the lungs is the most common cause of a greater than expected $P(A\text{-}a)o_2$ in chronic respiratory insufficiency. The extent of the $\dot{V}/\dot{Q}$ mismatching may be inferred from the size of the $P(A\text{-}a)o_2$, provided that excessive shunting (true venous admixture) has been ruled out. The amount of true venous admixture can be assessed qualitatively by sampling arterial blood while the patient is breathing 100% oxygen. Failure of the Pao_2 to rise above 500 mm Hg (at sea level) while the patient is breathing 100% oxygen indicates excessive shunting of blood, and a rise of the Pao_2 above 500 mm Hg while the patient is breathing 100% oxygen rules out excessive true venous admixture. One should remember that the Pao_2 may also fail to rise above 500 mm Hg while the patient is breathing oxygen if nonventilated lung lesions, such as atelectasis or consolidation, continue to be perfused.

In practice, the possibility of a diffusion defect is assessed by measurement of the single-breath diffusing capacity of carbon monoxide (DLco). A low DLco may be found when the alveolar surface available for diffusion is reduced as a result of parenchymal disease (fibrosis or emphysema) or surgical removal of considerable lung tissue. However, in the vast majority of cases, a low DLco reflects excessive $\dot{V}/\dot{Q}$ mismatching rather than a true diffusion defect, particularly when the inspired air is unevenly distributed.

ACID-BASE BALANCE

Assessment of acid-base status is an essential aspect of the investigation of patients with chronic respiratory insufficiency because the acid-base balance is affected by the $Paco_2$.

In patients with a restrictive disorder or in the earlier stages of obstructive disorders, the Pao_2 and $Paco_2$ are low and an alkalemia (pH over 7.45) is often present because of hypoxemia-induced hyperventilation. If the patient has been hyperventilating for some time, the arterial pH will usually be between 7.40 and 7.45 because of compensatory elimination of bicarbonate by the kidneys.

In severe chronic airflow obstruction, particularly when the work of breathing becomes excessive, the alveolar ventilation may be unable to cope with carbon dioxide production; thus the Pa_{CO_2} is elevated and the Pa_{O_2} is low. When this occurs acutely, the patient will be acidemic (pH under 7.35), but if the alveolar hypoventilation has been present for some time, the pH will be between 7.35 and 7.40 because of compensatory retention of bicarbonate by the kidneys.

Interpretation of the acid-base status may be difficult when patients with chronic respiratory insufficiency develop an acute disturbance or, as is often the case, have received varied medications. As a general rule, if the patient's pH is within the normal range and the Pa_{CO_2} is lower or greater than normal (i.e., under 35 or over 45 mm Hg at sea level), more than one disturbance is likely present. Under these circumstances, interpretation is based on the clinical evaluation, along with assessment of the duration of the problem and the therapy being administered. The level of the pH may also help: if the pH is below 7.40, an acidosis is likely the major disturbance; if it is above 7.40, it is likely an alkalosis.

· · ·

Assessment of respiratory function is an integral component of the clinical examination. Simple tests of function can be determined at the bedside or in the office. Provided basic principles of pulmonary physiology are kept in mind, evaluation of these simple parameters (along with those carried out in the pulmonary function laboratory) allows valid interpretation. Repeated assessments will allow the physician to follow the course of a disease process and to evaluate the impact of therapeutic regimens.

SUGGESTED READINGS

Cherniack, R.M.: Pulmonary function testing, Philadelphia, 1977, W.B. Saunders Co.
Cherniack, R.M., Cherniack, L., and Naimark, A.: Respiration in health and disease, ed. 2, Philadelphia, 1972, W.B. Saunders Co.
Comroe, J.H.: Physiology of respiration, ed. 2, Chicago, 1974, Year Book Medical Publishers, Inc.
Fenn, W.O.: Mechanics of respiration, Am. J. Med. **10:**77, 1951.
Filley, G.F.: Acid base and blood gas regulation, Philadelphia, 1971, Lea & Febiger.
Macklem, P.T.: Tests of lung mechanics, New Engl. J. Med. **293:**339, 1975.
West, J.B.: Respiratory physiology: the essentials, Baltimore, 1974, The Williams & Wilkins Co.
West, J.B.: Ventilation/blood flow and gas exchange, Oxford, 1965, Blackwell Scientific Publications.

Chapter 5

INFECTIOUS PNEUMONIAS
(excluding *M. tuberculosis* and fungi)

Frederick N. Hanson *and* **Michael D. Iseman**

Definition and background

Pneumonia or pneumonitis is an inflammatory process of the lung parenchyma. Many microbes, including bacteria, viruses, mycoplasmas, rickett-
siae, protozoa, and helminths, are known to produce pneumonia in humans.
This chapter will present a general approach to diagnosis and management
in adult patients with emphasis on establishing the specific etiologic
agent(s) responsible, since early diagnosis and specific therapy are the
cornerstones of successful treatment.

WHO GETS PNEUMONIA

To aid in diagnosing and treating pneumonia, physicians should consider
which individuals are apt to have which pneumonia in various settings.
Broadly speaking, patients with pneumonia may be divided into three main
categories.

The walking well

This group consists mostly of young individuals who have been in good
health until contracting an episode of respiratory illness. Pneumonia in this
setting may appear following a mild upper respiratory illness or may
abruptly manifest itself. The vast majority of such cases are pneumococcal in
etiology, but in situations conducive to epidemics, for example, military
camps and school dormitories, other organisms such as mycoplasma, adeno-
viruses, or influenza/parainfluenza viruses may be causative.

34

The walking but not-so-well

This group consists of individuals who contract their illnesses outside the hospital, but who have other health problems that predispose them to pneumonia. These include:

1. Disorders that, through interference with the normal upper airway function or esophagogastric integrity, promote apiration of bacterial contaminants and/or chemical irritants into the lower respiratory tract. Included would be primary neurologic diseases that involve bulbar cranial nerve function, conditions that result in loss of consciousness, such as alcoholism, drug abuse, epilepsy, trauma, and cerebrovascular accidents, and gastrointestinal disorders such as achalasia of the esophagus, esophageal cancer or strictures, gastroesophageal reflux with or without hiatus hernia, and gastric outlet obstruction.

2. Abnormalities of the lungs or thorax such as bronchiectasis, COPD, bronchogenic carcinoma, cystic fibrosis, recent lower respiratory tract viral illnesses (especially influenza), fractured ribs, and kyphoscoliosis.

3. Generally debilitating illnesses such as chronic alcoholism, uremia, congestive heart failure, diabetes, and sickle cell anemia, which predispose individuals to pneumonia through poorly understood mechanisms.

4. Diseases known to impair immunity such as lymphoma, leukemia, aplastic anemia, multiple myeloma, hypogammaglobulinemia, or therapy that is either intentionally (organ transplantation) or incidentally (antineoplastic or anti-inflammatory) immunosuppressive.[1-3] These agents include corticosteroids, cancer chemotherapy, irradiation, and antilymphocyte globulin.

In groups 1 to 3 the pneumococcus (streptococcus pneumoniae) has been and is still the predominant cause of pneumonia. However, other organisms are causative often enough to require critical and aggressive search for the etiologic agent. In general, situations that suggest that aspiration has occurred should raise the suspicion of involvement with anaerobic gram-negative bacilli of the *Bacteroides* and *Fusobacterium* species, aerobic gram-negative bacilli most commonly of the family Enterobacteriaceae, and anaerobic gram-positive organisms such as *Peptostreptococcus* and *Peptococcus*. Elderly persons with chronic alcoholism or diabetes are at increased risk of infection with *Klebsiella pneumoniae*. Patients with COPD and cystic fibrosis appear to be at relatively increased risk for *Haemophilus influenzae* infection. Pseudomonas infections are extremely common in patients suffering from cystic fibrosis. Recent viral lower respiratory tract illnesses significantly increase the risk for pneumonia with *Staphylococcus aureus*, *Streptococcus pyogenes*, and *Neisseria meningitidis*.

Patients in group 4, the immunosuppressed or compromised hosts, may be infected with a very wide variety of agents. In view of the potential dire consequences of erroneous diagnosis or delayed treatment, these patients should be evaluated diligently and promptly.

The hospitalized

Nosocomial or hospital-acquired infections have a special set of considerations in the evaluation and treatment of penumonias.[4] The predisposing conditions noted above (impaired upper airway defense mechanisms, general debility, chronic lung and thoracic conditions, and induced immunosuppression) also apply to the hospitalized patient. In addition to these problems, however, the hospitalized patient has certain risks unique to the institutional setting and the associated diseases. Such conditions include: (1) nonpulmonary medical or surgical conditions resulting in intraperitoneal, pelvic, or urologic sepsis, (2) burns involving the skin or respiratory tract, (3) mechanical invasions of the upper airway by endotracheal or tracheostomy tubes and nasotracheal suctioning, (4) aerosol invasion of the airways by nebulizing and ventilatory assistance devices, and (5) exposure to unusual microbes associated with altered endogenous flora or the selected organisms that colonize hospitals because of intensive antisepsis and antibiosis.

Patients with recent gastrointestinal sepsis are disposed to respiratory infections with Enterobacteriaceae and *Bacteroides* species and, less frequently, clostridia, pseudomonas, and enterococci. Pelvic sepsis should raise the index of suspicion for clostridial infection, while urologic infection or instrumentation may result in embolic pneumonia caused by Enterobacteriaceae (especially Escherichieae). Burn victims are at increased risk from *Pseudomonas aeruginosa* pneumonia, which may invade the lung either by colonizing the compromised respiratory tract or by septic embolization. Patients who are intubated and receiving nebulized humidification or assisted ventilation are at particular risk for pneumonia caused by *Serratia marcesens*, Enterobacteriaceae, and staphylococci. Patients who are receiving long-term, broad-spectrum antibiotics may develop pneumonitis caused by *Candida* or uncommon gram-negative species. Patients with badly infected gums (periodontitis) are more prone to anaerobic infections from the organisms that populate the oral cavity.

Individuals who contract pneumonia while hospitalized logically tend to be infected with the organisms that prevail in their environment. Although certain generalizations may be made about the microbes involved, each institution has its own profile of microflora. To aid in the search for the specific organism(s) involved or to assist in the empiric selection of antibiotics before a definite etiology is established, it is useful to know the pattern of organisms (and their usual antibiotic susceptibilities) recovered in nosocomial infections for that particular area of that hospital at that particular time. Such information should be available through the institution's infection control program.

Recently, attention has been called to epidemics of hospital-acquired pneumonia due to *Legionella pneumophila*. These outbreaks have been attributed most often to contaminated air-conditioning systems and constitute a unique epidemiologic challenge.

ESTABLISHING THE ETIOLOGIC AGENT

Using the information above as background, it is important to review other factors that are useful in identifying the causal agent(s).

History of present illness

Various signs and symptoms are common to many pneumonias regardless of the etiologic agent. Although certain combinations of these findings *may suggest* a specific infection, confirmation by culture is essential to establish the etiology. The onset of the pneumonia typically is marked by several or all of the following: fever, chills, sweats, pleuritic chest pains, cough, expectoration, hemoptysis, dyspnea, headache, and prostration.

Abruptness. An explosive onset before which the patient felt well and experienced sudden prostration is characteristic of gram-positive coccal pneumonias.

Chills. Although a vague sense of chilliness or "gooseflesh" is common to many infections, a frank shaking *rigor* is highly suggestive of a bacterial pneumonia with bloodstream invasion.

Pain. Sharp, stabbing pain over the lateral aspect of the chest that is markedly increased with breathing or coughing (as in pleurisy) is also typically associated with bacterial infections; it may cause voluntary restriction or splinting of chest motion in the affected region. Classic pleurisy is rarely seen with mycoplasmal or virus infections. More common with these infections is a burning or searing, midline, retrosternal pain that is also somewhat associated with respiration; it is believed to be caused by the tracheobronchitis common with these agents.

Cough and expectoration. It should be noted whether the cough is sporadic and productive of mucopurulent or sanguinopurulent (rusty) secretions that occur typically with bacterial infections or whether it is steady, barking, or hacking and productive of sparse amounts of mucoid or mucopurulent phlegm that usually occur in mycoplasmal or viral infections.

Dyspnea. Although shortness of breath is common in pneumonia, it is closely related to the extent of the pneumonia and to any underlying cardio-pulmonary disease. When dyspnea is disproportionate to these factors, the possibility of viral pneumonias with early interstitial involvement, *Pneumocystis carinii*, or pulmonary thromboembolism must be considered.

Headache. This is a common manifestation of general toxicity that, when very prominent, should increase consideration of viral, rickettsial, or mycoplasmal disease *or* a complicating meningitis.

Other findings. Obtundation disproportionate to the extent of the pneumonia has been noted commonly in cases of Legionnaire's disease (LD). Diarrhea may be prominent in LD or typhoidal pneumonia. Cutaneous abnormalities (i.e., various rashes) should call to mind such conditions as viral exanthem pneumonias (especially rubeola and varicella), rickettsioses, meningococcal pneumonia with septicemia, and the vasculitic pulmonary syndromes.

General history

Features to be developed in detail include:
1. Information suggesting that the illness is *not infectious pneumonia.* In particular, attention should be directed toward differentiating pneumonia from pulmonary thromboembolism, sarcoidosis, collagen vascular disease, cardiogenic or noncardiogenic pulmonary edema, inhalation of noxious gases or dusts, allergic or hypersensitivity reactions to drugs or other substances, hemoglobinopathies, neoplasia—both primary and metastatic, and pulmonary hemorrhage.
2. Contact with diseased individuals. This may be particularly helpful in suggesting viral pneumonias (including influenza, adenovirus, rubeola, and varicella), mycoplasma, and tuberculosis.
3. Exposure to animals. This should arouse suspicion of ornithosis, Q fever, histoplasmosis, cryptococcosis, leptospirosis, tularemia, and plague.
4. Travel to areas that present an increased risk of contracting specific infections (e.g., melioidosis in southeast Asia).[5]

Microbiologic studies

Examination of the secretions of the lower respiratory tract is of paramount importance. Sputum is usually readily accessible for smear and culture; however, the reliability of such studies has been questioned. Particular problems in sputum examinations include prior antibiotic therapy, contamination with the flora of the upper airways, and difficulty in culturing anaerobic organisms. If the gram stain of the sputum shows the presence of ciliated bronchial epithelial cells, a paucity of squamous upper airway epithelium, plentiful polymorphonuclear leukocytes, and a relatively pure population of morphologically similar organisms, it is reasonable to assume that the specimen will reflect the causal agent.

Washing and quantitative culture of expectorated sputum enhances the diagnostic accuracy of such specimens.[6] A technique of sputum liquefaction and quantitative culture also enhances the diagnostic value of expectorated sputum in aerobic pneumonia acquired outside of the hospital and not associated with bronchiectasis.[7] Counterimmunoelectrophoresis of the sputum has also been employed to establish the etiology of a case of pneumonia[8]; however, its role appears to be limited.[9]

When adequate sputum cannot be raised or when a strong consideration of anaerobic infection exists, a *transtracheal aspiration* (TTA) may be indicated. In this technique the cricorthyroid membrane is punctured percutaneously, and a catheter is introduced into the lower respiratory tract.[10] Caution should be observed in employing TTA in patients with deficient clotting factors, thrombocytopenia, hypoxemia, leukopenia, or the possible need for assisted ventilation; these individuals have increased hazards from bleeding, local infections, or subcutaneous emphysema. Despite these risks TTA can be a very useful method for obtaining valid diagnostic specimens.[11] TTA should not be employed indiscriminately but should be reserved for the circumstances cited above and in patients in whom the severity, rapidity or progression, or failure to respond to treatment are sufficiently compelling to outweigh the small but real risks and discomfort of the technique.

When these techniques fail to obtain adequate diagnostic material, more aggressive methods may have to be employed. Direct *transthoracic percutaneous lung aspiration* employing a syringe and a spinal needle may be particularly useful in the setting of a peripheral consolidating process, especially in the lower posterior lung fields. However, when the lesion(s) in question are poorly accessible, in juxtaposition to vital structures, or present in lungs with grossly altered mechanical or anatomic properties (e.g., emphysema, diffuse fibrosis), the risks may be unacceptably high. In patients who are receiving or may imminently need assisted ventilation, the risk of inducing a tension pneumothorax with this procedure virtually precludes its use. Finally, if a fungal infection is suspected, the possibility of inducing a difficult to manage empyema or bronchopleural fistula is a relative contraindication to this technique.

Recently, considerable interest has been expressed in the use of the flexible fiberoptic bronchoscope (FFB) either to aspirate secretions or to obtain endobronchial or transbronchial biopsy specimens.[12] Advantages of this technique are the promptness with which it can be employed, the low morbidity and mortality risk, the opportunity for direct visualization of the endobronchial anatomy to exclude the presence of neoplasms, strictures, or foreign bodies, and the opportunity to obtain separate specimens from both lungs. Drawbacks include difficulty in interpreting bacteriologic specimens caused by contamination from upper airway secretions, inhibition of culture specimens by the topical anesthetic agents, sampling error in interpreting very small biopsy specimens, and maintaining ventilation in patients with compromised pulmonary status. A new type of brush and catheter system has recently been developed that substantially reduces contamination from upper airway microbes.[13] This system entails a brush contained within a catheter that has a displaceable plug. First, the catheter is directed to the area to be cultured. The brush is advanced, pushing out the plug. After the physician brushes the area in interest, the brush is retracted back within the catheter and the catheter is withdrawn into the bronchoscope. Recent studies document a high degree of sensitivity and freedom from contamination with this technique (see also Chapter 3).[14]

The alternative to FFB is *open lung biopsy* performed by way of limited thoracotomy. This procedure is generally reserved for the critically ill and the compromised or immunosuppressed patient with diffuse lung disease in whom the range of possible causative agents is broad and the implications of missing the diagnosis are great. Advantages of open biopsy include larger specimens for microbiologic and histologic study, the ability to select tissue from variably involved areas, and the ability to control ventilation during the procedures. Shortcomings include postoperative discomfort, the small but real hazards of general anesthesia, and the inability to obtain specimens from both lungs.

The considerations involved in selecting these more aggressive diagnostic methods are complex and depend on the availability of resources, the abilities and preferences of the attending physicians and surgeons, and the patient's considerations.

Occasionally a definitive etiologic diagnosis in pneumonia can be made by means other than demonstrating or culturing the organisms from the lung. Examples include culturing an organism from the blood or pleural effusion, identifying an organism on stain of pleural fluid, or finding a diagnostic histologic picture on pleural biopsy, for example, the caseating granulomas of tuberculosis.

Radiographic features

In virtually all pneumonias, abnormalities are visible on the chest radiograph. By themselves these abnormalities are usually not sufficiently distinctive to permit an etiologic diagnosis. However, by careful analysis of the pattern, anatomic distribution, and progress of the changes, strong inferences may often be made regarding the causal agent.

Pneumonia may be radiographically manifested in the following ways:

1. *Alveolar or acinar* describes the fluffy shadows that result from fluid accumulation in the distal airspaces of the lung. They usually range from 0.5 to 1.0 cm in diameter and commonly are coalescent.
2. *Interstitial or reticular* describes the shadows that are a lacey network of linear markings that may reflect increased inflammatory material within the tissue surrounding the airspaces and/or vascular structures but most commonly represent chronic changes such as fibrosis. The linear changes may be the only abnormality or they may coexist with nodular shadows.
3. *Bronchopneumonia* describes scattered fluffy shadows that tend to be patchy and follow the distribution of the central conducting airways. These may become confluent but rarely produce the "air-bronchogram" effect.
4. *Lobar pneumonia* describes confluent shadows that usually terminate at pleural surfaces and usually but not always involve entire lobes or segments. A feature of lobar pneumonia is that the densities often surround the conducting airways, forming a highly visible contrasting interface, the "air-bronchogram" (Figs. 5-1 and 5-2).
5. *Necrotizing pneumonia* describes pneumonia in which necrosis of lung parenchyma results in cavity formation. Lung abscess is a variant of this process, distinguished from a necrotizing pneumonia by the relative paucity of surrounding pneumonic infliltration on the chest radiograph (see Chapter 18). The radiolucencies may be apparent at the outset or may evolve as the inflammatory process advances. It is important not to confuse prominent lucencies in a pneumonic shadow due to underlying emphysema with the true cavities of a necrotizing pneumonia.

Physical examination

Patients with mild pneumonia may have no abnormal physical findings. Those patients with lobar pneumonia frequently have signs of consolidation (see Chapter 2); those patients with bronchopneumonia usually have such signs only when the process is very extensive. Signs of fluid should not be overlooked. During the acute phase of severe pneumonia, patients are apt to reveal cyanosis, tachypnea, flaring of the alae nasi with inspiration, and severe prostration. As clearing and improvement occur, fine rales are replaced by coarse, bubbly rales and rhonchi.

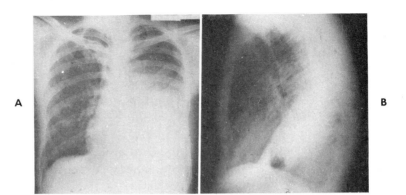

FIG. 5-1. Lobar pneumonia, left lower lobe. **A,** Posteroanterior, **B,** lateral. *(Courtesy Medical Illustration Service, Veterans Administration Hospital, Denver, Colorado.)*

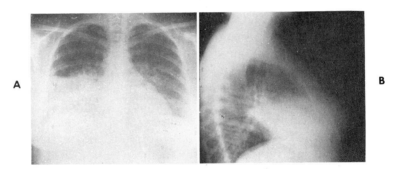

FIG. 5-2. Lobar pneumonia, right middle lobe. **A,** Posteroanterior, **B,** lateral. *(Courtesy Medical Illustration Service, Veterans Administration Hospital, Denver, Colorado.)*

GENERAL MANAGEMENT

Hypoxemia. Supplemental oxygen should be provided for patients with significantly reduced Pao_2. Caution should be exercised not to promote hypoventilation in patients with severe COPD ("CO_2 narcosis").

Pain. Analgesics should be given to control pleuritic pain, thus promoting adequate ventilation and cough. Salicylates or codeine may be adequate, but patients often require stronger agents. Care should be taken not to suppress cough or ventilatory drive, particularly in patients with COPD.

Dehydration. Prompt oral or intravenous replacement of fluids should be given to combat dehydration caused by poor intake, increased insensible loss from fever and hyperventilation, or both. Caution should be exercised in administering fluids to patients if rapidly progressive disease threatens the complication of adult respiratory distress syndrome (ARDS).

Paralytic ileus. Paralytic ileus is usually secondary to diaphragmatic pleurisy and contributes to already difficult ventilation. Rectal intubation and hot abdominal compresses often lead to decompression and considerable relief.

Empyema. If empyema is of sufficient degree to contribute to impaired ventilation or toxicity, it should be drained by needle, tube thoracostomy, or rib resection open drainage if necessary (see Chapter 19).

SPECIAL FEATURES AND TREATMENT OF SOME COMMON PNEUMONIAS[15,16]
Aerobic and anaerobic pneumonias

Pneumococcal pneumonia, caused by *Streptococcus pneumoniae*, an aerobic gram-positive diplococcus, is the most common of all community acquired pneumonias.[17,18] Clinical features include sudden onset, high fever, rigors, pleuritic chest pain, tachypnea, and cough productive of mucopurulent or rusty phlegm. Paralytic ileus is common. The chest radiograph usually reveals a lobar distribution; effusions occur in 10% to 20% of cases. Laboratory findings include leukocytosis to 20,000 with left shift, positive blood cultures in 25% to 30% of cases, frequent liver function derangement, and hypoxemia. Empyema is a common complication, especially with delayed therapy. Parapneumonic effusions that resolve spontaneously are even more common. Uncommon complications include meningitis, endocarditis, pericarditis, peritonitis, and septic arthritis. Leukopenia, hypotension, and multilobar involvement are unfavorable prognostic signs and may herald the onset of ARDS.[19] Treatment consists of procaine penicillin G 600,000 units intramuscularly every 12 hours, aqueous penicillin G 300,000 units intravenously every 4 hours, penicillin V 250 mg orally every 6 hours, cefazolin 500 mg intramuscularly or intravenously every 8 hours, or cephalexin 500 mg orally every 6 hours. The parenteral route is preferred in the more serious infections. Oral drugs are used to treat less ill patients and to follow initial parenteral treatment. Higher doses are reserved for complications only. Temperature should return to normal within 72 hours; if fever persists, complications or drug reactions are likely.

A polyvalent pneumococcal vaccine that provides protection for at least 3 years against 14 serotypes that cause some 75% of pneumococcal pneumonias became available in 1978. Its value in protecting the impaired host has recently been questioned.[20]

Staphylococcal pneumonia, caused by *Staphylococcus aureus*, an aerobic gram-positive coccus, is freqently seen in association with influenza. It may also be seen with right-sided bacterial endocarditis, particularly among intravenous drug abusers. It is rarely seen in the walking well patient. Clinical features are similar to those of pneumococcal pneumonia. The chest radiograph shows bronchial or lobar distribution, usually in both lungs. Other findings include a moderate leukocytosis with left shift and profound hypoxemia. Blood cultures are positive in 10% to 15% of cases. Complications include frequent empyema; less frequent ones are spontaneous pneumothorax and acute endocarditis. The cavities frequently become pneumatoceles or large, thin-walled, air-filled, rounded spaces in the clearing phase. Metastatic abscesses in the brain, kidneys, or other organs and meningitis and endocarditis are feared complications. Treatment consists of Oxacillin or Nafcillin 2 gm intravenously every 6 hours or cefazolin 0.5 gm intravenously every 4 hours (presume penicillin resistance until bacteriologic studies show otherwise). Chloramphenicol and Vancomycin are also effective against staphylococci.

Streptococcal pneumonia, caused by *Streptococcus pyogenes*, an aerobic gram-positive coccus, is a common postinfluenzal superinfection. Clinical features, chest radiographs, and laboratory findings are similar to those of staphylococcal pneumonia. The antistreptolysin-O titer may be elevated. Complications are common and include acute glomerulonephritis, empyema in over 50% of cases, occasional cavitation, and residual pleural thickening. Treatment consists of procaine penicillin G 1,200,000 units intramuscularly or intravenously every 8 hours. Higher doses are used in empyema.

Haemophilus influenzae pneumonia is commonly seen in elderly patients with COPD and/or chronic alcoholism.[21-23] The organism is a small, pleomorphic, aerobic gram-negative bacillus. The illness usually occurs as a bronchopneumonia with a predilection for the lower lobes. Because of *H. influenzae's* fastidious growth requirements, secretions should be plated on chocolate agar or blood agar with "staph-streak." Treatment should include ampicillin 1 to 2 gm intravenously every 6 hours or chloramphenicol 1 gm intravenously or intramuscularly every 6 hours.

Gram-negative pneumonias (GNPs) have become the most common type of nosocomial respiratory infection[24-26] through several factors: (1) the widespread use of broad-spectrum antibiotics, (2) the common use of assisted ventilation with the potential for respiratory equipment contamination, (3) compromised local host defenses that occur with the use of endotracheal tubes and tracheostomies, and (4) various causes of immunosuppression mentioned above under "Walking but not-so-well." Appropriate gram stains and cultures remain the best means of definitive diagnosis. Although GNPs classically present as an acute toxic illness, the onset is sometimes insidious with gradual progressive lung consolidation or necrosis with little fever or constitutional symptomatology. Clinical resolution of GNP is also often slow; mortality remains at a very high 50% to 80%, reflecting the seriousness of the underlying host disease.

Klebsiella (or Friedländer's) pneumonia is caused by *Klebsiella pneumoniae*, an aerobic gram-negative rod. It occurs especially in diabetic, elderly alcoholic, and hospitalized patients. It has the classic acute onset, but with severe cough productive of tenacious mucopurulent and bloody ("currant jelly") sputum. The patient often declines rapidly. The chest radiograph classically shows extensive lobar involvement, especially in an upper lobe in which secretions accumulate rapidly, producing the so-called bulging fissure sign more commonly than in other fulminant pneumonias. Leukopenia with marked left shift and hypoxemia are common. Caution in interpreting the gram stain of secretions is important, since *Klebsiella* may assume a coccobacillary form and be confused with over-decolorized pneumococci. Complications include empyema, cavitation, respiratory failure, and shock. Mortality is very high. Treatment should consist of a parenteral cephalosporin such as cefazolin 1 gm intramuscularly or intravenously every 4 to 6 hours and an aminoglycoside such as gentamicin 6 mg/kg/day intramuscularly or intravenously in divided doses every 8 hours. The dosage of aminoglycosides should be reduced in renal insufficiency.

Pseudomonas pneumonia, usually due to *P. aeruginosa*, is generally a hospital-acquired infection occurring in debilitated or immunocompromised patients. The organism has a particular propensity to grow in moist or liquid environments, and outbreaks have often been traced to contaminated inhalation therapy equipment. Most infections are due to inhalation or inapparent aspiration of the organism in patients with prior oropharyngeal colonization. The usual clinical presentation is not much different from other pneumonias. Relative bradycardia for the degree of fever, reversal of the usual temperature curve with the peak temperature occurring in the morning, and a predilection for lower lobe involvement, usually bilateral, are special features. Patchy infiltrates often progress rapidly despite therapy, resulting in massive consolidation. Abscesses, often very large, are common. Antibiotic treatment consists of an aminoglycoside plus either carbenicillin or ticarcillin.

Escherichia coli is an unusual cause of pneumonia in adults. In contrast to other GNPs, the route of *E. coli* infection is commonly a hematogenous spread from gastrointestinal or genitourinary infections. The clinical picture is nonspecific; special features include nausea, vomiting and abdominal pain, and a predilection for the lower lobes.

Mycoplasmal pneumonia is caused by *Mycoplasma pneumoniae*, an organism with a triple membrane and no cell wall; it has highly specialized growth requirements. It is common in young people and usually occurs as school or community epidemics, although it may appear episodically in all age groups.[18,27] The clinical picture includes a gradual onset with sore throat, rhinorrhea, malaise, nausea and vomiting, headache, hacking cough productive of sparse mucopurulent sputum, and fever.[28] Examination of the chest is frequently negative. Lymphadenopathy and a variety of mucocutaneous eruptions are commonly seen. The chest radiograph characteristically shows a mild scattered bronchopneumonia involving lower lobes, usually unilateral. Small effusions are frequent. High titers of IgM antibodies against erythrocyte I antigen (cold agglutinins) may occasionally produce hemolytic anemia with a positive direct Coombs test. Leukocytosis is usually mild, without left shift. Sputum typically shows many polymorphonuclear leukocytes but few organisms. Treatment should consist of erythromycin 250 to 500 mg orally every 6 hours or tetracycline 250 mg orally every 6 hours. Clearing of signs and symptoms occurs gradually, and prompt therapy is associated with a maximum response. Cough and malaise commonly persist for many weeks.

Anaerobic pneumonias are usually caused by *Bacteroides melaninogenicus, Bacteroides fragilis, Fusobacterium nucleatum, Peptostreptococcus, Peptococcus,* and combinations of these and other species (anaerobic gram-negative rods, gram-positive cocci, or both).[25,30] They are most common in hospitalized patients and in chronic alcoholics with infected gums and a predisposition to aspiration. One recent series observed an associated bronchogenic carcinoma in 17% of patients with anaerobic pneumonia.[31] The onset of symptoms is usually gradual over 1 to 2 weeks, with weight loss and cough that is productive of copious putrid sputum in less than half the patients. Roughly 20% of patients with anaerobic pneumonia develop lung abscesses. Patients with anaerobic pneumonia are generally less toxic and dyspneic than those with other acute bacterial pneumonias of comparable extent. The process predominantly involves the posterior and basilar gravity-dependent segments. Anemia and leukocytosis are common. Obtaining sputum specimens from which these fastidious organisms can be cultured may require transtracheal aspiration. Treatment consists of procaine penicillin G 1,200,000 units intramuscularly every 12 hours or aqueous penicillin G 500,000 units intravenously every 6 hours until fever, toxicity, sputum production, and leukocytosis have diminished. Treatment may then be changed to penicillin V 250 to 500 mg orally every 6 hours. The usual course of therapy is 6 to 8 weeks total. If the patient is allergic to penicillin or cultures yield *B. fragilis* resistant to penicillin, clindamycin 300 to 600 mg intravenously (given over a 30-minute period) every 8 hours may be used. Tetracycline 500 mg orally every 6 hours may also be used in subjects with penicillin allergy. Chloramphenicol 500 mg orally or intravenously every 4 hours should be used for *B. fragilis* infections in patients who cannot tolerate clindamycin.

Viral pneumonia

A large number of viruses are capable of causing pneumonias in adults and children. Most common causative viruses are associated with pharyngitis, bronchitis, bronchiolitis, or coryza, but other viruses such as rubeola, varicella, influenza, adenovirus, and cytomegalovirus can cause pneumonias in adults and children. Most viral pneumonias are community acquired; many, such as influenza, occur in epidemics. Secondary bacterial infection is often the factor responsible for the unusual mortality in viral pneumonias; rarely, the viral agent alone causes overwhelming respiratory failure. Adults with chickenpox (varicella-zoster virus) develop pneumonia in up to 50% of cases, in contrast to its rare occurrence in children. Immunosuppressed patients are particularly susceptible to pneumonia due to cytomegalovirus. Common symptoms in viral pneumonias include dry, nonproductive cough, chills, headache, fever, myalgias, malaise, and dyspnea. The chest radiograph varies from small patchy infiltrates to massive consolidation depending on the severity of the illness. The leukocyte count is usually below 12,000. Definitive diagnosis requires a significant rise in acute and convalescent viral titers or growth of the organism from properly obtained cultures. There is no specific therapy for most viral pneumonias, although amantadine has had limited success in treatment of one specific influenza strain.

Unusual pneumonias

Q fever, due to infection with the rickettsial organism *Coxiella burnetii,* results in a flulike illness that can also include pneumonia in up to 50% of patients. Most cases occur through inhalation of infected dust particles associated with infected livestock or from drinking unpasteurized milk. Tetracycline is the drug of choice.

Ornithosis (psittacosis) is caused by inhalation of infected dried excreta from birds of almost any type that are infected with *Chlamydia psittaci.* Usually a flulike illness occurs, but a more severe illness including severe pneumonia may occur. The antibiotic of choice is tetracycline.

Pneumocystis carinii is a parasite that causes infection almost exclusively in immunocompromised patients.[32] Physical signs are often minimal despite extensive pneumonia on chest radiograph. Pentamidine has been the only treatment available, but now trimethoprim-sulfa has been successful both for prophylaxis in susceptible patients and for the primary treatment of this infection.

Tularemia may cause either a primary pneumonia through inhalation of organisms or secondary pulmonary involvement from infection introduced through the skin. Most cases occur in hunters who have recently skinned wild rabbits. Regional and hilar lymph node enlargement is common. Streptomycin is specific for this infection.

Legionnaire's disease (LD) is a respiratory illness caused by a newly discovered gram-negative bacterium, *Legionella pneumophila*.[33] It was first recognized in an outbreak of severe respiratory illness at the 1976 American Legion Convention in Philadelphia. Retrospective serologic studies and current investigations indicate that LD is a persistent source of episodic and epidemic pneumonia that may cause up to 1% of community-acquired and 3% to 4% of sporadic, nosocomial pneumonia. Epidemiologically, the following characteristics have been observed for LD: (1) increased risk for middle-aged male smokers, (2) increased vulnerability with immunosuppression (including corticosteroid therapy), underlying COPD, diabetes, or alcoholism, (3) seasonal increase in summer and fall, and (4) epidemics in proximity to excavation sites, contaminated water systems, and contaminated air-conditioning systems.

The spectrum of illness associated with LD ranges from a flulike illness to overwhelming pneumonia. Typically, a prodrome of malaise, myalgias, and headache lasts for several days. Diarrhea with nausea and vomiting is also common early in the illness. Upper respiratory symptoms such as laryngitis, coryza, and sinusitis are noticeably *absent*. High fever (to 40° C), shaking chills, cough, dyspnea, and pleurisy herald the pneumonic phase. Altered mental status with delirium, emotional lability, and obtundation appears in 25% of patients.

The chest radiograph usually reveals a nondescript, patchy infiltrate in one or both lower lobes. Rapid spread to other lobes on the side of the initial infiltrates may occur. Small pleural effusions have been recorded. Other suggestive laboratory findings include an elevation of serum glutamic-oxalacetic transaminase (SGOT), microscopic hematuria, hyponatremia, and hypophosphatemia. Sputum gram stain typically reveals a modest number of polymorphonuclear leukocytes and a paucity of organisms. While *Legionella* are gram-negative, they stain weakly and are rarely identifiable on gram stain of sputum. Direct immunofluorescence staining of sputum is quick and specific but positive in only 25% of cases. The diagnosis is most readily made by demonstrating the organism in tissue. Dieterle's silver impregnation stain or immunofluorescence staining in lung tissue may be performed within 24 hours and returns the highest yield of any immediate study. Serologic studies are highly sensitive and specific but weeks are required to obtain and compare acute and convalescent sera. A diagnosis of LD must thus be made on a presumptive basis (unless direct immunofluorescence of sputum is available and positive, or lung tissue is obtained for histologic study). The decision whether to diagnose and treat empirically or to pursue definitive studies should be based on severity of the illness, potential of other infections or noninfectious causes, and rate of progression of the disease.

Erythromycin appears to be the treatment of choice: 1 gm intravenously every 6 hours for the seriously ill or 500 mg orally every 6 hours for the less ill. Rifampin has modest in vitro activity against LD and may be added if therapy is failing. Tetracycline is less effective than erythromycin but may be useful in the patient who does not tolerate erythromycin. Therapy should be continued for 2 to 3 weeks; relapses have been observed with early discontinuation. Untreated, LD mortality ranges from 25% to 75%. Erythromycin reduces mortality to approximately 15% for healthy individuals and 25% for immunocompromised patients.

Pittsburgh pneumonia agent (PPA), an organism similar to *Legionella*, was recently reported to cause an acute, severe pneumonic illness among immunocompromised patients, especially renal transplant recipients on high-dosage corticosteroid therapy.[34] The disease is marked by gradual onset, progressive fever, nonproductive cough, pleurisy, and lower zone bronchopneumonia or nodular infiltrates. Diagnosis is established by open lung biopsy with demonstration of the faintly gram-negative and *weakly acid-fast* organisms. Therapy is less well established than with LD; however, in vitro studies suggest efficacy with erythromycin, trimethoprim-sulfa, rifampin, and penicillin.

Recurrent pneumonia is a special problem.[35] It suggests underlying bronchiectasis and other predisposing conditions described in Chapter 2. Although it may arouse suspicion of a partially obstructing bronchogenic carcinoma, this condition is more often associated with failure to resolve rather than true recurrence.

REFERENCES

1. Williams, D.M., Krick, J.A., and Remington, J.S.: Pulmonary infection in the compromised host. I. Am. Rev. Respir. Dis. **114**:359, 1976.
2. Williams, D.M., Drick, J.A., and Remington, J.S.: Pulmonary infection in the compromised host. II. Am. Rev. Respir. Dis. **114**:593, 1976.
3. Bode, F.R., Pare, J.A.P., and Fraser, R.G.: Pulmonary diseases in the compromised host: a review of clinical and roentgenographic manifestations in patients with impaired host defense mechanisms, Medicine **53**:255, 1974.
4. Graybill, J.R., Marshall, L.W., Charache, P., et al.: Nosocomial pneumonia: a continuing major problem, Am. Rev. Respir. Dis. **108**:1130, 1973.
5. Everett, E.D., and Nelson, R.A.: Pulmonary melioidosis: observations in thirty-nine cases, Am. Rev. Respir. Dis. **112**:331, 1975.
6. Bartlett, J.G., and Finegold, S.M.: Bacteriology of expectorated sputum with quantitative culture and wash technique compared to transtracheal aspirates, Am. Rev. Respir. Dis. **117**:1019,1978.
7. Guckian, J.C., and Christensen, W.D.: Quantitative culture and gram stain of sputum in pneumonia, Am. Rev. Respir. Dis. **118**:997, 1978.
8. Leach, R.P., and Coonrod, J.D.: Detection of pneumococcal antigens in the sputum in pneumococcal pneumonia, Am. Rev. Respir. Dis. **116**:847, 1977.
9. Schmid, R.E., Anhalt, J.P., Wold, A.D., et al.: Sputum counterimmunoelectrophoresis in the diagnosis of pneumococcal pneumonia, Am. Rev. Respir. Dis. **119**:345, 1979.
10. Hahn, H.H., and Beaty, H.N.: Transtracheal aspiration in the evaluation of patients with pneumonia, Ann. Intern. Med. **72**:183, 1970.

11. Bartlett, J.G.: Diagnostic accuracy of transtracheal aspiration bacteriologic studies, Am. Rev. Respir. Dis. **115**:777, 1977.
12. Bartlett, J.G., Alexander, J., Mayhew, J., et al.: Should fiberoptic bronchoscopy aspirates be cultures? Am. Rev. Respir. Dis. **114**:73, 1976.
13. Wimberley, N., Faling, L.J., and Bartlett, J.G.: A fiberoptic bronchoscopy technique to obtain uncontaminated lower airway secretions for bacterial culture, Am. Rev. Respir. Dis. **119**:337, 1979.
14. Hayes, D.A., McCarthy, L.C., and Friedman, M.: Evaluation of two bronchofiberscopic methods of culturing the lower respiratory tract, Am. Rev. Respir. Dis. **122**:319, 1980.
15. Finland, M.: Pneumonia and pneumococcal infection with special reference to pneumococcal pneumonia, Am. Rev. Respir. Dis. **120**:481, 1979.
16. Lerner, A.M., and Jankauskas, K.: The classical bacterial pneumonias, Disease-A-Month 1-46, February, 1975.
17. Fekety, F.R., Jr., Caldwell, J., Gump, D., et al.: Bacteria, viruses, and mycoplasmas in acute pneumonia in adults, Am. Rev. Respir. Dis. **104**:499, 1971.
18. Foy, H.M., Wentworth, B., Kenny, G.E., et al.: Pneumococcal isolations from patients with pneumonia and control subjects in a prepaid medical care group, Am. Rev. Respir. Dis. **111**:595, 1975.
19. Van Metre, T.E.: Pneumococcal pneumonia treated with antibiotics. The prognostic significance of certain clinical findings, N. Engl. J. Med. **251**:1048,1954.
20. Broome, C.V., Facklam, R.R., and Fraser, D.W.: Pneumococcal disease after pneumococcal vaccination, N. Engl. J. Med. **303**:549, 1980.
21. Goldstein, E., Daly, A.K., and Seamans, C.: *Haemophilus influenzae* as a cause of adult pneumonia, Ann. Intern. Med. **66**:35, 1967.
22. Quintiliani, R., and Hymans, P.J.: The association of bacteremic *Haemophilus influenzae* pneumonia in adults with typable strains, Am. J. Med. **50**:781, 1971.
23. Hirschmann, J.V., and Everett, E.D.: *Haemophilus influenzae* infections in adults: report of nine cases and a review of the literature, Medicine **58**:80, 1979.
24. Johanson, W.G., Jr., Pierce, A.K., Sanford, J.P., et al.: Nosocomial respiratory infections with gram-negative bacilli: the significance of colonization of the respiratory tract, Am. Intern. Med. **77**:701, 1972.
25. Pierce, A., and Sanford, J.: Aerobic gram-negative bacillary pneumonia, Am. Rev. Respir. Dis. **110**:647, 1974.
26. Valdivieso, M., et al.: Gram-negative bacillary pneumonia in the compromised host, Medicine **56**:241, 1977.
27. Griffin, J.P., and Crawford, Y.E.: *Mycoplasma pneumoniae* in primary atypical pneumonia, J.A.M.A. **193**:1011, 1965.
28. Murray, H.W., Masur, H., Senterfit, L.B., et al.: The protean manifestations of *Mycoplasma pneumoniae* infection in adults, Am. J. Med. **58**:229, 1975.
29. Lorber, B., and Swenson, R.M.: Bacteriology of aspiration pneumonia: a perspective study of community and hospital acquired cases, Ann. Intern. Med. **81**:329, 1974.
30. Bartlett, J.G., and Finegold, S.M.: Anaerobic infections of the lung and pleural space, Am. Rev. Respir. Dis. **110**:56, 1974.
31. Bartlett, J.G.: Anaerobic bacterial pneumonitis, Am. Rev. Respir. Dis. **119**:19, 1979.
32. Walzer, P.D., Perl, D.P., Drogstad, D.J., et al.: *Pneumocystis carinii* pneumonia in the United States: epidemiologic, diagnostic, and clinical features, Ann. Intern. Med. **80**:83, 1974.
33. Balows, A., and Fraser, D.W., edtiors: International symposium on Legionnaire's disease, Ann. Intern. Med. **90**:489, 1979.
34. Myerowitz, R.L., et al.: Opportunistic lung infection due to "Pittsburgh Pneumonia Agent," N. Engl. J. Med. **301**:953, 1979.
35. Winterbauer, R.H., Bedon, G.A., and Ball, W.C., Jr.: Recurrent pneumonia: predisposing illness and clinical patterns in 158 patients, Ann. Intern. Med. **70**:689, 1969.

Chapter 6

BRONCHIAL ASTHMA

Charles Scoggin

Bronchial asthma is best defined as airflow obstruction characterized by episodic dyspnea and usually accompanied by wheezing associated with reactive airways. Asthma differs from COPD, emphysema, and chronic bronchitis in that its airflow obstruction is partially and at times totally reversible.

Asthma is one of the most common chronic pulmonary disorders. An estimated 10% of all people have some evidence of asthma during their lives. All age groups, every population, and both sexes are afflicted. Although asthma is more frequent in men than in women for reasons that are unclear, it tends to be more severe in women. The severity of asthma varies widely; some patients have only intermittent symptoms between long periods of good health, while others have unremitting symptoms and physiologic dysfunction. Even within a given patient, the severity of the illness may vary strikingly. A person may have seemingly stable asthma that quickly changes to a life-threatening attack. To the physician inexperienced with asthma, the disease's heterogeneous nature may be both confusing and intimidating. Fortunately, physicians' understanding and management of asthma is improving.

Etiology

A number of causes may precipitate an asthma attack. These include allergies, infection, exercise, emotional stress, environmental factors such as wind and cold, occupational exposures, and even pharmacologic agents (e.g., aspirin). Allergic asthma is particularly prominent in childhood. Individuals with allergic asthma often have accompanying atopy with skin rash, swelling of the nasal mucosa, and eosinophilia of the blood and sputum. Environmental factors include pets, plant pollens, and various dusts. Infections include bacteria and particularly viruses. A particularly intriguing precipitating cause is exercise. In fact, all asthmatics will manifest airways obstruction after hyperventilating subfreezing air. Occupational exposures include irritative substances such as cotton mill dust and ammonia.

Mechanisms of airway obstruction

Stimuli to the hyperirritable asthmatic airways accentuate the tracheobronchial tree's normal reactivity. The dynamic nature of the airways allows them to dilate normally when more air is needed, such as during exercise. Constriction of the airways, as with cough, limits the inhalation of irritative agents and facilitates their expulsion. The mechanism by which the caliber of the airways is altered is unknown; however, four factors appear to be important: (1) the parasympathetic or cholinergic nervous system, (2) the sympathetic nervous system, (3) irritant receptors within the lung, and (4) cellular mediators of airway reactivity.

The lung receives *parasympathetic* or cholinergic innervation through the vagus nerve. Stimulation of this system narrows the airways through smooth muscle constriction and excessive production of mucus. Atropine will block this reaction.

Bronchodilation is most effectively accomplished by stimulation of the β-adrenergic receptors of the *sympathetic nervous system*. The lung contains specific β_2-adrenergic receptors. Pharmacologic agents that selectively stimulate these receptors to the exclusion of the β_1-receptors of the cardiovascular system offer the advantage of promoting bronchodilation while minimizing cardiovascular side effects. β_2-selective drugs include isoetharine, metaproterenol, albuterol, and terbutaline.

Irritant receptors, when stimulated within the lungs, lead to cough and bronchoconstriction. It is probably in this way that maneuvers leading to distortion of the airways, for instance, coughing and laughing, may provoke reflex attacks of asthma.

Finally, cellular-mediated factors are of importance in promoting certain types of asthma. Allergy-mediated asthma is an example. When IgE molecules attached to mast cells are bridged by specific antigens, primary and secondary mediators of the allergic response are liberated. In asthma, these mediators cause bronchoconstriction. Primary mediators include histamine, platelet-activating factor, eosinophil and neutrophil chemotactic factors, serotonin, and heparin. Secondary mediators are slow-reactive substance of anaphylaxis (SRS-A) and arachidonic acid metabolites such as prostaglandins, thromboxins, and bradykinins.

It is important to remember that part of asthma's heterogeneous nature is reflected in the fact that the importance of each mechanism may vary among patients. Regardless of which factor predominates, clinical strategies are available to address each mechanism. It is important to avoid irritation of the airways, to try to prevent exposure to factors that may lead to the release of cellular mediators, to stimulate the β_2-adrenergic system, and, in some cases, to block the parasympathetic nervous system to prevent bronchoconstriction.

Many of the medications used to treat asthma are believed to modify the intracellular concentrations of cyclic nucleotides. "3,5' cyclic" adenosine monophosphate (cAMP) promotes bronchodilation by a mechanism not yet understood. It may have a direct effect on stimulating smooth muscle relaxation, and it may also prevent the release of mediators of the asthmatic attack from mast cells. β_2-adrenergic drugs increase its production, while the aminophylline-theophylline compounds prevent its breakdown. Regulation of intracellular levels of calcium ion may also be important in bronchodilatation.

Pathology

Patients who die of asthma show profound airways obstruction due to smooth muscle hypertrophy, mucosal edema, and extensive mucus plugging of the bronchioles. The mucus plugs or impactions are known as Curschmann's spirals when coughed out during life. Cellular infiltration, particularly with eosinophils, is a frequent finding. The lungs are hyperinflated but usually not emphysematous. These pathologic abnormalities of fatal asthma draw attention to the therapeutic aims in asthma.

Physiology

Airflow velocity is determined by airways conductance (Gaw) (reciprocal of Raw) and the elastic recoil properties of the lung. Resistance to flow is inversely proportional to the fourth power of airway caliber and normally is much higher in the larger airways, since the total cross-sectional area of these airways is much less than the total cross-sectional area of smaller airways; thus bronchoconstriction and mucus plugging in larger airways influence Raw considerably more than in small airways. In addition, the lungs of an asthmatic person have less elastic recoil than normal; this contributes to lower expiratory flow. To compensate for these two barriers to airflow, two main mechanisms are operative:

1. The lungs enlarge and increase airways caliber. Since narrowed, constricted airways close early during expiration, air is trapped in the lungs. The resulting increase in lung size causes interstitial forces to pull on airways and distend them. The degree of increase in caliber depends on the balance between distending and bronchoconstrictive forces. In addition, at a larger lung volume, the recoil pressure contributing to expiratory flow may be greater. The enlargement of the

lungs in asthma thus partially compensates for the bronchoconstriction and loss of elastic properties.

2. Accessory muscles of respiration are recruited to assist in inspiratory lung distention and to increase driving pressure during expiration. This latter mechanism helps maintain expiratory flow against narrowed airways.

The FEV_1, FVC, FEV_1/FVC ratio, and $\dot{V}_{max}$ decrease in asthma, but these tests do not define the relative contribution of loss of elastic recoil or increased Raw to the decreased flows. Spirometric pulmonary function tests often worsen before symptoms occur in exacerbating asthma. Changes in Raw can be detected by the body plethysmograph. This method is extremely sensitive to changes in large airway caliber, but extensive bronchoconstriction of airways less than 2 mm diameter is required to increase Raw.

Residual volume and total lung capacity are increased, even to some extent during remissions; these changes may worsen before other evidence of airways obstruction is apparent. Since the residual volume often increases more than the total lung volume, the vital capacity may also decrease. This decrease in vital capacity may be misinterpreted as evidence of restrictive lung disease unless flow rates and lung volumes are also measured.

Partial or complete improvement in ventilation is often seen after inhalation of a bronchodilator. However, it is inadvisable to rely too much on this test to define the reversibility that may exist, since this reversibility varies among individuals and may be delayed until after treatment has become maximally effective.

Early in the course of asthma the obstruction to airflow leads to two physiologic abnormalities. First, Raw increases; this is perceived by the patient, through receptors within the lung, as dyspnea. Secondly, the obstruction to airflow leads to a mismatching of ventilation with perfusion—a V/Q disturbance. This disturbance leads to varying degrees of arterial hypoxemia. As the asthma becomes very severe, true alveolar hypoventilation occurs, ultimately causing an increase in $Paco_2$ and respiratory acidosis. If untreated, airway obstruction increases the work of breathing and muscular activity and results in the production of excessive lactic acid. This contributes a metabolic component to the respiratory acidosis when present. Thus in life-threatening asthma, such as is seen in the emergency room or intensive care unit, the pathophysiologic abnormalities are reflected in blood hypoxemia with systemic acidosis. If untreated, these abnormalities may cause death.

Clinical picture

The common symptoms of asthma reflect the irritable nature of the asthmatic airways and the consequences of airway obstruction. Cough, breathlessness, and wheezing are the major symptoms. The breathlessness of patients who have asthma is sometimes identifiable by difficulty in both inspiration and expiration. At times patients with asthma may have no symptoms, the illness being detectable only by inhalation challenge.

All precipitating factors should be sought out in taking the history. Since asthma tends to have a hereditary aspect, the family history is important. The natural history of asthma varies greatly. In some, it wanes and disappears permanently. At the other end of the spectrum, some cases become chronic and convert into COPD. Emphysema is said not to be a complication, but some 15% of patients dying of COPD with morphologic evidence of both emphysema and chronic bronchitis gave histories of having had an asthma-like illness at the outset. Most cases fall between these two extremes.

The physical findings of asthma vary greatly. When the patient is asymptomatic, the physical examination is usually entirely normal. Wheezing or rhonchi are frequently the only findings in mild cases. During an acute attack, respiratory distress will be obvious. Although wheezing is the classic sign of asthma, airflow in acute severe asthma may be so limited that the chest is virtually silent. Skin rash, nasal mucosal edema, and nasal polyps are common findings in allergic asthma. *Triad asthma* is the combination of nasal polyps, aspirin intolerance, and asthma.

Differential diagnosis

All wheezing is not asthma; other disease processes that can include wheezing are as follows:

1. Incomplete endobronchial obstruction caused by either a tumor or a foreign body may present with an isolated wheeze that is likely to intensify during lateral recumbency on the side of the lesion. Resultant air trapping may be detected with inspiratory and expiratory chest radiography and especially by fluoroscopy.
2. Cardiogenic pulmonary edema may cause small airway compression (i.e., *cardiac asthma*).
3. Carcinoid syndrome (gastrointestinal or pulmonary carcinoids) may release bronchoconstrictive mediators.
4. Pulmonary embolism may lead to subsequent release of bronchoconstrictive mediators from injured pulmonary tissue.
5. Bronchoconstriction may occur in polyarteritis nodosa, pulmonary infiltration with eosinophilia and asthma, and extrinsic allergic alveolitis. (See Fig. 6-1 for a compilation of these factors.)

Laboratory findings

The chest radiograph may be normal or show hyperinflation. Rarely, fine stippling in the midlungs is seen in very severe attacks, due presumably to

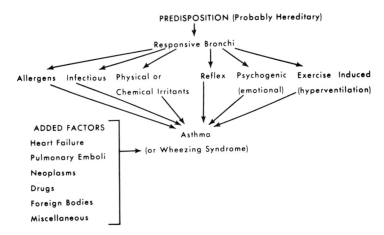

FIG. 6-1. Relationship of bronchodilator drugs to the cAMP system.

bronchiolar mucus plugging (see Fig. 10-3). Examination of blood and sputum in asthma may show eosinophilia, but the absence of eosinophils does not exclude the diagnosis. Purulence of sputum may be due either to infection or eosinophilia.

MODES OF TREATMENT

The treatment of asthma revolves principally around two axes: environmental control and bronchodilator therapy. Environment control to minimize factors that may precipitate asthma attacks is essential. Here, a careful history is invaluable. It is important, however, to balance reason with practicality. For example, getting rid of the family pet may do both good and harm: good by reducing precipitating allergens and harm by inducing emotional turmoil. The use of hyposensitization in individuals with allergic asthma is controversial, being beneficial mostly in children and young adults; therapy is unquestionably beneficial for some allergic rhinitis but is much less reliable in the prevention of asthmatic attacks.

The bronchodilator drugs used to manage asthma are basically of two classes: those used to prevent attacks and those used to prevent *and* treat attacks. The purely preventive drugs are disodium cromoglycate (cromolyn) and inhaled corticosteroids. Those that both prevent and treat are the aminophylline-theophylline compounds, β-adrenergic stimulators, antimuscurinic drugs, and oral and parenteral corticosteroids.

Before a physician uses any pharmacologic agent in asthma, familiarity with its clinical application and knowledge of situations in which it may be useful are essential.

Aminophylline-theophylline compounds

Aminophylline-theophylline compounds are thought to work by inhibiting the enzyme phosphodiesterase, which breaks down cAMP. Aminophylline, which is approximately 80% theophylline, is used intravenously. A loading dose of 5 to 6 mg/kg is given over 20 minutes; this is followed by a maintenance dosage of 0.5 to 0.9 mg/kg/hr. In patients who have been taking a theophylline preparation before receiving intravenous therapy, no loading dose is given. Since this drug is metabolized by the liver, half the normal loading dose and maintenance dosage should be given to patients with liver disease or congestion of the liver due to heart failure. The dosage of aminophylline-theophylline should also be reduced in patients with pneumonia.

Oral theophylline is usually given in a dosage of 10 to 15 mg/kg/day in 4 doses. Compounds of theophylline that have sustained release have recently become available; they are usually given every 12 hours and have the major advantage of increased tolerance and compliance. Toxic effects of theophylline include gastrointestinal upset, seizures, and cardiac arrhythmias; they almost always occur with blood concentrations of greater than 20 μg/ml. Since both patient metabolism and absorption of the drug may be erratic, theophylline serum concentrations are sometimes necessary in order to monitor dosage. Young children are more susceptible to seizures than adults and should be closely monitored for signs of CNS stimulation. Hypoxemia and acidosis are said to aggravate the toxicity of the theophylline compounds.

β-adrenergic drugs

β-adrenergic agents promote bronchodilatation by stimulating the production of cAMP.

Epinephrine. Epinephrine is a well-proven agent for the management of acute bronchial asthma. It may be given subcutaneously or by inhalation. When given subcutaneously for the treatment of acute asthma, the dosage varies from 0.2 to 1 ml. Epinephrine is also available in metered dose inhalers. Epinephrine has two major disadvantages: a relatively short duration of action and the risk of causing cardiac excitation. It must be used with caution in patients who have heart disease, who are elderly, and who have heart rates in excess of 120 beats/min.

Isoproterenol. Isoproterenol is usually given by inhalation; rarely, in severe cases of asthma, it is given intravenously. It stimulates both the β_1-receptors of the cardiovascular system and the β_2-receptors of the tracheobronchial tree. Because of this, tachycardia and vasodilatation are major side effects. This vasodilatation may alter the V/Q balance within the lung and lead to paradoxical arterial hypoxemia along with bronchodilatation. When given as an aerosol mist by a nebulizing device, the usual dosage is 3 to

7 deep inhalations of a 1:100 or 1:200 solution. Isoproterenol is also available in a metered dose device that delivers approximately 125 μg/puff of the bronchodilator in a mist form. The usual dosage in adults is 1 to 2 puffs every 3 to 4 hours. A similar dosage is used for children.

An epidemiologic association between the occurrence of sudden death in asthma and the use of metered dose aerosol devices has been reported. Some patients do "abuse" their inhalers. However, this so-called abuse reflects two other things: an inhaled β-adrenergic agent provides rapid readily available relief of bronchospasm; frequent, sometimes excessive, use is therefore understandable. On the other hand, if a patient relies heavily upon inhaled drugs, it means that other, especially oral, medications are probably not being employed correctly to control bronchospasm. Often in this situation, the physician should reassess the entire therapeutic program to improve relief of bronchospasm.

Ephedrine. Ephedrine is an oral sympathomimetic drug that promotes the release of endogeneous epinephrine. It is most frequently found as one ingredient in compound formulations of asthma remedies. These compounds usually combine ephedrine, theophylline, and phenobarbitol. The major disadvantage of these compounds is the inability to modify the dosage of the various drugs to each patient's needs.

Isoetharine. Isoetharine is a selective β_2-adrenergic stimulator. As mentioned previously, these compounds have the advantage of decreasing stimulation of the β_1-receptors in the cardiovascular system, while stimulating the β_2-bronchodilator receptors of the tracheobronchial tree. Because the β_2-receptors are also found in skeletal muscle, tremor is a common side effect. Isoetharine is only available by inhalation and is usually given in the dosage of 1 to 3 puffs every 4 hours. It is available both in a metered dose device and in solution for nebulizers.

Metaproterenol. Metaproterenol is a selective β_2-adrenergic stimulator that is available by inhalation (metered dose device and solution), tablet, and syrup. The oral dosage is 10 to 20 mg every 6 hours; the inhaled dosage is 2 to 3 puffs every 4 to 6 hours.

Terbutaline. Terbutaline is a compound similar in action to metaproterenol. It may be given subcutaneously as a substitute for epinephrine. The tablet form of the drug is given in a dosage of 2.5 to 5 mg every 6 to 8 hours.

Albuterol. Albuterol is similar to metaproterenol. It is the most frequently prescribed β-adrenergic compound in the world. It has only recently been released in the United States. In this country it is only available by metered dose inhalation. It appears to have a longer duration of action as compared to other β_2-adrenergic stimulator medications.

Corticosteroids

Corticosteroids can give dramatic relief to patients with asthma. The mechanism of action is complex but relates at least in part to their nonspecific anti-inflammatory effect. Potentiation of the action of the β_2-adrenergic drugs is also apparently involved. Corticosteroids can be given either intravenously or by mouth for both treatment and prevention. When inhaled, corticosteroids are effective only in preventing attacks. The dosage of steroids both orally and intravenously must be tailored to the individual patient. The customary dosage used for the immediate control of asthma is 30 to 60 mg prednisone orally; the dosage is tapered down in a few days. In acute situations where asthma cannot be controlled by intravenous aminophylline, 125 mg hydrocortisone or some other equivalent steroid compound is administered every 4 to 6 hours. After the acute attack has been controlled the patient receives oral corticosteroids, and the daily dosage is progressively reduced.

The major disadvantage of corticosteroids is their many side effects, some of them serious. For this reason, patients who require long-term corticosteroid therapy should, if possible, be converted to corticosteroids every other day; the use of inhaled corticosteroids, disodium cromoglycate, or both may reduce or abolish the need for oral corticosteroids. Acute exacerbations of asthma frequently necessitate a temporary return to either oral or even intravenous corticosteroids.

Inhaled corticosteroids in the form of beclomethasone have the advantage of delivering the drug locally and minimizing systemic effects. The usual dosage varies between 400 and 1200 μg/day in 4 divided doses. The major side effect of inhaled steroids is irritation of the airways and possible oral candidiasis. The irritation may induce acute bronchospasm; pretreatment with an inhaled β-adrenergic agent may block this response. If oral candidiasis does develop, treatment with a mycostatin (Nystatin) oral solution may be necessary.

Disodium cromoglycate

Disodium cromoglycate (Intal) is a water-insoluble micronized powder that can only be inhaled. Its mechanism of action is thought to inhibit the release of mediators of the asthmatic attack from mast cells. In patients with asthma that only corticosteroids have controlled, the substitution of cromolyn may allow discontinuation or reduction in corticosteroid dosage. Given in this setting cromolyn must be taken on a regular basis; it may take at least 4 weeks for it to help prevent acute asthmatic attacks. The usual dosage is 20 to 40 mg (1 to 2 capsules) 4 times daily using a Spinhaler device. For maintenance therapy it is occasionally possible to reduce the dosage to twice daily. Cromolyn is of no value in treating acute asthma attacks.

Chronic administration of cromolyn is not necessary to prevent exercise-induced asthma; the cromolyn need only be used once before the exercise.

Atropine

As mentioned above, one of the mechanisms producing bronchoconstriction in asthma is stimulation of the cholinergic nervous system. Inhaled atropine may help block this effect. Inhaled atropine is particularly useful in patients with cough as a major symptom of their asthma. Surprisingly, when given by inhalation, drying of the mouth appears to be the only major side effect; drying of secretions, tachycardia, and other muscurinic side effects are usually not troublesome. Atropine must be used in a 1 to 3 mg dose in solution, delivered by a handbulb nebulizer. Patients must be cautioned against spraying atropine into their eyes.

SELECTION OF DRUGS FOR THE TREATMENT OF ASTHMA
Acute asthma

Acute asthma is usually treated with β-adrenergic drugs and theophyllines. If the patient has an acute attack, only brief history and examination should be performed initially. Inquiry should be made as to what possible factors may have triggered the attack, what medications the patient has been taking, and if any coexisting illness such as heart disease would complicate the use of therapeutic agents. Since hypoxemia is almost a universal finding in attacks severe enough for medical attention, oxygen should be routinely administered. Although not necessary in every patient with acute asthma, the $Paco_2$ and Pao_2 may help determine whether carbon dioxide retention and respiratory acidosis are present. Simple spirometry may be helpful in gauging response to therapy after control of the acute attack. In patients who have not been receiving medication before their acute attack, 0.2 to 1 mg subcutaneous epinephrine should be administered. If relief of bronchospasm is not accomplished within 15 to 30 minutes, the dose may be repeated. If the attack appears to be worsening, intravenous aminophylline should be started; when an adequate amount of theophylline, β-adrenergic stimulants, or both have been taken before the attack, the patient should be considered to be in *status asthmaticus*. β-adrenergic drugs, either subcutaneously or by inhalation, should be given along with intravenous aminophylline, hydrocortisone, or both.

In treating acute asthma, the physician must remember to avoid certain forms of therapy. Because of the irritable nature of the airways in acute asthma, inhaled steroids and cromolyn are not recommended. Likewise, micronized mist from ultrasonic generators should not be used. Acetylcysteine (Mucomyst) may also irritate airways. Compounds containing aspirin should be avoided in all forms of asthma. β_2-blocking agents such as pro-pranolol are also contraindicated. Because of the reported risk of sudden death, the intermittent positive pressure breathing (IPPB) device should not be used in treating acute asthma.

Status asthmaticus

Status asthmaticus is a life-threatening asthma attack refractory to the use of theophyllines and β-adrenergic agents. It is at this point that intra-venous corticosteroids are required. Hydrocortisone or its equivalent is given in a dosage of 125 mg every 6 hours. Larger dosages are sometimes used, but their value remains controversial. It is important to remember that status asthmaticus may progress to respiratory failure and even death. For this reason, treatment must be aggressive and therapeutic decisions must be made promptly. On occasion, before medical management can be instituted and rarely in spite of good management, patients may develop respiratory failure requiring mechanical ventilation. The chart below lists the indica-tions for use of mechanical ventilation in status asthmaticus and the princi-ples to follow in the management of patients requiring ventilatory assistance for status asthmaticus.

INDICATIONS FOR MECHANICAL VENTILATION IN STATUS ASTHMATICUS

1. Cardiopulmonary arrest
2. Retention of carbon dioxide with respiratory acidosis as determined by serial blood gases
3. Clinical deterioration of the patient as denoted by fatigue and hyper-somnolence

PRINCIPLES OF MANAGEMENT OF PATIENTS WITH STATUS ASTHMATICUS REQUIRING MECHANICAL VENTILATION

1. Use large diameter endotracheal tube and prestretched soft cuff
2. Employ volume ventilator
3. Ensure adequate humidification
4. Use lowest possible ventilator cycling pressure
5. Keep respiratory rate slow on the ventilator
6. Avoid hypocapnia
7. Paralyze and suppress respirator drive if necessary

Table 6-1. Pharmacologic treatment of asthma

Drug	Dosage	Comment
Isoetharine	2-3 puffs metered aerosol or solution delivered by nebulizer	β_2 selective Available only by inhalation Tremor is major side effect
Metaproterenol	*Inhalation:* 2-3 puffs metered aerosol or solution delivered by nebulizer *Oral:* 10-20 mg q6h	β_2 selective Same side effects as isoetharine and terbutaline
Terbutaline	*Subcutaneous:* 1 mg *Oral:* 2.5-5 mg q8h	Essentially the same as with isoetharine and metaproterenol
Albuterol	2-3 puffs metered aerosol	Essentially same side effects as with isoetharine, metaproterenol, and terbutaline
Corticosteroids	*Oral:* 10-30 mg q AM or q.o.d. (varies from patient to patient) *Intravenous:* High dosage in acute phase *Inhaled:* Beclomethasone 400-1200 mg in 4 daily divided doses	Reserved for patient not controlled with aminophylline-theophylline and B_2-adrenergic agents
Cromolyn	10-20 mg by inhaler q6h	May block allergic and exercise-induced asthma
Atropine	1-3 mg by inhalation	
Aminophylline	*Initial:* 3-5 mg/kg *Maintenance:* 0.6-0.9 mg/kg/hr	Toxicity if blood level greater than 20 μl/ml No loading dose if patient already taking aminophylline-theophylline Give ½ loading and maintenance dose if patient has heart disease, liver disease, or pneumonia Major toxic effects are seizures and cardiac arrhythmias
Theophylline	200-300 mg q6h in adults	Available as sustained released compounds May cause nausea, vomiting, diarrhea, inability to sleep, arrhythmias, and seizure
Isoproterenol	2-3 puffs metered aerosol or solution delivered by nebulizer	Short acting More cardiovascular side effects than selective β_2-adrenergic drugs May be associated with paradoxical bronchial constriction
Epinephrine	0.2-1 mg sc	Used to treat airway bronchospasm Caution in patients who are elderly, who have heart disease, or who have a heart rate >120 beats/min

Chronic persistent asthma

Patients with chronic persistent asthma are those with persistent airflow obstruction and frequent acute attacks necessitating continuous therapy. A combination of theophyllines and beta adrenergic agents is useful in these patients (Table 6-1). A common regimen would be 200 mg of a theophylline compound given orally every 6 hours plus an inhaled or oral β-adrenergic agent such as isoetharine, metaproterenol, albuterol, or terbutaline. In those who fail to do well with this approach, corticosteroids should be given orally and followed by either inhaled cromolyn or steroids, in an attempt to replace the patient's need for oral steroids. Frequent use of simple spirometry is helpful in validating the patient's symptoms with objective information.

SPECIAL CONSIDERATIONS IN ASTHMA

Surgery. Surgery, both elective and emergent, in the asthmatic patient can usually be accomplished without difficulty. In fact, many of the anesthetic agents given by inhalation are bronchodilators (e.g., halothane). The major concern is to avoid complications. It is important to continue the administration of all medications being taken before surgery. Inhaled β-adrenergic agents can be delivered by the usual method; if the patient is intubated, they can easily be delivered by in-line nebulizer. Patients receiving oral steroids should receive stress dosages of steroids in the preoperative and postoperative periods.

Pregnancy. Asthma during pregnancy is managed in much the same way as in the nonpregnant asthmatic. The theophylline and β-adrenergic agents are smooth muscle relaxers and thus present no danger of premature delivery. The fetus is likewise at no risk of danger from these agents. However, the hypoxemia of acute asthma presents a distinct threat to the fetus. Corticosteroids have not been shown to be teratogenic in humans and thus may be used as usual. Iodine and tetracycline should be avoided because of the risk of fetal damage.

Cough. Occasionally patients with asthma may have no symptoms other than cough. Cough in asthmatics is often successfully treated by the usual antiasthma treatment.

Exercise. Exercise, particularly in cold weather, may provoke bronchospasm in many asthmatics, which is probably caused by the excessive exchange of heat and water from the airways into the inspired air. A cold weather mask may be quite effective in this situation. Inhaled β-adrenergic agents or inhaled cromolyn have also been used with success.

Allergic aspergillosis. The airways of some asthmatics may become infected with aspergilli, leading to an immediate and delayed hypersensitivity reaction characterized by poorly controlled asthma, fleeting infiltrates on the chest radiograph, fever, and even weight loss. The diagnosis is made by recovering the organisms from the sputum, elevated serum titers of antibodies to aspergilli, and positive aspergillus skin tests. The use of antimicrobial agents is of no benefit here; however, corticosteroid therapy may be effective in controlling this disorder.

SUGGESTED READINGS
Pathogenesis of asthma

Gross, N.J.: What is this thing called love?—or, defining asthma, Am. Rev. Respir. Dis. **121**:203, 1980.

McFadden, E.R.: Asthma: airway reactivity and pathogenesis, Semin. Respir. Med. **1**:287, 1980.

Boushey, H.A., Holtzman, M.J., Sheller, J.R., et al.: Bronchial hyperreactivity, Am. Rev. Respir. Dis. **121**:389, 1980.

Charkin, L.W., and Krell, R.D.: Pathophysiology and pharmacotherapy of asthma: an overview, J. Pharm. Sci. **69**:236, 1980.

Messer, J.W., Peters, G.A., and Bennett, W.A.: Causes of death and pathological findings in 304 cases of bronchial asthma, Dis. Chest **38**:616, 1960.

Goldberg, N.D., Haddox, M.K., Nicol, S.E., et al.: Biologic regulation through opposing influences of cyclic GMP and cyclic AMP: the Yin Yang hypothesis, Adv. Cyclic Nucleotide Res. **5**:307, 1975.

Gold, W.M.: The role of the parasympathetic nervous system in airways disease, Postgr. Med. J. (London) **51** (7 Suppl.):53, 1975.

Samter, M., and Beers, R.F., Jr.: Concerning the nature of intolerance to aspirin, J. Allergy **40**:281, 1967.

Diagnosis of asthma

Parker, C.D., Bilbo, R.E., and Reed, C.E.: Methacholine aerosol as test for bronchial asthma, Arch. Intern. Med. **115**:452, 1965.

McFadden, E.R., Jr.: Exertional dyspnea and cough as preludes to acute attacks of bronchial asthma, N. Engl. J. Med. **292**:555, 1975.

McFadden, E.R., and Lyons, H.A.: Arterial blood gas tension in asthma, N. Engl. J. Med. **278**:1029, 1968.

Conrad, W.M., Braman, S.S., and Irwin, R.S.: Chronic cough as the sole presenting manifestation of bronchial asthma, N. Engl. J. Med. **300**:633, 1979.

Williams, M.H., Jr.: Evaluation of asthma (editorial), Chest **76**:3, 1979.

Treatment of asthma

Paterson, J.W., Woolcock, A.J., and Shenfield, G.M.: Bronchodilator drugs, Am. Rev. Respir. Dis. **120**:1149, 1979.

Weinberger, M.W., Matthay, R.A., Ginchansky, E.J., et al.: Intravenous aminophylline dosage: use of serum theophylline measurements for guidance, J.A.M.A. **235**:2110, 1976.

Collins, J.V., and Jones, D.: Corticosteroid mechanism and therapeutic schedules. In E.B. Weiss, editor: *Status Asthmaticus*, Park Press, Baltimore, 1978, University Park Press, pp. 235-253.

McCombs, R.P., Lowell, F.C., and Ohman, J.L.: Myths, morbidity and mortality in asthma, J.A.M.A. **242**:1521, 1979.

Scoggin, C.S., Sahn, S.A., and Petty, T.L.: Status asthmaticus: a nine year experience, J.A.M.A. **238**:1158, 1977.

Karetzky, M.S.: Asthma mortality associated with pneumothorax and intermittent positive-pressure breathing, Lancet **1:**828, 1975.

Weinstein, A.M., Dubin, B.D., and Podleski, W.K., et al.: Asthma and pregnancy, J.A.M.A. **241:** 1161, 1979.

Konig, P.: Conflicting viewpoints about treatment of asthma with cromolyn: a review of the literature, Ann. Allergy **43:**293, 1979.

Slavin, R.G.: Asthma in adults. III. Occupational asthma, Hosp. Prac. **13:**133, 1978.

Chapter 7

ADULT RESPIRATORY DISTRESS SYNDROME (ARDS)

Thomas L. Petty

The adult respiratory distress syndrome (ARDS) is best defined as a clinical-pathophysiologic state characterized by severe dyspnea, hypoxemia, loss of pulmonary compliance, and diffuse, bilateral pulmonary infiltrations following acute lung injury in previously healthy persons, usually with no prior major lung disease. This chapter describes the clinical presentation, discusses the current state of medical knowledge of pathogenesis, and presents an approach to systematic, physiologically oriented management of ARDS.

Historical perspective

ARDS is not new to medicine. Physicians' original characterization of ARDS[1,2] cited earlier descriptions of the pathologic conditions related to ARDS, previously termed *congestive atelectasis*.[3] Today ARDS is recognized as an important clinical state and is better understood and better managed, although substantial problems with management remain. Rapidly growing interest in ARDS has resulted in an increasing number of editorial comments, some using other names for the syndrome,[4-6] and some controversy over the appropriateness of the term as a proper designation of the clinical syndrome has surfaced.[7,8]

Two multidisciplinary conferences concerning ARDS have served to indicate that it occurs following a variety of unrelated lung injuries[9,10] and that many loosely used clinical terms actually refer to the same entity. (See the accompanying chart.)

ARDS was first described as a clinical syndrome[1] in 1967. In 12 patients clinical features were reported that were believed "remarkably similar to the infantile respiratory distress syndrome [IRDS]." Ventilatory management with PEEP was also first reported in ARDS in that article, although the technique of PEEP had been described earlier.[11] Five patients survived.

PRESENTATION OF ARDS

A. *Clinical signs following catastrophic event (e.g., shock from any cause)*
   1. Pronounced dyspnea
   2. Tachypnea
   3. Labored respirations
   4. Intercostal retractions
   5. Cyanosis, refractory to oxygen therapy
B. *Radiographic and physiologic signs*
   1. Diffuse bilateral pulmonary infiltrates
   2. Reduced lung and chest wall compliance $\Delta V/\Delta P$ (measured on ventilator)
   3. Increased alveolar or inspired to arterial oxygen tension difference
   4. Improved pulmonary oxygen transport with PEEP
   5. High minute ventilation (spontaneous or with a ventilator)
C. *Conditions to be excluded*
   1. Advanced chronic pulmonary disease
   2. Left heart failure
D. *Pathology*
   1. Heavy lungs, usually > 1000 gm
   2. Congestive atelectasis
   3. Hyaline membranes
   4. Fibrosis (after 72 hours)

OTHER TERMS FOR ARDS

1. Shock lung
2. Traumatic wet lung
3. White lung syndrome
4. Capillary leak syndrome
5. Acute alveolar failure
6. Postperfusion lung
7. DaNang lung
8. Congestive atelectasis
9. Adult hyaline membrane disease

POSSIBLE CAUSES OF ARDS

1. Complement activation
2. Leukocytic enzymes
3. Platelets
4. Humoral agents
5. Immunologic reactions
6. Neurogenic shock
7. Oxygen
8. Microemboli
9. Toxins
10. Overhydration
11. Viral infections

Autopsy findings in the seven who died showed striking alveolar atelectasis, engorgement of capillaries, and hyaline membrane formation.[1]

The mechanisms of acute lung injury were and remain unknown, but speculations regarding toxic factors or vasoactive substances, the pulmonary effects of fat embolization, lung ischemia, surfactant abnormalities, hemodynamic factors, and exogenous factors such as overtransfusion of fluids were considered as possibly involved in the pathogenesis of ARDS. Current research focuses on proteolytic mechanisms of damage possibly mediated by enzymes released from leukocytic aggregates following complement activation. It is believed that complement activation may be a final pathway of various insults including sepsis, shock, and acute pancreatitis.[12]

Clinical setting and presentation

The clinical onset of ARDS may be sudden or insidious. Often there is a latent period between the initial injury (e.g. shock, multiple trauma) and the subsequent full development of the clinical, radiographic and pathophysiologic features.

Since ARDS occurs following a variety of direct and indirect lung insults the clinical presentation as well as the manifestations of the clinical syndrome itself will be a consequence of the type of injury. These findings are summarized in the chart on p. 67. Respiratory distress, labored respirations, diffuse monotonous bilateral infiltrates, and profound hypoxemia are hallmarks of the syndrome. The respiratory rate and minute ventilation are high.[13]

Interestingly, the physical examination is often not very revealing. The patient's labored respirations are obvious, and cyanosis, known to be an unreliable sign of hypoxemia, may or may not be present. On auscultation of the lungs very few abnormal sounds are heard in spite of the pronounced respiratory distress and massive pulmonary infiltrations of the fully developed syndrome. Specifically, the bubbling rales of cardiogenic pulmonary edema, the rhonchi caused by secretions in large airways, and the crackling rales of pulmonary fibrosis are not heard. One generally hears a harsh short inspiratory phase and a rather normal expiratory phase during mechanical ventilation. Cardiac sounds are usually normal, with no third or fourth heart sound and no valvular murmurs unless there is associated myocardial trauma.

Pathophysiology

Laboratory determinations measured at the bedside with the patient receiving mechanical ventilation help to elucidate the pathophysiology in a clinically useful way. Overall pulmonary compliance—the sum of lung and chest wall compliances—is notably decreased. This can be easily measured in patients receiving mechanical ventilation by dividing the delivery pressure of the ventilator into the tidal volume delivered by the machine. Maintaining static pressure on the lungs and thorax by holding the lungs at end inspiration, by occluding the exhalation manifold, or by using the inflation hold control available on some respirators allows a static compliance measurement to be made. Overall compliance measurements by this method are usually 15 to 40 cc/cm; normal values are 75 to 100 cc/cm. This is evidence of the notably impaired overall compliance due to "stiff lungs." High minute ventilation (which is many times more than 20 L/min) is present and can be measured with a simple hand spirometer (Wright, for example) or calculated from ventilator rate and tidal volume. Profound hypoxemia is usually present despite high inspired oxygen fractions, with accompanying hypocarbia due to the high minute ventilation.

The difference between inspired and arterial oxygen tensions is indicative of the difficulty with oxygen transfer across the lung; it is probably a more useful bedside test than the measurement of alveolar to arterial tension difference during ventilation with 100% oxygen, as is commonly done in some intensive respiratory care units. I prefer this method of assessing the impairment in oxygen transfer across the lungs because it deals with the arterial tension at which the patient is receiving mechanical ventilation and avoids the artifact of increasing the alveolar arterial tension difference on 100% oxygen breathing, which converts low V/Q regions into shunt regions.[2] The underlying physiologic basis for the gas transfer abnormality is severe V/Q[14] mismatch and wasted ventilation, which affect arterial oxygenation a great deal more than carbon dioxide elimination. A true diffusion defect may also be present due to interstitial edema, hyaline membrane formation, and a reduced capillary blood volume.[15,16]

The causes of the mechanical derangement of the lungs in ARDS are not clearly known. Increased elastic and surface forces are present and are considered in the discussion of surfactant below.

Chest radiographs

The features seen on chest radiographs are monotonously similar despite the many different pathways to the development of ARDS. Generally, diffuse, bilateral, dense alveolar infiltrates are present without pleural effusions or enlargement of the cardiac silhouette unless a related myocardial injury or pericardial effusion resulted from the original lung injury (Fig. 7-1, *B*). It must be stressed that the radiographic features are not specific for the nature or degree of acute pulmonary insult and do not correlate with the degree of physiologic abnormality present. Radiographic clearing occurs much more slowly than in cardiogenic pulmonary edema (Fig. 7-2).

Possible factors in pathogenesis

It is apparent that the lung can be injured by insults delivered either by way of the airways or the circulation.[17] Causes leading to these remarkably similar clinical features include shock from any cause (hemorrhagic, cardiogenic, septic, or even anaphylactic),[18] multiple trauma including massive fat

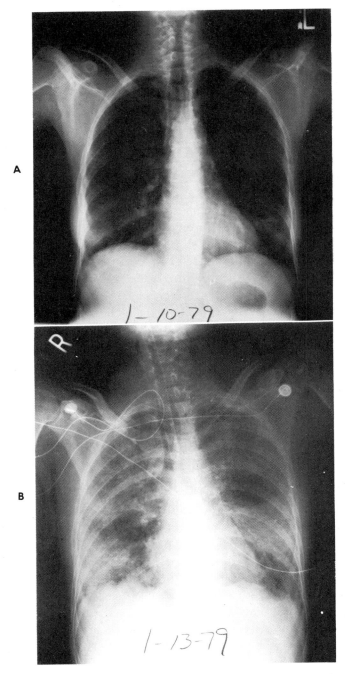

FIG. 7-1. A, Initial chest radiograph from a patient 44 years of age seen in an emergency room for flulike syndrome including cough and myalgias. **B,** Film on admission to hospital with acute respiratory distress. Patient required mechanical ventilation, F_{IO_2} 1.0, and PEEP 12 cm for adequate arterial oxygenation at 62 mm Hg.

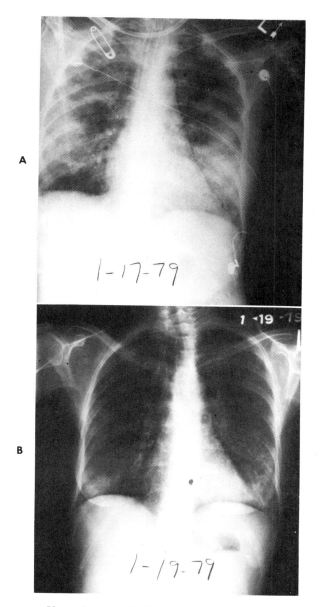

FIG. 7-2. Subsequent films showing little clearing 4 days after entry, **A,** and nearly complete clearing after extubation, **B.** The patient made a complete recovery.

embolization,[19] diffuse intravascular coagulation,[20] endotoxemia,[21] paraquat poisoning,[22] drowning,[23] overwhelming viral pneumonia,[24] massive aspiration,[25] CNS injury[26] including both trauma and drug intoxication (especially narcotic drugs),[27,28] and acute fulminant pancreatitis.[29] Many possibilities concerning the exact mechanism of injury exist. Possible agents or mechanisms involved in diffuse lung injury are cited on the chart on p. 67. A "final common pathway" must occur following these diverse insults that injure the lung either by way of the inhaled route or the circulation. There is strong evidence to support the hypothesis of increased capillary permeability leading to "capillary leak."[25,30,31] As mentioned earlier, complement activation may be operative in the final common pathway.[12]

Pathologic findings

The lungs are heavy, airless, and appear like liver in cut sections. Alveoli are collapsed, and a hemorrhagic infiltration with debris and hyaline membranes is found lining alveolar spaces. These pathologic features are nonspecific and represent the final common pathway of massive diffuse lung injury.[1,9]

Role of surfactant abnormalities

The increased elastic recoil of ARDS, the shared features with IRDS,[32] and the suggestion of surfactant abnormalities in some experimental models have focused attention on possible surfactant abnormalities in ARDS. A primary surfactant abnormality cannot, of course, be implicated, but the possibility of surfactant inactivation in states of pulmonary edema has been raised.[33] Secondary surfactant abnormalities could then contribute to the pathogenesis of ARDS.[34] The hypothesis is that alveolar atelectasis would augment the transudation of pulmonary edema and hemorrhage, thereby leading to massive focal atelectasis. The fact that a latent period of 12 to 24 hours or more often occurs between acute lung injury and the development of ARDS is intriguing in this regard, since it is known that surfactant half-life (on release from the type II pneumocyte) is approximately 18 to 24 hours after experimental pulmonary embolization and recovery.[35] Considerable evidence exists that type II cells and probably surfactant production can be damaged by high oxygen concentrations, which are often required for life support in severe states of ARDS.[36,37]

Although our original report suggested surfactant abnormalities from observations made on minced lung specimens,[1] it was not until recently that we were able to show abnormalities in surfactant compressibility and in the isopycnic density of the alveolar lipoprotein aggregates in a fresh specimen from a patient with ARDS following severe hemorrhagic shock.[38] Shortly thereafter we found similar abnormalities in surfactant function in five additional ARDS cases due to septicemia and narcotic overdose with aspiration alone and hemorrhagic shock, respectively.[39]

Therefore, although the role of surfactant abnormalities remains speculative, the existence of surfactant abnormalities is now strongly suggested. The role of surfactant in the evolution of ARDS following the initial injury, and its role in the mechanical improvement that can be observed clinically (see below) on recovery, parallels the necessary time for recovery and regeneration of type II cells. Both the experimental and clinical observations, therefore, have credibility in relation to the pathogenesis of ARDS.

Incidence

The true incidence of ARDS in the United States today is not known. This is due largely to lack of uniformity and agreement on definition and lack of an effective reporting mechanism. The task force of the Lung Division of the National Heart, Lung, and Blood Institute has estimated that at least 150,000 cases are identified and treated each year.[40] The true incidence is probably much greater.

Management

Prevention. Ideally, ARDS should be both anticipated and prevented. This means the avoidance of fluid overload whenever possible, of the lowest possible oxygen fraction in oxygen therapy use for adequate tissue oxygenation, and, at least in the case of multiple long bone fractures, the institution of corticosteroid drugs to prevent or minimize the adverse effects of free fatty acids on the lung in the dramatic syndrome of fat embolization.[19] Other considerations for steroids are discussed below.

Supportive management. In brief, the treatment of the full-blown syndrome is primarily supportive and requires the placement of a definitive airway and mechanical ventilation using a ventilator with high pressure and flow capabilities. An endotracheal tube can be placed initially and is suitable for short-term management, that is, 2 to 4 days. Endotracheal tubes can be left in place longer, but they have the disadvantage of comparatively poor patient tolerance, may be an inferior route for suctioning, and usually prevent the patient from taking nourishment by mouth.

A volume ventilator providing high pressure and flow capabilities and accurate control of the inspired oxygen fraction is required. The ventilator provides mechanical work and allows modification of pressure wave forms. The Bennett MA-1 and MA-2, Bourns Bear, and Ohio Critical Care Ventilator are four that offer the necessary pressure and flow capabilities required in most cases of ARDS. To avoid possible oxygen toxicity, it is important to reduce the inspired oxygen fraction as rapidly as possible while maintaining adequate oxygen transport across the lungs commensurate with tissue demands. The possibility of further oxygen-induced injury must be minimized with the use of the lowest possible oxygen fraction. Most modern ventilators have accurate control of oxygen fraction delivery. These have been summarized in various textbooks. The time-dose threshold in producing oxygen toxicity in humans remains unknown. An extensive review considers this subject.[41,42]

PEEP also improves oxygen transport across the lung by reducing shunting.[1,2,13,42-47] Lung units are very likely recruited with the use of PEEP. Functional residual capacity is clearly increased.[45,46] Since pressures on the order of 5 to 15 cm water are generally all that is required, it is unlikely that cardiac output is significantly reduced.[47]

In some circumstances tissue oxygen transport may, in fact, be reduced by PEEP,[48] and the possibility of barotrauma may be increased with high levels of PEEP. Therefore, a concept of optimal PEEP is emerging.[49,50] Optimum PEEP, as judged by systemic oxygen transport, usually occurs within the best compliance region ($\Delta V/\Delta P$) of mechanical ventilation.[49,50]

Initially, the mechanical ventilator is adjusted with a fairly high tidal volume of 12 to 14 ml/kg, and the machine is used in the assister-controller mode. The routine measurement of pressure-volume curves of lungs and thorax is recommended in order to establish the tidal volume and PEEP level that exist within the region of best overall compliance.[49-51]

It is preferable whenever possible not to paralyze patients requiring ventilation. Even with crush injuries of the chest many patients will allow the ventilator to provide the work of breathing in the combined assister-controller mode with an appropriate rate. The application of the modern ventilator must of course by guided by frequent arterial blood gas determinations.

Fluid management

Proper fluid management is essential in maintaining an adequate circulation and in avoiding further complications. Whereas aggressive fluid therapy was the rule in shock management before the characterization of ARDS,[52] it subsequently became clear that fluid overload is an important complicating factor in ARDS.[1,2,13] Fluid sequestration in the lung is probably facilitated by increased capillary permeability. In addition, fluid retention as a response to ventilator management by way of excessive antidiuretic hormone activity is a likely complicating factor.[53] Nonetheless, adequate systemic perfusion is mandatory in order to maintain organ integrity.[54]

The choice of replacement fluid remains somewhat controversial. Albumin replacement to restore the delicate Starling relationship between hydrostatic and colloid pressure has been suggested in patients with ARDS and those with interstitial edema who are hypoproteinemic.[55] Other experimental evidence indicates, in contrast, that lung water may be increased with the use of colloid compared with crystalloid infusions.[56] For this reason and on the basis of bedside clinical experience, I now prefer the use of crystalloid solutions. Diuretics such as furosemide or ethacrynic acid are also employed if overt evidence of fluid overload exists and systemic circulation is satisfactory. In the most difficult cases one often must balance between fluid administration, monitoring evidence of adequate perfusion such as systemic blood pressure, adequate urine flow (such as 25 to 30 ml/hr), and the avoidance of overhydration using the pulmonary capillary wedge pressure measured through a Swan-Ganz catheter.[57] Renal function may become a relatively low priority during this period; mild to moderate azotemia is common. Even advancing renal failure should not demand a pronounced increase of fluid infusion.

Adjunctive pharmacologic management

Certain groups of drugs are commonly used during the ventilatory support phase of ARDS care. A brief commentary on corticosteroids, antibiotics, and fluid management according to contemporary knowledge is therefore appropriate.

Corticosteroids have a theoretic benefit in their ability to prevent or reduce aggregation of leukocytes that may cause damage by the release of proteolytic enzymes within the lung. Steroids also prevent complement activation of leukocytes.[12] Some authors think that corticosteroids are protective in the face of endotoxic shock by reducing the activity of lysosomal enzymes.[58,59] Methylprednisolone has increased the survival rate in dogs with lung injury induced by oleic acid.[60] It has also been suggested from observations in humans and in experimental animal models that corticosteroids are effective in treating fat embolization.[19,61]

Against the use of steroids in their potential effect of reducing lung bacterial clearance, as shown in experimental studies.[62] We have reported that sepsis complicating ARDS remains an unsolved enigma.[63] Whether steroids have other therapeutic benefits or disadvantages is not known. In practice, I use methylprednisolone sodium succinate (30 mg/kg of body weight, given intravenously in divided dosage) for the first 24 to 48 hours. In theory, this dosage will capitalize upon the beneficial effects and minimize long-term side effects such as sepsis and oxygen toxicity.

The use of prophylactic *antibiotics* is to be condemned. In a review of our earlier experience the use of prophylactic antibiotics failed in any way to prevent infection with dangerous gram-negative bacilli.[63] Use of antibiotics should be reserved for identified infections and then guided by culture and drug susceptibility tests.

Strategies of care

Management priorities are: (1) adequate arterial oxygenation (for example, arterial oxygen saturation [Sa_{O_2}] 90%) and adequate circulating hemoglobin to maintain oxygen content; (2) adequate cardiac output (for example, sufficient for mixed venous oxygen pressure [P_{O_2}] greater than 30 mm Hg) and (if possible to observe) adequate mentation or integrated central nervous system responses, warm extremities, and some renal flow; and (3) lowest possible fraction of inspiratory oxygen ($F_{I_{O_2}}$), ideally to 0.6 or less within 24 hours and to 0.5 or less after 2 or 3 days. Naturally there are trade-offs in these strategies and, of course, the bottom line is adequate oxygenation and maintenance of brain function.

Weaning

Mechanical ventilatory support is required until the patient recovers sufficiently to support his or her own ventilation and to adequately transfer oxygen without PEEP. Briefly, the chest must be stable, the patient alert and cooperative, and PEEP no longer required. PEEP should not be reduced until the inspired oxygen concentration can be reduced to 40% ($F_{I_{O_2}}$ less than 0.4); then PEEP should be reduced in 3 cm water increments with repeated monitoring of blood gases both initially and 1 hour after each reduction. At this stage, if oxygen transport is adequate, short trials with a T-piece attached to the endotracheal tube or tracheostomy collar are made with arterial blood gas monitoring at 30- to 60-minute intervals. If blood gases are maintained and the patient remains comfortable, the ventilatory assistance is no longer needed and the endotracheal tube or tracheostomy can be removed if it is not needed as an independent airway. Further details of useful weaning techniques in ARDS are cited elsewhere.[64]

Prognosis

The immediate patient outcome in ARDS involves three basic factors: (1) the degree of original lung injury, (2) the success of initial resuscitation and support of the patient, and (3) the avoidance of complications and further injury. Certainly, lung injury is so severe in some patients that survival is not possible. These patients often die shortly after reaching the hospital. Properly applied support methods will generally permit the immediate survival of most patients in spite of severe lung injury. Modern mechanical ventilators provide sufficient work capability to support the ventilation of even severely damaged lungs. In most patients, adequate oxygenation can be accomplished

TABLE 7-1. Survival in ARDS

Year	1967[1]	1972[63]	1975
Patients	12	51	100
Survived	5	21	44
%	42	41	44

at the onset with high inspired oxygen fractions (tensions); however, this is at the cost of potential further lung injury from oxygen toxicity. It must be emphasized again that it is extremely important to minimize the likelihood of oxygen toxicity by carrying out mechanical ventilation with the lowest possible inspired oxygen fraction (see **Principles of management**). Avoidance of septic complications is equally important.

Observations made at the bedside can be good prognostic indicators. Patients with the best compliance and the best and most prompt blood gas response to PEEP are most likely to recover.[65] Open lung biopsy studies in those with more unfavorable physiologic findings showed the greatest cellular and fibrotic changes.[65]

The comparison of survival rates from various institutions is difficult because of different selection criteria. Our own experience in 100 consecutive patients managed at Colorado General Hospital from 1966 to 1975, beginning with our first case, is cited in Table 7-1. It is evident that the overall survival is not improving, but is must be stressed that 8 patients in whom liver transplantation was done, all of whom died with sepsis, are included in the last 50 cases. Without these special cases the survival rate in our overall series is 49%, which is similar to that in other series.[40]

Sequelae on recovery

Late sequelae are surprisingly infrequent. In a series of 10 patients with ARDS who required mechanical ventilation for 3 to 36 days (mean 13.5 days) from an F_{IO_2} greater than 0.6 for 2 to 13 days (mean 4.6 days), 4 were entirely asymptomatic and 6 had only mild to moderate symptoms when carefully evaluated 4 to 42 months after recovery (mean 23 months).[66] The physiologic abnormalities were only mild to moderate and included both obstructive and restrictive ventilatory abnormalities, a moderate diffusion defect that tended to improve with time, and normal blood gas values at rest (except for slight hypoxemia during exercise). A reevaluation in 9 of our original patients (follow-up 39 to 83 months after ARDS) showed a further improvement in patients with a restrictive ventilatory defect and stable minimal airflow obstruction or normal lung function, except in 1 person with underlying

COPD.[67] Interestingly, airway hyperreactivity with increased response to methacholine was found in 2 of 7 patients tested.

The morphologic basis for lung recovery from severe diffuse injury is suggested by the work of Bachofen and Weibel,[16] who have shown that the type I alveolar lining cell is geometrically too complex to replicate and, therefore, if injured, dies. Type II, or so-called metabolically active cells, however, can proliferate and differentiate into type I cells to reestablish the alveolar capillary membrane.[16] That this occurs is strongly suggested by the gradual improvement shown in forced vital capacity, functional residual capacity, single breath diffusion tests, and arterial blood gas studies on recovery.[66,67]

The future

Physicians need to understand mechanisms of disease, how the lung responds to injury, and how repair may occur without fibrosis. We desperately need markers of injury by which we can detect ARDS before the advanced syndrome is recognized clinically. Physicians must find ways to induce oxygen tolerance, protect the lung from sepsis, and learn the role of surfactant abnormalities in the pathogenesis of ARDS. So far, new approaches to support using an extracorporeal oxygenator for partial oxygenation of severely injured patients have not proved more successful than conventional means of support; a few long-term survivors have been reported, however.[68,69] It is possible that this form of support would be more successful if applied to less severe cases. The key to success is to protect the lung from further injury during the life-support period; the challenge is to reduce the risk of sepsis and oxygen toxicity.

REFERENCES

1. Ashbaugh, D.G., Bigelow, D.B., Petty, T.L., et al.: Acute respiratory distress in adults, Lancet **2**:319, 1967.
2. Petty, T.L., and Ashbaugh, D.G.: The adult respiratory distress syndrome: clinical features, factors influencing prognosis and principles of management, Chest **60**:233, 1971.
3. Jenkins, M.T., Jones, R.F., Wilson, B., et al.: Congestive atelectasis; complications of intravenous infusion of fluids, Ann. Surg. **132**:327, 1950.
4. Adult respiratory distress syndrome (editorial), Med. J. Aust. **1**:865, 1974.
5. Pietra, G.G.: The lung in shock, Hum. Pathol. **5**:121, 1974.
6. Fishman, A.P.: Shock lung: a distinctive nonentity, Circulation **47**:921, 1973.
7. Petty, T.L.: The adult respiratory distress syndrome: (confessions of a lumper), Am. Rev. Respir. Dis. **111**:713, 1975.
8. Murray, J.F.: The adult respiratory distress syndrome: (may it rest in peace), Am. Rev. Respir. Dis. **111**:716, 1975.
9. Eiseman, B., and Ashbaugh, D.G. Eds.: Pulmonary effects of non thoracic trauma, J. Trauma **8**:621, 1968.
10. Petty, T.L., and Hudson, L.D.: Proceedings of the 16th Aspen Lung Conference, Chest **65** (Suppl):1S, 1974.

11. Frumin, M.J., Bergman, N.A., Holaday, D.A., et al.: Alveolar-arterial O_2 differences during artificial respiration in man, J. Appl. Physiol. **14**:694, 1959.
12. Hammerschmidt, D.E., Weaver, L.J., Hudson, L.D., et al.: Association of complement activation and elevated plasma-C5a with adult respiratory distress syndrome, Lancet **1**:947, 1980.
13. Ashbaugh, D.G., Petty, T.L., Bigelow, D.B., et al.: Continuous positive-pressure breathing (CPPB) in adult respiratory distress syndrome, J. Thorac. Cardiovasc. Surg. **57**:31, 1969.
14. Wagner, P.D., Laravuso, R.B., Uhl, R.R., et al.: Distributions of ventilation-perfusion ratios in acute respiratory failure, Chest **65**(Suppl):32S, 1974.
15. King, T.K.C., Weber, B., Okinaka, A., et al.: Oxygen transfer in catastrophic respiratory failure, Chest **65**(Suppl):40S, 1974.
16. Bachofen, M., and Weibel, E.R.: Basic pattern of tissue repair in human lungs following unspecific injury, Chest **65**(Suppl):14S, 1974.
17. Petty, T.L., and Ashbaugh, D.G.: Intensive and rehabilitative respiratory care, ed. 2, Philadelphia, 1974, Lea & Febiger.
18. Edde, R.R., and Burtis, B.B.: Lung injury in anaphylactoid shock, Chest **63**:636, 1973.
19. Ashbaugh, D.G., and Petty, T.L.: The use of corticosteroids in the treatment of respiratory failure associated with massive fat embolism, Surg. Gynecol. Obstet. **123**:493, 1966.
20. Blaisdell, F.W., Lim, R.C., and Stallone, R.J.: The mechanisms of pulmonary damage following traumatic shock, Surg. Gynecol. Obstet. **130**:15, 1970.
21. Gemer, M., Hirsch, E.F., Hayes, J.A., et al.: Controlled endotoxemia and the lung, Chest **65**(Suppl):47S, 1974.
22. Kimbrough, R.D.: Toxic effects of the herbicide paraquat, Chest **65**(Suppl):65S, 1974.
23. Martin, C.M., and Barrett, O.: Drowning and near-drowning: a review of ten years' experience in a large army hospital, Milit. Med. **136**:439, 1971.
24. Ferstenfeld, J.E., Schlueter, D.P., Rytel, M.W., et al.: Recognition and treatment of adult respiratory distress syndrome secondary to viral interstitial pneumonia, Am. J. Med. **58**:709, 1975.
25. Robin, E.D., Cross, C.E., and Zelis, R.: Pulmonary edema, N. Engl. J. Med. **288**:239, 292, 1973.
26. Moss, G., and Stein, A.A.: The centrineurogenic etiology of the respiratory distress syndrome: protection by unilateral chronic pulmonary denervation in hemorrhagic shock, J. Trauma **16**:361, 1976.
27. Frand, U.I., Shim, C.S., and Williams, M.H.: Heroin-induced pulmonary edema: sequential studies of pulmonary function, Ann. Intern. Med. **77**:29, 1972.
28. Frand, U.I., Shim, C.S., and Williams, M.H.: Methadone-induced pulmonary edema, Ann. Intern. Med. **76**:975, 1972.
29. Interiano, B., Stuard, I.D., and Hyde, R.W.: Acute respiratory distress syndrome in pancreatitis, Ann. Intern. Med. **77**:923, 1972.
30. Pontoppidan, H., Geffin, B., and Lowenstein, E.: Acute respiratory failure in the adult, N. Engl. J. Med. **287**:690, 743, 799.
31. Webb, W.R., Wax, S.D., Kusajima, K., et al.: Microscopic studies of the pulmonary circulation in situ, Surg. Clin. North Am. **54**:1067, 1974.
32. Farrell, P.M., and Avery, M.E.: Hyaline membrane disease, Am. Rev. Respir. Dis. **111**:657, 1975.
33. Said, S.I., Avery, M.E., Davis, R.K., et al.: Pulmonary surface activity in induced pulmonary edema, J. Clin. Invest. **44**:458, 1965.
34. Hopewell, P.C., and Murray, J.F.: The adult respiratory distress syndrome, Ann. Rev. Med. **27**:343, 1976.
35. Greenfield, L.J., Pearce, H.J., and Nichols, R.T.: Recovery of respiratory function and lung mechanics following experimental pulmonary embolectomy, J. Thorac. Cardiovasc. Surg. **55**:160, 1968.
36. Katzenstein, A.A., Bloor, C.M., and Leibow, A.A.: Diffuse alveolar damage—the role of oxygen, shock, and related factors, Am. J. Pathol. **85**:210, 1976.
37. Bowden, D.H., and Adamson, I.Y.R.: Reparative changes following pulmonary cell injury:

ultra structural, cytodynamic and surfactant studies in mice after oxygen exposure, Arch. Pathol. **92:**279, 1971.

38. Petty, T.L., Reiss, O.K., Paul, G.W., et al.: Characteristics of pulmonary surfactant in adult respiratory distress syndrome associated with trauma and shock, Am. Rev. Respir. Dis. **115:**531, 1977.

39. Petty, T.L., Silvers, G.W., Paul, G.W., et al.: Abnormalities in lung elastic properties and surfactant function in adult respiratory distress syndrome, Chest **75:**571, 1979.

40. Murray, J.F.: Mechanisms of acute respiratory failure, Am. Rev. Respir. Dis. **115:**1071, 1977.

41. Winter, P.M., and Smith, G.: The toxicity of oxygen, Anesthesiology **37:**210, 1972.

42. Kapanci, Y., Tosco, R., Eggerman, J., et al.: Oxygen pneumonitis in man, Chest **62:**162, 1972.

43. Ashbaugh, D.G., and Petty, T.L.: Positive end-expiratory pressure—physiology, indications, and contraindications, J. Thorac. Cardiovasc. Surg. **65:**165, 1973.

44. Leftwich, E.I., Witorsch, R.J., and Witorsch, P.: Positive end-expiratory pressure in refractory hypoxemia: a critical evaluation, Ann. Intern. Med. **79:**187, 1973.

45. Wayne, K.S.: Positive end-expiratory pressure (PEEP) ventilation, J.A.M.A. **236:**1394, 1976.

46. McIntyre, R.W., Laws, A.K., Ramachandran, P.R.: Positive expiratory pressure plateau: improved gas exchange during mechanical ventilation, Can. Anaesth. Soc. J. **16:**477, 1969.

47. Nicotra, M.B., Stevens, P.M., Viroslav, J., et al.: Physiologic evaluation of positive end-expiratory pressure ventilation, Chest **64:**10, 1973.

48. Lutch, J.S., and Murray, J.F.: Continuous positive-pressure ventilation: effects on systemic oxygen transport and tissue oxygenation, Ann. Intern. Med. **76:**193, 1972.

49. Suter, P.M., Fairley, H.B., and Isenberg, M.D.: Optimum end-expiratory airway pressure in patients with acute pulmonary failure, N. Engl. J. Med. **292:**284, 1975.

50. Demers, R.R., Irwin, R.S., and Braman, S.S.: Criteria for optimum PEEP, Respir. Care **22:**596, 1977.

51. Bone, R.C.: Compliance and dynamic characteristic curves in acute respiratory failure, Crit. Care Med. **4:**173, 1976.

52. Hardaway, R.M., James, P.M., Jr., Anderson, R.W., et al.: Intensive study and treatment of shock in man, J.A.M.A. **199:**779, 1967.

53. Sladen, A., Laver, M.B., and Pontoppidan, H.: Pulmonary complications and water retention in prolonged mechanical ventilation, N. Engl. J. Med. **279:**448, 1968.

54. Shoemaker, W.C.: Pattern of pulmonary hemodynamic and functional changes in shock, Crit. Care Med. **2:**200, 1974.

55. Giordano, J.M., Joseph, W.L., Klingenmaier, C.H., et al.: The management of interstitial pulmonary edema—significance of hypoproteinemia, J. Thorac. Cardiovasc. Surg. **64:**739, 1972.

56. Holcroft, J.W., and Trunkey, D.D.: Extravascular lung water following hemorrhagic shock in the baboon: comparison between resuscitation with Ringer's lactate and plasmanate, Ann. Surg. **180:**408, 1974.

57. Swan, H.J.C., Ganz, W., and Forrester, J.: Catheterization of the heart in man with use of a flow-directed balloon-tipped catheter, N. Engl. J. Med. **283:**447, 1970.

58. Massion, W.H., Rosenbluth, B., and Kux, M.: Protective effect of methylprednisolone against lung complications in endotoxin shock, South. Med. J. **65:**941, 1972.

59. Wilson, J.W.: Treatment or prevention of pulmonary cellular damage with pharmacologic doses of corticosteroid, Surg. Gynecol. Obstet. **134:**675, 1972.

60. Jones, R.L., and King, E.G.: The effects of methylprednisolone on oxygenation in experimental hypoxemic respiratory failure, J. Trauma **15:**297, 1975.

61. Wertzberger, J.J., and Peltier, L.F.: Fat embolism: the effect of corticosteroids on experimental fat embolism in the rat, Surgery **64:**143, 1968.

62. Skornik, W.A., and Dressler, D.P.: The effects of short-term steroid therapy on lung bacterial clearance and survival in rats, Ann. Surg. **179:**415, 1974.

63. Ashbaugh, D.G., and Petty, T.L.: Sepsis complicating the acute respiratory distress syndrome, Surg. Gynecol. Obstet. **135:**865, 1972.

64. Sahn, S.A., Lakshminarayan, S., and Petty, T.L.: Weaning from mechanical ventilation, J.A.M.A. **235**:2208, 1976.
65. Lamy, M., Fallat, R.J., Koeniger, E., et al.: Pathologic features and mechanisms of hypoxemia in adult respiratory distress syndrome, Am. Rev. Respir. Dis. **114**:267, 1976.
66. Lakshminarayan, S., Stanford, R.E., and Petty, T.L.: Prognosis after recovery from adult respiratory distress syndrome, Am. Rev. Respir. Dis. **113**:7, 1976.
67. Simpson, D.L., Goodman, M., Spector, S.L., et al.: Long-term follow-up and bronchial reactivity testing in survivors of the adult respiratory distress syndrome, Am. Rev. Respir. Dis. **117**:449, 1978.
68. Hill, J.D., Ratliff, J.L., Fallat, R.J., et al.: Prognostic factors in the treatment of acute respiratory insufficiency with long-term extracorporeal oxygenation, J. Thorac. Cardiovasc. Surg. **68**:905, 1974.
69. Kolobow, T., Stool, E.W., Sacks, K.L., et al.: Acute respiratory failure: survival following ten days' support with a membrane lung, J. Thorac. Cardiovasc. Surg. **69**:947, 1975.

Chapter 8

RESPIRATORY FAILURE

Thomas M. Hyers

Respiratory failure occurs when the respiratory system cannot supply adequate oxygen to maintain metabolism, eliminate sufficient carbon dioxide to avoid respiratory acidosis, or both. This definition emphasizes that respiratory failure always causes other organ dysfunction as well. Clinically, respiratory failure is recognized when the patient's Pa_{O_2} is less than 50 mm Hg or when the Pa_{CO_2} is greater than 50 mm Hg with associated symptomatic abnormalities.

Pathophysiology

Alveolar gas pressure or tension is formed by the sum of the partial pressures of nitrogen, oxygen, carbon dioxide, and water vapor. Since total alveolar gas pressure and the partial pressures of nitrogen and water vapor are fixed, the alveolar partial pressures of oxygen and carbon dioxide tend to vary inversely. This simplified version of the alveolar gas equation shows the inverse relationship:

$$P_{A_{O_2}} = \text{inspired } P_{O_2} - \frac{P_{A_{CO_2}}}{\text{Respiratory quotient}}$$

The respiratory quotient is the ratio of carbon dioxide production divided by oxygen uptake and is determined by tissue metabolism in the steady state. The ratio usually takes a value of approximately 0.8, which means that an increase in P_{CO_2} will result in a slightly larger decrease in P_{O_2}. Since carbon dioxide is highly soluble in liquids and freely diffusible, alveolar and arterial tensions of this gas are nearly always equal. Therefore, when the Pa_{CO_2} rises, the cause is a widespread inability to ventilate alveoli. This state is called *diffuse alveolar hypoventilation* and is the only important cause of an elevated Pa_{CO_2}. Diffuse alveolar hypoventilation can occur in intrinsic lung diseases (usually COPD or chronic bronchitis and emphysema), in disorders of the neuromusculature and chest wall, and with abnormalities of central ventilatory drive as described below. From the alveolar gas equation it is clear that when the Pco_2 rises, the Po_2 must fall unless oxygen is added to the inspired air.

The transport of oxygen is more complicated than carbon dioxide elimination. Oxygen is both less soluble in liquids and less diffusible than carbon dioxide, which means that the Pao_2 will always be 10 to 20 mm Hg less than the Pao_2, even in normal lungs. In abnormal lungs the *gradient* between the Pao_2 and the Pao_2 can be much larger. The most common disorder that enlarges this gradient is seen in COPD, where regions of decreased alveolar ventilation do not keep pace with capillary blood flow (V/Q disturbance or mismatch). The extreme example of V/Q mismatch is *shunt*, which is a region of no alveolar ventilation without impairment of blood flow. Shunt is seen often in pneumonia and pulmonary embolism. The third disorder that can cause an enlarged gradient and hypoxemia is impaired *diffusion*, which results when the alveolar-capillary distance is widened or when there is widespread destruction of the capillary bed. This problem is often encountered in interstitial lung diseases and, somewhat paradoxically, in advanced emphysema. Thus, hypoxemia may occur in V/Q mismatch, shunt, impaired diffusion, and, of course, diffuse alveolar hypoventilation.

Minute ventilation (tidal volume × respiratory rate) is regulated by neurologic, metabolic, and chemoreceptor input. Of these factors, chemoreceptor input is best understood; it is composed of a Pao_2 sensor in the carotid body and $Paco_2$ sensors in the carotid body and brain stem. Either a fall in Pao_2 or a rise in $Paco_2$ can stimulate ventilation in the healthy individual. In a few people, abnormalities in this central ventilatory drive mechanism may lead to diffuse alveolar hypoventilation with both elevated $Paco_2$ and decreased Pao_2.

Low oxygen tension or elevated carbon dioxide tension may cause increased pulmonary artery pressure by a direct constriction of pulmonary arterioles. The usefulness of this reflex in adults is unclear; it may simply be a vestigial fetal reflex. Chronic elevation of pulmonary artery pressure can eventually cause right ventricular failure analogous to the way systemic hypertension causes left ventricular failure. This state is called *cor pulmonale*, that is, heart failure caused by lung disease.

Causes

Intrinsic diseases of the lung, disturbances of the chest wall or neuromusculature, and disorders of the central ventilatory drive can all lead to respiratory failure (see the chart on p. 84).

Of the intrinsic lung diseases, COPD is easily the most frequent cause of respiratory failure. Severe viral and bacterial pneumonias, interstitial lung

CAUSES OF RESPIRATORY FAILURE

A. *Intrinsic lung diseases*
1. COPD (e.g., chronic bronchitis and emphysema)
2. Interstitial lung diseases
3. Infections
4. Inhalation of toxic gases
5. Drowning
6. Chest trauma

B. *Neuromuscular and chest wall*
1. Neuromuscular blocking agents (e.g., curare)
2. Cervical spinal cord injuries
3. Diseases (e.g., myasthenia gravis, amyotrophic lateral sclerosis, myotonic dystrophy, Guillain-Barré syndrome, poliomyelitis, botulism)
4. Kyphoscoliosis

C. *Central ventilatory drive*
1. Drug overdose (e.g., opiates, barbiturates, tranquilizers, alcohol)
2. Obesity-related hypoventilation (pickwickian syndrome)
3. Myxedema
4. Stroke, brain trauma

D. *Other causes*
1. Carbon monoxide inhalation
2. Upper airways obstruction (e.g., foreign body, tumor, micrognathia)
3. Adult respiratory distress syndrome (see Chapter 7)

diseases, drowning, and inhalation of toxic substances such as nitrogen dioxide can also be causative. In this setting the chest wall and central ventilatory drive are usually normal; the lung architecture itself is the deterrent to effective oxygen transport (see Chapter 7). Some of these causes of respiratory failure can be either acute or chronic, and the degree of *renal* bicarbonate retention in compensation for any respiratory acidosis present ($Paco_2$ elevation) often furnishes the clue to chronicity (Table 8-1).

Disturbances of the chest wall or neuromusculature are less frequent than intrinsic lung diseases but important to recognize. Acute causes include neuromuscular blocking agents used in anesthesia; more chronic causes are cervical spinal cord injuries, myasthenia gravis, Guillain-Barré syndrome, amyotrophic lateral sclerosis, myotonic dystrophy, and, rarely, poliomyelitis and botulism.

Central ventilatory drive can be suppressed acutely by overdoses of opi-

TABLE 8-1. Blood gas patterns in respiratory failure

	Pao$_2$	Paco$_2$	pH	HCO$_3$ (meq/L)
Acute hypoxemia	≤50	≤40	7.44*	24
Acute hypoxemia and hypercapnia	≤50	≥50	≤7.30	24
Chronic hypoxemia and hypercapnia, with renal compensation	≤50	≥50	7.38	≥30

*Approximate.

ates, barbiturates, or tranquilizers. Stroke and brain trauma can also cause respiratory failure by suppressing central ventilatory drive, and some individuals seem to have a genetic insensitivity to elevated Paco$_2$ and lowered Pao$_2$. Obesity-related hypoventilation is a well-known cause of chronic respiratory failure in this group.

Inhalation of carbon monoxide causes a unique form of respiratory failure by inhibiting the access of oxygen to hemoglobin. Since only the binding of oxygen to hemoglobin is affected, the Pao$_2$ can be normal even with massive carbon monoxide inhalation. Thus the problem can be difficult to recognize and must be suspected in any type of smoke inhalation. The treatment is high-flow oxygen supplementation that speeds the clearance of carbon monoxide from the blood.

Diagnosis

No matter what the cause, respiratory failure can be difficult to recognize. Symptoms include altered mentation, malaise, difficulty with sleep, headache, weakness, weight loss or gain, palpitations, breathlessness, and cough—all deceptively nonspecific. Cardiovascular manifestations include tachycardia, arrhythmias, cyanosis, ascites, and edema. CNS manifestations vary from mild personality changes to stupor and coma. When respiratory failure is suspected, arterial blood gases and pH must be measured immediately to confirm the diagnosis.

Treatment

Acute respiratory failure can often be a medical emergency, and two priorities of therapy must be committed to memory. Adequate oxygenation is always the first priority. Oxygen can be administered by nasal prongs or by a tight-fitting mask with attached reservoir bag if manual assistance in breathing is required. These methods are usually adequate until the arrival of someone trained to perform endotracheal intubation.

The second priority is reversal of respiratory acidosis. Carbon dioxide retention, signifying diffuse alveolar hypoventilation, frequently accompanies acute respiratory failure and is quickly corrected by increasing alveolar ventilation. Rarely is administration of intravenous sodium bicarbonate necessary to correct respiratory acidosis, and in some instances sodium bicarbonate may be detrimental by overloading an already compromised cardiovascular system. The proper initial therapy of acute respiratory failure is thus maintenance of an adequate airway, supplemental oxygen, and assisted ventilation as necessary to correct Pao_2 and acid-base abnormalities.

Proper treatment ultimately depends on correctly identifying the underlying cause. With this knowledge in mind the clinician selectively treats infection if present, administers antidotes as available to counteract ingested drugs or toxins, initiates controlled oxygen therapy, and begins chest physiotherapy to assist in the removal of obstructing secretions.

The use of IPPB lacks proven benefit in acute respiratory failure. In general, inhaled drugs can be nebulized as effectively with powered but nonpressurized nebulizers. Furthermore, IPPB frequently can tire a patient and lead to pneumothorax and air swallowing with massive gastric distension.

The decision to perform endotracheal intubation and initiate mechanical ventilation is based both on clinical evaluation and on blood gas abnormalities. Many individuals with respiratory failure caused by COPD may be treated with judicious oxygen therapy, chest physiotherapy, bronchodilators, and antibiotics without use of intubation and mechanical ventilation, although arterial blood gases interpreted alone might dictate ventilation, although arterial blood gases interpreted alone might dictate otherwise. In contrast, some individuals with massive pneumonia or drug overdose require immediate mechanical ventilation. General indications for endotracheal intubation and mechanical ventilation in acute respiratory failure include (1) unconsciousness, (2) copious secretions that cannot be cleared by coughing, and (3) severe hypoxemia or respiratory acidosis that does not respond promptly to lesser measures.

A hospital in which endotracheal intubation and mechanical ventilation are performed must have an adequately staffed intensive care unit, a physician skilled in the care of the critically ill and the use of mechanical ventilators, and a laboratory capable of accurate and immediate arterial blood gas analysis. Endotracheal intubation must be performed by an experienced physician, and the position of the tube checked with a portable chest radiograph. The end of the tube should be 3 to 4 cm above the carina. A prestretched, high compliance cuff is important to avoid extensive ischemia to the tracheal mucosa and cartilaginous rings. The internal diameter of the tube must be large enough ($\geqslant 7\frac{1}{2}$ mm) to allow easy passage of a suction catheter. In general, endotracheal tubes are left in place from 3 to 10 days, after which a tracheostomy is performed if intubation is still necessary.

Mechanical ventilators used today are mostly of the *volume* delivery type; that is, they will deliver a preset volume of gas limited only by a very high airway pressure (60 to 100 cm water) that, upon being reached, opens a safety valve. Some ventilators are *pressure* regulated and deliver gas only until a preselected pressure of 20 to 30 cm water is reached. Pressure-regulated ventilators are subject to the vagaries of pulmonary compliance in that as lung compliance decreases because of pulmonary edema, pneumonia, or fibrosis, delivered tidal volume also decreases. All ventilators must be used with an in-line audible alarm system sensitive to changes in airway pressure or flow. Large tidal volumes are used (10 to 15 ml/kg body weight) to help prevent atelectasis, and when possible the machine is adjusted so that the patient's breathing effort will trigger the machine. When a patient is apneic, the rate is set to achieve a Pao_2 between 60 and 90 mm Hg and a pH between 7.35 and 7.50. A minute ventilation between 5 and 10 L will usually approach this pH and oxygen tension. Because of the physical characteristics of oxygen-hemoglobin affinity, a Pao_2 higher than 90 mm Hg does not result in an appreciable increase in blood oxygen content but can cause lung damage from hyperoxia. In all instances, oxygen tension and acid-base status must be monitored by repeated arterial blood gas determinations. Other maneuvers may be necessary. These include sedation, the addition of respiratory dead space if the patient is markedly hyperventilating, and the use of PEEP in certain types of ARDS when oxygenation is difficult (see Chapter 7 and the accompanying checklist).

CHECKLIST FOR ENDOTRACHEAL INTUBATION AND MECHANICAL VENTILATOR THERAPY

A. *Endotracheal tube*
1. Type—7½ mm or greater internal diameter with prestretched high compliance cuff (cuff pressure < 30 mm Hg)
2. Position—check with portable chest radiograph

B. *Mechanical ventilator*
1. Tidal volume—12 to 15 ml/kg body weight
2. Rate—as set by the patient or to maintain the Pao_2 and pH listed below (usually a minute ventilation of 5 to 10 L is sufficient)
3. Alarm—in-line, pressure or flow sensitive, continuous use

C. *Patient*
1. Arterial blood gases—Pao_2: 60 to 90 mm Hg; pH: 7.35 to 7.50
2. Vital signs—frequent monitoring aimed at normalizing (fast pulse and low blood pressure can be caused by a pneumothorax or a large tidal volume interfering with venous return)
3. Cardiac rhythm—should be continuously monitored
4. End organ function—especially mentation, urine output

Adequate oxygen supply to tissues is the treatment goal in respiratory failure, and one must remember that tissue oxygenation depends on both blood oxygen content and cardiac output. Careful attention must be paid to pulse, blood pressure, and cardiac rhythm during mechanical ventilation. In some instances determination of cardiac output is necessary.

Nosocomial pneumonia is the primary complication of acute respiratory failure. This problem is caused not only by the patient's weakened condition, but also by the common use of antibiotics in high dosages in the intensive care unit.

The direct complications of intubation and mechanical ventilation are iatrogenic and can be lethal. These include inadvertent intubation of the right mainstem bronchus, respiratory acidosis or alkalosis caused by improper use of the ventilator, pneumothorax, and tracheal damage and stenosis.

Weaning procedures

Endotracheal intubation and mechanical ventilation cannot be viewed as specific therapy for respiratory failure but rather as support until reversible abnormalities (e.g., pneumonia, bronchitis, pulmonary edema) are resolved. Once the patient appears to be responding to treatment for the underlying cause of respiratory failure, the following criteria should be met before discontinuing ventilatory support: (1) adequate arterial oxygen (a Pao_2 above 60 mm Hg with an Fio_2 of 0.4 or less), (2) a spontaneous minute ventilation less that 10 L as measured with a Wright respirometer, (3) a maximal voluntary ventilation at least twice the resting minute ventilation, and (4) a vital capacity at least 2 to 3 times the resting tidal volume. When these criteria are met, the ventilator may be removed and spontaneous breathing allowed through the endotracheal tube. The Fio_2 should be the same or slightly higher than that delivered with the ventilator, and adequate humidity must be added to the inspired air. The patient must remain in the intensive care unit for close observation. If alveolar ventilation decreases (i.e., the $Paco_2$ rises) or other signs of respiratory failure appear (restlessness, tachycardia, diaphoresis, confusion), ventilation is started again and weaning postponed. If the patient remains stable and arterial blood gases remain satisfactory for more than 30 minutes, the endotracheal tube can usually be safely removed.

Chronic respiratory failure

COPD is also the principal cause of chronic respiratory failure. Less common causes include interstitial lung diseases, neuromuscular disorders and obesity-related dysfunction of central ventilatory drive. In chronic respiratory failure the work of breathing can become a significant part of total body metabolism because of inefficiency of the respiratory system. The patient tends to respond to this marginal situation either by decreasing ventilation relative to metabolic demand to allow a higher blood $Paco_2$ and a lower Pao_2 or by shedding lean body mass. Both responses can be considered compensatory because each leads to decreased work of breathing relative to the metabolic demands of the body. The former compensation is seen typically in the "blue bloater" and the latter in the "pink puffer" COPD patient. The basis for selection of one of these responses is not clear but may depend in part on a genetic predisposition. Neither response is completely compensatory, and each leads to further problems. The "blue bloater" hypoventilates with a resultant respiratory acidosis and more hypoxemia, both of which increase pulmonary hypertension, hastening the onset of cor pulmonale. The "pink puffer" frequently develops cachexia severe enough to suggest neoplastic disease (see Chapter 10).

The administration of supplemental oxygen has potential hazard in the individual with chronic respiratory failure and elevated $Paco_2$. The chemoreceptor drive to breathe is directed by hypoxemia here, and the sudden introduction of high-flow oxygen can cause increased hypoventilation or even apnea by suppressing the hypoxemic drive. In practice this is rarely seen with nasal oxygen flows of 3 L/min or less, and these flow rates are usually sufficient to raise the Pao_2 to an acceptable level. When someone with chronic respiratory failure is given ventilatory therapy, one must avoid the temptation to correct an elevated $Paco_2$ when the pH is nearly normal. In these patients the pH approaches normal because of previous renal conservation of bicarbonate ion, and a rapid lowering of $Paco_2$ can lead to severe metabolic alkalosis with seizures, hypotension, and arrhythmias. In fact, it is usually better to ventilate to the $Paco_2$ to which the patient has previously compensated the pH with bicarbonate ion retention.

In patients with chronic respiratory failure and cor pulmonale, the administration of continuous low-flow (1 to 2 L/min) nasal oxygen can frequently correct or alleviate pulmonary artery hypertension, correct or prevent congestive right heart failure, and return the patient to a more functional life.

SUGGESTED READINGS

Asmundsson, T., and Kilburn, K.H.: Survival after acute respiratory failure: 145 patients observed 5 to 8½ years, Ann. Intern. Med. **80:**54, 1974.

Petty, T.L.: Intensive and rehabilitative respiratory care, ed. 2, Philadelphia, 1974, Lea & Febiger.

Sahn, S.A., and Lakshminarayan, S.: Bedside criteria for discontinuation of mechanical ventilation, Chest **63:**1002, 1973.

Tillotson, J.R., and Finland, M.: Bacterial colonization and clinical superinfection of the respiratory tract complicating antibiotic treatment of pneumonia, J. Infect. Dis. **119:**597, 1969.

Wynne, J.W., Block, A.J., Hemenway, J., et al.: Disordered breathing and oxygen desaturation during sleep in patients with chronic obstructive lung disease, Am. J. Med. **66:**573, 1979.

Zwillich, C.W., Pierson, D.J., Creagh, C.E., et al.: Complications of assisted ventilation: a prospective study of 354 consecutive episodes, Am. J. Med. **57:**161, 1974.

Chapter 9

RESPIRATORY THERAPY INCLUDING CARDIOPULMONARY RESUSCITATION

James T. Good, Jr., *and* **H. Dennis Waite**

Respiratory therapy has experienced tremendous expansion in the 1960s and 1970s. Much of the expansion has resulted from economic rather than scientific considerations. As a result, much therapy is prescribed without proper consideration for indications or desired results. The first conference examining the scientific basis of respiratory therapy occurred in 1974; the indications and efficacy of all forms of therapy were reviewed.[1] Many questions emanated from this conference, especially regarding the efficacy of IPPB and continuous oxygen administration. Results of a multicenter study of oxygen therapy favor continuous rather than nocturnal administration. In addition, another study is reviewing the efficacy of IPPB versus aerosolized bronchodilator therapy. The American College of Chest Physicians has recently outlined its recommendations for organizing and administering hospital respiratory care services.[2]

THERAPEUTIC OXYGEN

Oxygen[3] is one of the most frequently used forms of medical therapy. Tissue oxygenation depends on: (1) alveolar oxygen concentration, (2) diffusion of oxygen at the alveolar-capillary membrane, (3) V/Q relationships within the lung, (4) the quantity and carrying capacity of hemoglobin, and (5) cardiac output. Disturbances of any of these functions may result in tissue hypoxia. In most situations, supplemental oxygen increases the alveolar oxygen concentration and tissue delivery of oxygen.

Because therapeutic oxygen is potentially harmful, the dosage must be written as *liters per minute* or *percent concentration in inspired air*. The indication for supplemental oxygen is hypoxemia (Pao_2 below 50 mm Hg), which may be manifested by any of the following physical findings: cyanosis,

90

diaphoresis, tachycardia, confusion, and, at times, erythremia. Skin color must be evaluated with care; it is best assessed in bright daylight. Erythremia tends to accentuate or even simulate cyanosis; anemia tends to obscure it. Arterial blood gases, ear oximetry, and patient assessment are the major ways of evaluating the adequacy of oxygen therapy.

Individuals with chronic respiratory insufficiency frequently need continuous oxygen therapy for the duration of their lives. In past years it was thought that 12 hours oxygen therapy (especially nocturnal administration) was as effective therapeutically as continuous 24-hour administration. The recent nocturnal oxygen therapeutic trial, however, strongly supports the concept that continuous 24-hour oxygen is more effective because it significantly reduced patient mortality at both 1- and 2-year follow-up periods.[4] The goal of supplemental oxygen is to raise the Pao_2 to approximately 60 mm Hg, thus reducing hypoxic vasoconstriction of the pulmonary vascular bed and pulmonary artery pressure and improving right ventricular function and tissue delivery of oxygen.

The nasal cannula is the most commonly used (and most comfortable) device for administering oxygen. Mouth breathing will not affect the Fio_2 during nasal oxygen administration as long as the nasal passages are patent. The maximum acceptable flow rate is 7 L/min, which yields an Fio_2 of approximately 0.35. An alternative method of oxygen delivery is the simple oxygen mask, without reservoir bag or valve, which *fits loosely* over the nose and mouth. Two large ports allow for entrainment of room air and exhalation of inspired air. At flow rates of 4 to 12 L, an Fio_2 ranging from 0.25 to 0.45 may be achieved. The long-term use of masks interferes with eating, drinking, and talking. When the nasal cannula alone will not provide an adequate Fio_2, the simple oxygen mask may be used in conjunction with it.

The *venturi mask* delivers a precise low concentration of oxygen. It has no advantage over the nasal route and has the disadvantages of all other masks.

The *partial rebreathing mask* is a simple oxygen mask with an open circuit to a reservoir bag. This mask is used to increase the Fio_2, not the $Fico_2$. Proper functioning of the bag depends on gas flow and a tight fit. Flow rates adequate to prevent the bag from collapsing on inspiration (8 to 16 L/min) should be maintained at all times. The maximum Fio_2 obtainable with this mask is 0.40 to 0.70.

The *nonrebreathing mask* has a one-way valve leading to the oxygen reservoir bag and a one-way valve on the exhalation port. These valves prevent the entrainment of room air and the flow of exhaled air from entering the bag. With a porperly fitting mask of this type, an Fio_2 as high as 0.8 to 0.9 may be obtained. It is almost impossible to deliver an Fio_2 of 1.0 without intubating the patient. Such high oxygen concentrations should be used only in life-threatening situations and then only for the briefest possible time because of the dangers of oxygen toxicity and, in COPD, of "CO_2 narcosis."

BRONCHIAL HYGIENE

Cleansing of the bronchial tree improves or maintains airway patency in obstructive and restrictive lung disease, neurologic and neuromuscular diseases, and preoperative and postoperative patients. The techniques available to accomplish bronchial hygiene are (1) inhaled bronchodilator aerosol with or without IPPB, (2) inhaled moisture therapy to loosen secretions, (3) controlled coughing and postural drainage with or without percussion, and (4) vibrations to aid in the removal of secretions (see Chapters 7, 8, and 10).

When prescribing bronchial hygiene the physician must clearly define the clinical problem and therapeutic goals and then select only the techniques necessary to achieve these goals. Generally, patients who have respiratory diseases characterized by production of large amounts or excessively sticky mucus and secretions will benefit most from bronchial hygiene programs. Specifically, patients with bronchiectasis, cystic fibrosis, Kartagener's syndrome, chronic bronchitis, and asthma need a regular program of bronchial hygiene. A recent study evaluating the efficacy of chest physiotherapy and IPPB in the resolution of pneumonia, on the other hand, indicated that these therapeutic maneuvers did not hasten resolution.[5]

Medication nebulizers, used to deliver *aerosolized bronchodilators* to patients with asthma or COPD, are hand-bulb nebulizer, metered-dose device, and powered sidestream nebulizer in conjunction with IPPB. The choice of delivery system depends on the patient's manual dexterity and ability to take a deep breath. IPPB therapy is indicated when a patient is incapable of an effective inspiratory effort and sometimes when coordination of the aerosol generation and inspiration is lacking. Patients may be evaluated by vital capacity measurements with and without IPPB.[6] If the volume is not considerably greater when IPPB is used, it is not beneficial except when patients are psychologically dependent on it. When IPPB is used, the physician's orders should include tidal volume and maximum pressure desired, type and amount of bronchodilator (for patients with asthma and COPD), and maximum length of treatment.

Moisture therapy (aerosol or humidity) assists in liquifying and mobilizing secretions. Heated large reservoir nebulizers should not be relied on for supplemental oxygen because the patient frequently removes the mask for eating, walking, and talking. Inhalation of moisture should always follow the inhalation of a bronchodilator and precede measures for removing secretions.

Heated large reservoir nebulizers (e.g., Puritan All-Purpose) and heated humidifiers (e.g., Cascade) with a tracheostomy collar or an endotracheal tube adapter must provide 100% body humidity to replace the function of the bypassed upper airways. To prevent drying of secretions and subsequent complications, supplemental humidity must be delivered continuously.

The ultrasonic nebulizer can deliver a large volume of water or normal saline solution but should be limited to use in patients with very tenacious secretions. Ultrasonic nebulizers can precipitate bronchospasm and hypoxemia in patients with asthma or COPD and should always be preceded by inhaled bronchodilators.

Chest physiotherapy helps to mobilize retained secretions, improves breathing efficiency, and may improve distribution of ventilation.[7] *Postural drainage* aids mucus clearance by positioning the body to drain specific areas by gravity. This technique is enhanced with the addition of chest percussion in the drainage positions. The vibrations from percussion are transmitted to the lung tissue, thus loosening mucus. Postural drainage with or without percussion should be considered whenever the patient's cough is weak or ineffective, large amounts of secretions are present, or both. Postural drainage and percussion are not without hazards, and the benefits from these techniques must be carefully weighed against the potential risks.

In many patients *deep breathing* and *segmental breathing* seem to improve the distribution of inhaled air and increase the efficiency of breathing. The use of incentive spirometry may be a more efficient method of reducing postoperative respiratory complications and atelectasis than IPPB.[9] Many of the incentive spirometers are disposable, and treatments are more economical.

Coughing, a natural defense of the lungs, aids in removing foreign particles and secretions. Patients with an ineffective cough such as occurs in severe COPD, postoperative abdominal and thoracic procedures, or neuromuscular diseases or abnormalities must be instructed and assisted in proper coughing maneuvers.

PREOPERATIVE AND POSTOPERATIVE RESPIRATORY CARE

It has been well established that patients at high risk for postoperative pulmonary complications can be identified preoperatively. Patients with COPD, asthma, obesity, or a history of smoking or exposure to polluted air who are scheduled for thoracic or abdominal surgery are at high risk. Patients with suspected restrictive or obstructive lung disease should have bedside spirometry (FVC and FEV_1) and arterial blood gases included in their preoperative work-up.

It is known that patients with an FEV_1 of 60% or less of their vital capacity will have fewer pulmonary complications if they receive aggressive pulmonary hygiene for at least 3 to 4 days before surgery. The program should include abstinence from smoking, the use of systemic and inhaled bronchodilators, and bronchial hygiene. Asthmatic patients should usually receive an intravenous aminophylline drip (0.5 to 0.9 mg/kg/hr) and have a bolus of corticosteroid (the equivalent of 50 to 60 mg methylprednisolone) 4 to 6 hours before surgery.

All patients will benefit greatly from preoperative counseling on the importance of postoperative deep breathing and coughing despite the pain involved.

Ventilators

Occasionally a patient will have a profound defect in ventilatory capacity or oxygen transport that requires total ventilatory support. The decision to use a ventilator can be very difficult. Deteriorating blood gas values (i.e., a falling Pao_2 despite supplemental oxygen or a rising $Paco_2$ despite maximum therapeutic effort) are good indicators. Clinical signs of worsening respiratory failure are also useful; restlessness, diaphoresis, confusion, and tachycardia are the most common. Once the decision to provide support is made, the physician must: (1) establish an airway, (2) choose the most appropriate ventilator and the correct machine settings to meet the patient's needs, (3) determine the adequacy of the ventilatory support system after its initiation, and (4) wean the patient from ventilatory support in due course.[9] (See Chapter 8 for details.)

Because intubated patients have greatly impaired clearance mechanisms (e.g., an ineffective cough and an endotracheal tube within the airway), all intubated patients will benefit from periodic aerosolized bronchodilators to augment suctioning. Sometimes the addition of an aminophylline drip (even in the absence of wheezing) will improve bronchopulmonary clearance.

Cardiopulmonary resuscitation[10]

Basic life support is undertaken as an emergency first aid procedure in all patients with recognized cardiac or respiratory arrest. In a collapsed or unconscious patient adequate ventilation and circulation must be established very quickly (usually within 10 seconds). This can be done by taking the following steps:

1. Determine consciousness by shaking the person's shoulder.
2. If the patient does not respond, open the airway by placing one hand beneath the patient's neck and the other on his or her forehead.

Then lift the neck and push back on the forehead in one maneuver.

3. Check for spontaneous breathing by listening over the mouth and watching to see if the chest rises and falls. This is important, since simply opening the airway solves the ventilation problem in many unconscious patients.

4. If no spontaneous breathing occurs, begin breathing support. Maintain an open airway by continuation of upward pressure on the neck and backward pressure on the forehead with the heel of the other hand. Using the thumb and forefinger of that hand, pinch the nostrils closed. Take a deep breath, make a tight seal over the patient's mouth with your mouth, and blow. Watch to see that the chest rises, and listen for the escape of air when your mouth is removed. Repeat this four times in rapid succession.

5. If no spontaneous ventilation begins, check the carotid pulse. Feel in the groove between the larynx and the neck muscles (sternocleido-mastoid) for at least 10 seconds. Maintain an open airway with the other hand at all times.

6. If the airway remains obstructed the following manual maneuvers should be performed in the following sequence until airway patency is established:

   a. Back blow: four sharp blows delivered with the heel of the hand over the spine between the shoulder blades;

   b. Manual thrusts: a series of four thrusts to upper abdomen or lower chest; and

   c. Finger sweep: the tongue is grabbed and the index finger of the other hand is placed deeply in the throat to attempt to dislodge a foreign body.

7. If no pulse is felt, proceed with artificial circulatory support. Place the victim on a hard surface in a horizontal position. Locate the xiphoid process with one hand; place the heel of the second hand over the sternum 1 to 2 inches above the xiphoid; place the first hand on top of the second; keep elbows locked and depress the sternum 1½ to 2 inches by rocking forward over the chest. Keep the compressions adequate but not too forceful (broken ribs are frequent), and keep the *fingers* off the chest wall.

8. If alone, give 15 compressions at a rate of 80/min, then 2 quick ventilations. If another person is helping, give 5 compressions at a rate of 60/min and interpose 1 breath.

9. Continue these steps until advanced life support personnel arrive or until spontaneous breathing and circulation resume.

REFERENCES

1. Pierce, A.K., and Saltzman, H.A.: Proceedings of the conference on scientific basis of respiratory therapy, Am. Rev. Respir. Dis. **110**(6 Pt 2):1, 1974.
2. Miller, W.F., and Plummer, A.L.: Guidelines for organization and function of hospital respiratory care services, Chest **78**:79, 1980.
3. Shapiro, B.A., Harrison, R.A., and Trout, C.A.: Clinical Application of Respiratory Care, Chicago, 1979, Year Book Medical Publishers, Inc.
4. Nocturnal Oxygen Therapy Trial Group: Continuous or nocturnal oxygen therapy in hypoxemic chronic obstructive lung disease, Ann. Intern. Med. **93**:391, 1980.
5. Graham, W.G.B., and Bradley, D.A.: Efficacy of chest physiotherapy and intermittent positive-pressure breathing in the resolution of pneumonia, N. Engl. J. Med. **299**:624, 1978.
6. Powers, W.E., and Morrison, D.R.: Evaluation of inspired volumes in postoperative patients receiving volume-oriented IPPB, Respir. Care. **23**:39, 1978.
7. May, D.B., and Munt, P.W.: Physiologic effects of chest percussion and postural drainage in patients with stable chronic bronchitis, Chest **75**:29, 1979.
8. Dohi, S., and Gold, M.I.: Comparison of two methods of postoperative respiratory care, Chest **73**:592, 1978.
9. Sahn, S.A., Lakshminarayan, S., and Petty, T.L.: Weaning from mechanical ventilation, J.A.M.A. **235**:2208, 1976.
10. Standards and guidelines for cardiopulmonary resuscitation (CPR) and emergency cardiac care (ECC), J.A.M.A. **244**:453, 1980.

Chapter 10

CHRONIC OBSTRUCTIVE PULMONARY DISEASE (COPD)

Roger S. Mitchell *and* Thomas L. Petty

Definitions

Chronic obstructive pulmonary disease (COPD) is a clinical syndrome of dyspnea on exertion with objective evidence of reduced airflow not explained by specific or infiltrative lung or heart disease. Productive cough is often present. Reduced airflow is detected on physical examination by diminution in the sounds of air movement, especially on expiration, throughout both lungs. Reduced airflow may be measured by the standard ventilation tests (MVV, FEV_1, FEV_1/FVC, and PEF_{25-75} [formerly MMEF]) or by measuring increased Raw (in the body plethysmograph). Synonyms include chronic obstructive pulmonary emphysema, chronic obstructive lung disease, chronic airways obstruction, diffuse obstructive pulmonary syndrome, emphysema, chronic bronchitis, and others.

Emphysema is defined morphologically as a state of the lungs in which the air spaces distal to the terminal bronchioles are abnormally increased in size and undergo destructive changes in their walls. The Ciba Symposium in 1958 took the position that increase in the size of the air spaces may result either from dilation or destruction; in other words, in its view, overinflation alone (i.e., dilatation without destruction as in one lung after removal of the other) may be regarded as emphysema. The view accepted by most observers, however, is that overinflation alone should be labeled simply as overinflation and not as emphysema.

Chronic bronchitis is defined clinically; it is characterized by excessive mucus secretion in the bronchial tree with chronic or recurrent productive cough on most days for a minimum of 3 months a year for not less than 2 successive years. The diagnosis can only be made after excluding the presence of specific diseases of the lungs or bronchi such as tuberculosis, abscess, tumor, bronchiectasis, and others that may cause identical symptoms.

97

Pathology and physiology

COPD is almost always a mixture of emphysema and chronic bronchitis, plus, at times, elements of bronchiolitis and asthma. Emphysema has been classified as *centrilobular* (CLE) or *centriacinar* involving initially the respiratory bronchioles, *panlobular* (PLE) or *panacinar* involving the entire acinus, *paraseptal*, and *irregular* or "scar" emphysema. As CLE progresses, it becomes increasingly difficult to distinguish it from PLE, and it may be labeled *mixed* or *endstage*. CLE is predominantly a disease of bronchitic patients who smoke cigarettes, whereas PLE, the type associated with α_1-antitrypsin deficiency (zz type), is also often found in bronchitic patients who smoke cigarettes. The airway tissues, especially the cartilaginous tissue, have often become atrophic, resulting in flabbiness and premature collapse on expiration. Physiologically, advanced emphysema is most commonly identifiable by loss of elastic recoil, increased total lung capacity, and impaired oxygen diffusion. The impaired diffusion tends to be balanced by the destruction of the capillary bed; V/Q imbalance is therefore often slight or absent.

Chronic bronchitis is characterized morphologically by hypertrophy and hyperplasia of the mucous glands lining the bronchi, chronic leucocytic and lymphocytic infiltration of the bronchial walls, increase in mucous-secreting goblet cells, loss of cilia, and squamous metaplasia. These changes often extend to the noncartilage-bearing bronchioles that may be almost or totally occluded by inflammation, exudate, or dried mucus plugs (as in bronchiolitis and asthma).

In normal lungs most of the normal resistance to airflow lies in airways more than 2 mm in diameter, because the total cross-sectional diameter of the smaller ones is so much greater than those larger than 2 mm in diameter. Involvement of the small airways therefore must be extensive before MVV, FEV_1, FEV_1/FVC, and PEF_{25-75} will be abnormal. As chronic bronchitis progresses over the years, small airways disease impairs ventilation, while perfusion remains normal or only slightly impaired; this produces a V/Q imbalance resulting in hypoxemia. The hypoxemia gradually induces pulmonary hypertension, cor pulmonale, and episodes of right heart failure.

COPD in its advanced stages may present as the "pink puffer" syndrome—intense dyspnea, marked weight loss, hyperlucent lungs, small heart, and a tendency to normal blood gases, or as the "blue bloater" syndrome—relatively mild dyspnea, no weight loss, large heart, episodes of right heart failure, erythremia, hypercapnia, and hypoxemia. Untreated, the "pink puffer" tends to show severe emphysema and relatively little inflammatory airway disease; the "blue bloater" tends, on the other hand, to show severe airways disease and less emphysema. The majority of cases, however, generally fall between these two extremes.

COPD is much more common in men than in women and in smokers than in nonsmokers. It is also more common in urban than in rural dwellers and in socioeconomically disadvantaged than in economically privileged persons. Cigarette smoking is the most important known risk factor in the pathogenesis of COPD, whether it is manifested by emphysema, chronic bronchitis, or both. Cigarette smoke contains numerous irritants that stimulate mucus production, impair and ultimately destroy ciliary function, induce cough, and cause alveolar wall damage. Persons who regularly smoke cigarettes are also more susceptible to recurrent deep respiratory infections, which appear to play a contributory role in the evolution of COPD. Cigarette smoke contains high concentrations of carbon monoxide, which can aggravate the hypoxemia that is a frequent problem late in the course of the disease. Urban air pollution plays a role in COPD similar to that of cigarette smoke but to a lesser degree.

Severe chronic cough may cause further damage to already partially damaged bronchial, bronchiolar, and alveolar walls. This opinion is supported by the clinical observation that progression of disability tends to slow down when coughing disappears or is controlled in the not too severely ill patient. Microscopic pulmonary thromboemboli, possibly induced by nicotine, carbon monoxide, or other ingredients of cigarette smoke, may also play a role in causing alveolar wall damage.

Finally, certain tissue defects and increased susceptibility to injury appear to be involved in the pathogenesis of COPD. How else can some individuals live in an industrial, heavily polluted city and inhale cigarette smoke regularly all their lives and still not develop the severe symptomatic disease? These defects may be acquired or genetically determined. A small number of individuals with deficiency of α_1-antitrypsin (zz type) tend to have early onset PLE emphysema. Patients with the heterozygous deficiency who also smoke cigarettes *may* have a higher than expected risk of emphysema and COPD. The mechanism of this form of alveolar damage appears to be a failure of protection against protein digestion from enzymes released from disintegrating macrophages and leukocytes. Recent evidence indicates that cigarette smoke also enhances this mechanism of alveolar wall damage. A forme fruste of mucoviscidosis in the adult has been proposed as an underlying tissue defect by some observers. Airway clearance becomes severely impaired in advanced COPD; healthy young persons and persons with mild disease have a spectrum of airway clearance from rapid to slow. It is thus possible that impaired clearance, genetic or acquired, may also be an important predilection factor.

The mechanisms of airways obstruction are somewhat better understood than the etiology. These mechanisms include (1) inflammatory swelling of the bronchial and bronchiolar walls, causing them to narrow, (2) the presence of excessive and viscid mucus obstructing airflow, especially in the bronchioles, (3) atrophy of airway walls, presumably a complication of prior inflammation, together with loss of the normal supporting elastic structure and elastic recoil (i.e., emphysema), causing them to kink and collapse prematurely on expiration, and (4) bronchioles no longer patent because of prior obliterative inflammation.

Clinical picture

COPD at times appears to have its origin in repeated chest infections in childhood. About two thirds of cases, however, begin in individuals aged 30 to 50 with chronic productive cough and repeated "colds" or deep chest infections. Approximately 15% of patients give a history of episodic, noneffort-dependent, wheezing dyspnea (i.e., presumably bronchial asthma) generally during childhood, before the onset of effort-dependent dyspnea. Some 20% of patients insist that dyspnea on exertion was their first symptom, but when closely questioned, most of these add that chronic cough started at the same time or soon after. Some 5% of patients deny the presence of chronic cough at any time throughout the course of their disease. A few patients begin with a *sudden* awareness of dyspnea and cough; others report a sudden and persistent worsening of their dyspnea at some time during the course of the disease. These sudden episodes, sometimes devastating to exercise tolerance, are often labeled *pneumonia* by the attending physician. They often are no doubt episodes of some form of pneumonia, but some may be episodes of *acute* bronchiolar inflammation, which may become chronic or result in irreversible obliteration of many bronchioles; some may be episodes of extensive microscopic thromboembolism. Most such episodes, however, probably simply represent an acute awareness of a little more damage to an already damaged respiratory system. It has been suggested that progressive alveolar destruction provides collateral ventilation distal to simultaneously occurring bronchiolar obliteration—in other words, a temporary *advantage* induced by some emphysema. It is a fact that a considerable amount of disease may be present with little subjective dyspnea and no or only mild airways obstruction as measured by the FEV_1, so that a superimposed deep respiratory infection may be enough to make an individual abruptly and permanently symptomatic.

The *appearance of the sputum* is important in the evaluation of patients with COPD. When it is purulent, a readily treatable and potentially reversible aspect of the disease has been identified.

The physical findings vary with the type and severity of the airways obstruction. A relatively immobile chest with shoulders carried high, suppressed breath sounds (especially on expiration), and decreased cardiac dullness are common findings in severe emphysema. An apparent increase in the anteroposterior diameter, scattered rhonchi, occasionally a few fine basal rales, accentuated second heart sound in the pulmonic area, palpable P_2 in the second left intercostal space, gallop rhythm, right ventricular lift, cyanosis, and dependent edema may all be observed in the advanced stage of COPD.

The chest radiograph may be helpful when properly interpreted (Figs. 10-1 to 10-4). Radiographic signs suggesting emphysema are flattening of the hemidiaphragms, hyperinflation and avascularity of the lungs, the presence of bullae, and increased retrosternal space. Indications of chronic bronchitis include increased bronchovascular markings, increase in the size of the main and branch pulmonary arteries, and an enlarged heart. Chest fluoroscopy may be useful in estimating the speed of expiratory airflow; this dynamic measure of air trapping cannot be reliably predicted from an inspiratory film, not even when accompanied by an expiration film, since some patients can empty their lungs fully if given enough time. Complicating bronchiolitis may be manifest radiographically by a fine stippling in both midlung fields (Fig. 10-3). A bronchogram, if performed, may reveal bits of contrast medium in dilated bronchial mucous gland ducts, especially under the left main bronchus. It may also reveal a failure of the bronchi to taper peripherally and thus look like scattered "leaves on a winter tree," a finding that has been labeled *bronchiolectasis* (Fig. 10-5). A bronchogram is seldom needed in these cases; when used, it should be performed with great care (i.e., including one side at a time). The information it provides is of academic interest rather than practical value.

Bronchoscopy in severe chronic airways obstruction will show easy collapsibility of all the visible major airways including the trachea. In chronic bronchitis the mucosa has a red velvety appearance, and secretions may be seen bubbling up from the involved airways.

The electrocardiogram is useful in detecting the presence of cor pulmonale and pulmonary hypertension. Various findings are associated with right ventricular enlargement:

1. Right axis deviation (most common)
2. Terminal forces rightward, inferiorly and anteriorly directed (most reliable)
3. Tall 0.04 sec R in V_3R or V_1
4. R/S ratio $V_1 = >1$; R/S ratio $V_6 = <1$
5. rsR' or rSR', in V_3R with R' >5 mm or >½ of S
6. RAD of terminal forces with shallow notched sV_1 or rSr • V_1 and prominent SV_{5-6} (early RVH)

Text continued on p. 106.

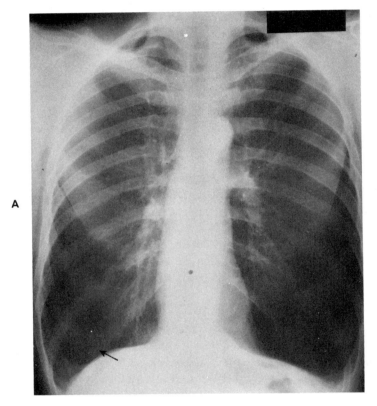

FIG. 10-1. COPD with diffuse emphysema, severe. **A,** Posteroanterior: note right hemi-diaphragm at seventh anterior rib. No pneumothorax is present despite absence of lung markings.

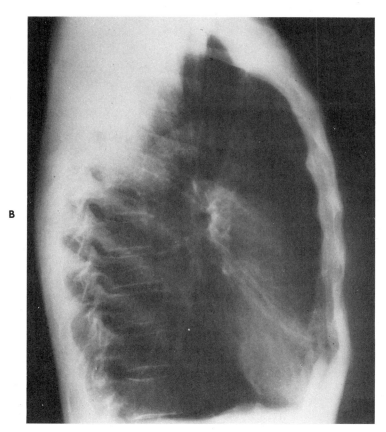

FIG. 10-1, cont'd. B, Lateral. (**A** and **B** *courtesy Medical Illustration Service, Veterans Administration Hospital, Denver, Colorado.*)

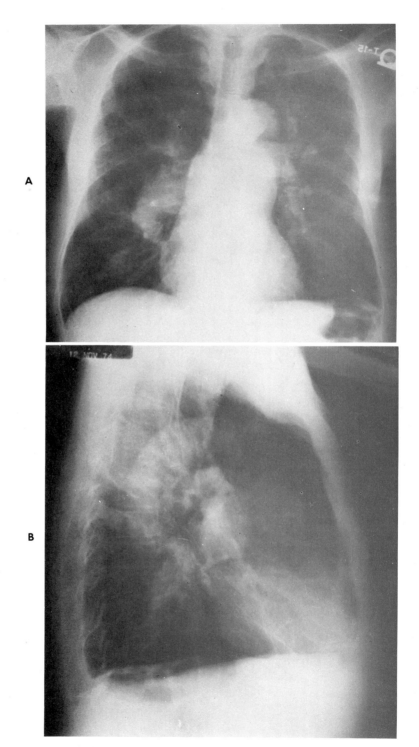

FIG. 10-2. COPD with predominant chronic bronchitis and cor pulmonale. **A,** Postero-anterior. Note huge pulmonary arteries. **B,** Lateral. *(Courtesy Medical Illustration Service, Veterans Administration Hospital, Denver, Colorado.)*

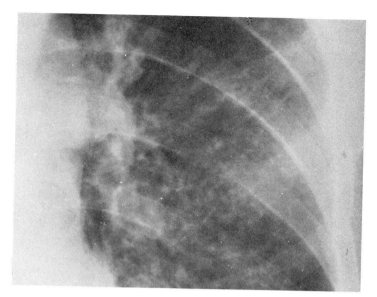

FIG. 10-3. Bronchiolitis manifested by scattered, nonuniform, fine, "soft" nodulation. A complication of severe COPD and asthma. *(Courtesy Medical Illustration Service, Veterans Administration Hospital, Denver, Colorado.)*

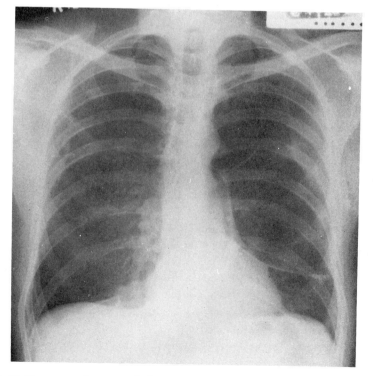

FIG. 10-4. Bullous emphysema, bilateral, left more than right. *(Courtesy Medical Illustration Service, Veterans Administration Hospital, Denver, Colorado.)*

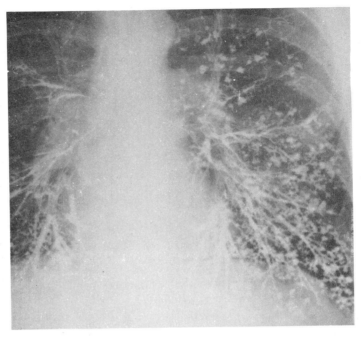

FIG. 10-5. Bronchiolectasis—"leaves on a winter tree"—a bronchographic indication of centrilobular emphysema. *(Courtesy Medical Illustration Service, Veterans Administration Hospital, Denver, Colorado.)*

7. S_1, S_2, S_3 syndrome
8. R in a VR >5 mm
9. With RBBB
   a. RAD of unblocked QRS forces
   b. $R'V_1$ >15 mm

An elevated hematocrit is useful as an indicator of secondary erythremia and chronic hypoxemia.

The course of COPD is commonly punctuated by exacerbations, usually caused by infections or by the inhalation of noxious fumes and by trauma, but sometimes apparently unrelated to any identifiable event. When an exacerbation is complicated by right heart failure, the outlook is likely thereafter to be poor. Progressive weight loss is also a poor prognostic sign. The causes of death in COPD are respiratory failure, congestive heart failure secondary to cor pulmonale, pneumonia, bronchitis, pulmonary thromboembolism, perforation or hemorrhage of a peptic ulcer, and spontaneous pneumothorax, in approximately that order of frequency.

Differential diagnosis

The differential diagnosis of COPD should include other causes of congestive heart failure, other causes of erythremia, and the various specific causes of chronic cough and expectoration such as tuberculosis, bronchiectasis, and fungus diseases.

One unusual cause of chronic cough and, at times, of recurrent patchy pneumonia is reflux of usually acidic stomach contents into an esophagus that has impaired motility, with resultant recurrent aspiration of irritant material, usually at night. Based on personal observations, postpoliomyelitic or encephalitic impairment of pharyngeal constrictors may also cause inadvertent inhalation of nasal mucus or saliva and thus lead to cough.

Principles of management

Patient knowledge. COPD is a lifelong illness. Patients must be completely informed of (1) the nature of their disease, (2) the extreme importance of cessation of smoking, (3) the avoidance of respiratory irritation, and (4) the understanding of principles of care. Properly informed patients can participate in their own care. Self-care has been quite effective in other chronic diseases such as diabetes mellitus and renal disease. It is really the backbone of all COPD therapy. Simple pamphlets and a brief monograph* have been valuable in helping patients learn how to cope with this problem.

Bronchial hygiene. After the avoidance of smoking and irritants, probably one of the most important principles of maintenance management is daily *bronchial hygiene.* Patients with chronic airflow obstruction have impaired clearance of mucus, which further aggravates the obstruction phenomenon in the conducting airways. Those with smooth muscle narrowing (bronchospasm) have an additional problem of increased Raw. The systematic inhalation of bronchodilating aerosols such as isoetharine, isoproterenol, albuterol, or metaproteranol should become a daily habit in patients with COPD.

Nebulization devices. A variety of methods for inhaling bronchodilating aerosols can be used. These include metered-dose devices (probably the simplest method), hand-bulb nebulizers, pump-driven nebulizers, and IPPB devices. The physician should consider the patient's physiologic resources when prescribing bronchodilator therapy. Generally, patients who can take a reasonably deep breath (i.e., those with a vital capacity of greater than 2 L and those with an FEV_1 of greater than 1 L) do not need the assistance of positive pressure for the delivery and deposition of therapeutic aerosols. Also, there is some evidence that IPPB devices are less efficient in aerosol

---

*Petty, T.L., and Nett, L.M.: For those who live and breathe (a manual for patients with emphysema and chronic bronchitis) ed. 2, Springfield, Ill., 1972, Charles C Thomas, Publisher.

delivery than simple nebulizers. For these and other reasons IPPB devices are being used much less frequently, and their efficacy is a matter of current study. Metered-dose devices and pump-driven nebulizers are most convenient. Also, many patients find that simple hand-bulb nebulizers (e.g., De-Vilbiss No. 40 glass or No. 45 plastic) are quite convenient and effective.

Drug dosage. The dosage of bronchodilating aerosol varies greatly among patients. In the metered-dose device, 1 or 2 puffs (350 μg isoetharine/puff) every 4 to 6 hours is usually sufficient. The average dosage of bronchodilator for either the hand-bulb, pump-driven, or IPPB nebulizer is approximately 1 drop isoetharine or isoproterenol/10 kg body weight, often diluted with equal or greater amounts of water. Patients should continue to inhale their bronchodilator to the point of relief but not to the point of toxicity. Symptoms of toxicity include palpitation, nervousness, and lightheadedness. It should be stressed that the dosage of bronchodilator drug must be adjusted to each patient's needs, short of serious side effects.

After the inhalation of bronchodilating aerosols, patients with retained secretions often benefit from the inhalation of moisture. Again, this can be accomplished by simple methods such as the inhalation of steam through simple devices. Moisture helps thin secretions. Following this, expulsive coughing and/or postural drainage over pillows in bed help remove the retained secretions.

Experimental studies suggest that sympathomimetic bronchodilating aerosols also stimulate mucociliary activity to more rapidly propel the mucus. The true clinical significance of this finding in humans is not certain, but most patients are aware of increased mucus production after the use of a bronchodilating aerosol and moisture.

Pharmacologic agents

Antibiotics. Antibiotics are among the most important drugs for patients with COPD. They are mainly useful in combating the bacterial invasion that often follows viral infections in exacerbations of chronic bronchitis. The two most common organisms involved are *S. pneumoniae* and *H. influenzae;* tetracycline, ampicillin, and trimethoprim-sulfa are most useful. Common regimens are (1) 2 gm tetracycline daily for 2 days followed by 1 gm daily for 5 to 7 days, (2) 1 gm trimethoprim-sulfamethoxazole twice daily for 7 to 10 days, and (3) 2 gm ampicillin daily for 7 to 10 days. Generally, antibiotics can be started empirically at the first sign of a deep chest infection, that is, with the appearance of purulent sputum, increasing cough, and fever. In fact, patients are often given a supply of antibiotics to use on their own when infection develops. If response is not immediate, patients on a home-maintenance program should then consult their physician. It is not necessary to culture sputum each time. The most common organisms may or may not be revealed, and it is also possible that so called normal flora such as anaerobic streptococci become involved in the pathogenesis of chronic bronchitis. Antimicrobial drugs should be used singly and liberally to treat infection and prevent the further damage that comes from recurrent inflammatory processes caused by bacteria.

Corticosteroid drugs. Corticosteroid drugs remain somewhat controversial in COPD. They are extremely useful in asthma even though the mechanism of benefit is not clearly understood. Corticosteroids are also effective in what is commonly termed *reversible bronchitis*. The patients most apt to benefit from corticosteroid drugs are those with a background of asthma in childhood, patients with a relatively short duration of disease, and patients with marked ups and downs in their clinical course. Also benefited are patients with a significant bronchodilator response in the laboratory and those whose clinical background includes wheeze, either uncovered by questioning or observed on examination.

In addition, corticosteroid drugs are even effective in patients without these features. We think that any patient not doing well with a complete bronchial hygiene regimen should receive a clinical trial of corticosteroid drugs guided by the patient's symptom complex and the expiratory spirogram. Generally, 30 mg prednisone is given daily for approximately 1 week; the dosage is then reduced. If the patient experiences marked improvement, the steroids should be continued. Very often, extremely modest dosages such as 10 mg daily or slightly higher dosages every other day will maintain the clinical benefit appreciated during the clinical trial. The dreaded problems of peptic ulcer, osteoporosis, and cataract formation are quite uncommon on low dosages, particularly on alternate-day steroid therapy. Inhaled beclomethasone may be useful in steroid-responsive patients as a maintenance drug.

Digitalis and diuretics. Both digitalis and diuretics are useful in the heart failure associated with cor pulmonale. The role of digitalis in cor pulmonale has been controversial in the past, but it is now generally accepted that the cardiac glycosides are mostly useful for arterial tachycardias and associated left heart failure, if present (see below). Short-acting digitalis preparations such as digoxin are preferable. Generally, the thiazide diuretics are preferable when edema formation is not controlled by salt restriction.

Oral bronchodilators. Theophylline or theophylline salts (methylxanthines) are commonly used if tolerated (by the gastrointestinal tract) and if there is a reversible bronchospastic component in COPD. A common dosage is 200 mg 3 or 4 times a day. β-agonists such as terbutaline or metaproterenol may be added to the baseline theophylline for a possible additional effect. Combination tablets, often containing ephedrine and a barbiturate or other sedative drug, are less desirable.

Other methods. Influenza virus vaccine should be given to patients with

COPD each fall for whatever protection it affords. Pneumonia vaccine should be given every 2 or 3 years. Patients with COPD are extremely susceptible to pulmonary infections, and any protection is desirable. During epidemic periods the use of the new antiviral agent amantadine also affords protection against many A strains, including the Hong Kong influenza A-2 strain.

Phlebotomy is useful only in symptomatic patients with advanced COPD and very high hematocrits (over 60). The expanded red cell mass is an adaptive response to hypoxemia and generally does not cause serious symptoms such as headache or mental clouding unless very high hematocrit levels are reached.

Breathing retraining. Breathing retraining is another extremely important therapy modality. Patients with advanced COPD often breathe in a rapid inefficient fashion. They tend to hyperinflate the chest with their accessory muscles and try to force air in with their abdominal muscles. This is an extremely awkward way to breathe. The patients need to relax the abdomen and lower chest, encouraging the abdomen to protrude on inspiration, thus allowing maximum descent of the diaphragm. Exhalation against pursed lips, as in whistling, also promotes more complete emptying of the lungs and improved gas transport across the alveolar membrane. Many patients gain immense relief while employing this breathing pattern during exercise; some patients learn to follow this pattern while at rest and even while asleep.

Physical reconditioning. General muscular reconditioning is another extremely important form of therapy. Patients with severe COPD become progressively unfit, do less and less, and therefore find themselves in a downhill spiral of dyspnea, muscular impairment, progressive disability, and weight loss. Following breathing retraining, graded walks, sometimes with the use of supplemental oxygen, are useful. The vicious cycle of inactivity and disability thus may be interrupted. Recent studies suggest that muscular conditioning improves cardiovascular responses and coordination in these patients.

Supportive measures

Home oxygen. Patients with marked hypoxemia, often associated with cor pulmonale, benefit by the long-term use of oxygen. The knowledge that oxygen can reverse pulmonary hypertension is fundamental to the management of cor pulmonale; oxygen may also improve myocardial function in patients with severe hypoxemia. The most important effect of oxygen, however, is improved brain function, improved exercise tolerance, and overall improved quality of life in patients with advanced COPD and sustained severe hypoxemia.

By no means do all patients with advanced COPD require oxygen, however. A Pao_2 under 55 mm Hg is generally taken as a sign that oxygen may be necessary. In most patients, however, this degree of hypoxemia accompanies an exacerbation of chronic bronchitis, pneumonia, incipient heart failure, episodic bronchospasm, or even an occult pulmonary embolus. It is important to identify the cause of hypoxemia and to treat it appropriately and specifically, if possible, before embarking on long-term home oxygen with its attendant cost and inconveniences. If sustained hypoxemia is present despite therapy directed at underlying causes, all evidence points to improved survival with oxygen. A recent multicenter study has demonstrated that continuous (i.e., nearly 24 hr/day) oxygen was more effective than 12 hr/day, including the hours of sleep (see Chapter 9).

Home oxygen tanks used with a long (50-foot) tubing allow mobility. In addition, patients with profound hypoxemia requiring oxygen-supported exercise can have portable devices that will allow oxygen to be used outside the home. Various portable oxygen systems are now available, including simple transfilling oxygen bottles that provide about a 2-hour oxygen supply. Liquid portable oxygen devices remain very popular and provide up to 9 hours of oxygen at a 2 L flow (weight is approximately 4 kg). Lighter weight devices that provide up to 5 hours supply are now available. The flow rates can be controlled on both the compressed gas and liquid systems. The latest oxygen delivery system is a home oxygen concentrator that concentrates oxygen from the air. It is currently being evaluated as an efficient and less expensive method of home oxygen therapy.

Clinical approaches

The above modalities must be applied individually to each patient depending upon the patient's problems and physiologic resources in order to develop a realistic medical care program. The details of care listed above will be applied by different means to each patient, depending in part on the severity of the disease.

The incipient or early case. Very likely, patients with cough, expectoration, and relatively mild expiratory airflow obstruction can be effectively managed simply by the cessation of smoking, the careful use of antibiotics during each specific chest infection, and possibly the use of a bronchodilating aerosol by a metered-dose device or a hand-bulb nebulizer each morning. These patients are also urged to be active and encouraged to enjoy life. They must report any complications to their physician such as chest infections that do not respond to antibiotic therapy. Patients with an FEV_1 over 2 L who follow these simple measures may have a nearly normal prognosis.

Patients with unexpected reversibility. This is an extremely important group of patients because objective pulmonary function improvement may follow effective, systematic therapy including corticosteroids. Detailed bronchial hygiene and corticosteroid drugs will identify these patients, who, with reversibility, may also have a nearly normal prognosis.

Moderately advanced cases. These patients require more aggressive daily therapy, particularly with vigorous bronchial hygiene and physical reconditioning. It is likely that the prognosis of patients with an FEV_1 of 1 to 1½ L can be improved, although it must be admitted that patients with this degree of disease tend to progress slowly and that a normal life expectancy is unlikely. Nonetheless, systematic care greatly improves the quality of life for these patients.

Severely afflicted, home-bound patients. Even these individuals' lives can be improved by application of the measures listed above. Often these patients require home oxygen as a measure of support and to improve the quality of life. Nonetheless, physicians should approach their management with a great degree of enthusiasm because recent studies have indicated that at least in some cases, particularly in patients with cor pulmonale, prognosis may be improved.

THE FUTURE

Systematic and comprehensive care allows patients to live with the least possible interference with normal activities. Once patients understand the disease process, they are no longer anxious about the unknown. If the disease is caught early or is partly reversible, the prognosis is generally favorable. Even with greater degrees of impairment, patients can live outside the hospital and often be able to work.

Certainly, the solution to the COPD problem is early identification and management. This important strategy is based on office spirometry, using new, practical, and accurate devices. An enlightened public must learn how to protect the lungs from smoking and air pollution. Identification of genetic background factors will help determine patients at highest risk, and genetic counseling will be important in the future. New antiviral drugs will also very likely become available and help prevent infections that can damage the lungs. Earlier methods of identification will also become available to help physicians find the very earliest signs of COPD and thus institute preventive and therapeutic measures.

SUGGESTED READINGS

Burrows, B., editor: Symposium on chronic respiratory disease, Med. Clin. N. Am. **57**:545, 1973.
Burrows, B., and Earle, R.H.: Course and prognosis of chronic obstructive lung disease; a prospective study of 200 patients, N. Engl. J. Med. **280**:397, 1969.
Camner, P., Philipson, K., Friberg, L., et al.: Human tracheobronchial clearance studies: with fluorocarbon resin particles tagged with ¹⁸F, Arch. Environ. Health **22**:444, 1971.

Falk, G.A., and Smith, J.P.: Chronic bronchitis: a seldom noted manifestation of homozygous alpha₁-antitrypsin deficiency, Chest **60:**166, 1971.

Gelb, A.F., Bruch, H., Wright, R.R., et al.: Physiologic diagnosis of clinically unsuspected pulmonary emphysema, Am. Rev. Respir. Dis. **103:**891, 1971.

Hodgkin, J.E., Balchum, O.J., Koss, L., et al.: Chronic obstructive airway diseases: current concepts in diagnosis and comprehensive care, J.A.M.A. **232:**1243, 1975.

Hogg, J.C., Macklem, P.T., and Thurlbeck, W.M.: Site and nature of airway obstruction in chronic obstructive lung disease, N. Engl. J. Med. **278:**1355, 1968.

Macklem, P.T., Thurlbeck, W.M., and Fraser, R.G.: Chronic obstructive disease of small airways, Ann. Intern. Med. **74:**167, 1971.

Mitchell, R.S., Silvers, G.W., Dart, G.A., et al.: Clinical and morphological correlations in chronic airways obstruction, Am. Rev. Respir. Dis. **97:**54, 1968.

Mitchell, R.S., et al.: The morphology of the bronchi, bronchioles, and alveoli in chronic airways obstruction: a clinicopathologic study, Am. Rev. Respir. Dis. **114:**137, 1976.

Mitchell, R.S., et al.: The right ventricle in chronic airways obstruction: a clinicopathologic study, Am. Rev. Respir. Dis. **114:**147, 1976.

Mittman, C., Lieberman, J., Morasso, F., et al.: Smoking and chronic obstructive lung disease in alpha₁-antitrypsin deficiency, Chest **60:**214, 1971.

Petty, T.L., Stanford, E.R., and Neff, TA.: Continuous oxygen therapy in chronic airway obstruction: observations on possible oxygen toxicity and survival, Ann. Intern. Med. **75:**361, 1971.

Petty, T.L., Stanford, E.R., and Neff, T.A.: Continuous oxygen therapy in chronic airway obstruc-bronchitis and chronic airway obstruction, Am. Rev. Respir. Dis. **114:**881, 1976.

Petty, T.L.: Pulmonary rehabilitation, Continuing Education **9:**28, 1978.

Petty, T.L., editor: Chronic obstructive pulmonary disease, New York City, 1978, Marcel Dekker, Inc.

Reid, L., and Millard, F.J.C.: Correlation between radiological diagnosis and structural lung changes in emphysema, Clin. Radiol. **15:**307, 1964.

Thurlbeck, W.M.: Chronic obstructive lung disease: correlation of structure and function. In Lane, D.J., editor: Tutorials in postgraduate medicine: diseases of the respiratory system, London, 1973, William Heineman Medical Books Ltd.

Thurlbeck, W.M.: Chronic bronchitis and emphysema—the pathophysiology of chronic obstructive lung disease, Basics Respir. Dis. Am. Thorac. Soc. **3:**1, 1974.

Chapter 11

PULMONARY THROMBOEMBOLISM AND PULMONARY HYPERTENSION

Thomas A. Neff

PULMONARY THROMBOEMBOLISM

Pulmonary thromboembolism (PTE) presents a very real diagnostic and therapeutic challenge. Autopsies of hospitalized patients and adult outpatients reveal that PTE is one of the most frequent immediate causes of death. It is a further unhappy fact that the majority of cases of pulmonary thromboembolism are not diagnosed before death.

Etiology and pathophysiology

Careful autopsy studies have revealed that the majority of pulmonary emboli come from the leg and pelvic veins and from the inferior vena cava. Approximately half the patients with pulmonary thromboembolism, however, have no clinically manifest venous disease.

Clots form in the peripheral venous system and pass downstream into and through the right heart chambers and then become wedged or impacted in the first pulmonary arteries that are small enough to arrest them. Three basic factors are related to the development of thromboembolism: (1) venous stasis, (2) endophlebitis, and (3) hypercoagulability.

Venous stasis and phlebitis often coexist in hospitalized patients. Classic settings are postoperative states, especially those involving the lower extremities and pelvis and postoperative immobilization as with casts. Patients immobilized with congestive heart failure, myocardial infarction, coma, or for any cause have an increased incidence of these complications. Patients with overt lower extremity thrombophlebitis are at special risk in the early stages of its development. Patients with an increased number of platelets, as in polycythemia vera, or an "activated coagulation cascades system" accompanying visceral neoplasms, as in mucin-secreting adenocarcinoma

114

of the pancreas, are also at increased risk. Finally, certain drugs—notably birth control medications—may induce a hypercoagulable state.

Clinical picture

Depending on the size of the clot or clots, the clinical picture may range from no signs or symptoms at all to sudden collapse and almost immediate death as a result of a "saddle embolus" at the bifurcation of the main pulmonary artery blocking the entire outflow of the right ventricle.

In patients without underlying cardiopulmonary disease approximately 25% to 30% or more of the pulmonary arterial bed (total) must be occluded to produce an altered hemodynamic response (i.e., increased pulmonary artery pressure). Since the lung parenchyma receives oxygen delivered by the bronchial (systemic) arteries as well as the pulmonary arteries, plus possibly some directly from the airways, the frequency of true infarction (tissue necrosis, which heals by scarring) is rare in the patient without accompanying congestive heart failure or other underlying cardiopulmonary disease. A so-called reversible pulmonary infarction has been described, wherein the lung distal to the occlusion becomes consolidated without frank necrosis and heals by resolution without scarring.

Diagnosis

PTE can be one of the most pernicious, difficult, and deadly diseases known. Syphilis and tuberculosis were the great mimics of other diseases of past years; PTE is the major mimic of other diseases today. It is always essential to think of PTE in any acute, obscure, and, especially, serious lung disease. Even after careful consideration PTE is often impossible to prove or rule out with certainty.

Table 11-1 lists the major symptoms and signs of PTE in comparison with those of pneumonia, with which it is so often confused. Early in the course of PTE, dyspnea, tachypnea, tachycardia, and restlessness seem to be out of proportion to the meager physical or radiographic findings of the chest; on the other hand, in typical bacterial pneumonia, the chest radiographic findings are generally more consistent with the symptomatology. Evidence of toxicity such as high fever and leukocytosis of $15,000/mm^3$ or more is frequent in pneumonia. A frank shaking chill seldom if ever occurs with an uninfected pulmonary embolism or infarction. Careful examination of the heart (including the electrocardiogram) and the extremities is more helpful in distinguishing PTE from pneumonia than is examination of the lungs. The ability to diagnose deep venous thrombosis on clinical grounds alone is unreliable; however, three new, relatively noninvasive tests—the Doppler ultrasonic examination, impedance plethysmography, and fibrinogen uptake

TABLE 11-1. PTE contrasted with bacterial pneumonia

	PTE	Pneumonia
Symptoms		
Pain: Onset	Usually sudden	Sudden or gradual
Character	Often pleuritic	Usually pleuritic
Location	Usually lateralized	Usually lateralized
Severity	Variable	Variable
Cough	Uncommon until infarction	Usually present early
Dyspnea*	Mild to severe	Mild to severe
Sputum	More bloody	More purulent or rusty
Fever	None to moderate	Usually high
Chills	Rare	Common†
Collateral history	Immobilization; previous phlebitis; post-operative, especially leg, hip, and pelvis; birth control medication; erythremia; malignancy; congestive heart failure; prior PTE	Chronic alcoholism, COPD, bronchiectasis, diabetes, immunodeficient states
Signs		
Respiratory rate*	Rapid	Rapid
Pulse*	Rapid	Rapid
Chest examination	Often normal, especially early	Usually consolidated
Friction rub	±	±
Pleural effusion	±	± (may be empyema)
Heart examination	Normal to frank failure†	Usually normal
Extremities	Calf tenderness, + cuff test in 50%‡	Normal

*These symptoms and signs are more severe than would be suggested by chest film findings in PTE and more equal to the severity of pneumonia on chest film.
†Very helpful, if present, in identifying pneumonia.
‡Very helpful, if present, in identifying PTE.

labeled with I125—are available and increasingly useful. In selected cases, deep venous phlebography of the lower extremities, although invasive, is most reliable.

As soon as the diagnosis of PTE is suspected, pulmonary perfusion and sometimes ventilation scanning should be carried out. Since "cold" areas can be simulated by pneumonia, emphysematous bullae, pleural effusions, asthma, congestive heart failure, and various infiltrative diseases, a pulmonary angiogram (the most definitive test) may be necessary and should be carried out promptly, especially in patients who are quite ill.

The white blood count may be low, normal, or only sightly increased in virus pneumonia and in some overwhelming bacterial pneumonias, especially with bacteremia.

In PTE, lactic acid dehydrogenase levels (LDH) and serum bilirubin levels may be elevated with normal SGOT levels; however, this combination occurs too often in other situations to be as diagnostic as previously believed.

The Pa_{CO_2} is low or low normal. The Pa_{O_2} is often below normal, but the same is just as true of pneumonia and numerous other acute pulmonary diseases.

The sputum in PTE is generally scant, nonpurulent, and blood stained, especially with accompanying pulmonary infarction. In pneumonia, on the other hand, the sputum is purulent, sometimes "rusty," and usually shows numerous organisms on smear and pathogens on culture. In short, careful gross and microscopic examination of sputum is essential when PTE is suspected.

If pleural fluid is present, it should be obtained before giving the patient anticoagulant therapy to avoid the risk of bleeding induced by thoracentesis. With PTE the presence of fluid is generally an indication of accompanying infarction; the fluid is generally an exudate with 1000 to 10,000 leukocytes and contains blood varying from grossly imperceptible to frankly sanguinous. The pleural fluid in PTE is often indistinguishable from that in pneumonia unless the latter is an empyema. A pleural transudate, even if serosanguinous, strongly suggests the diagnosis of congestive heart failure without PTE. A pleural fluid containing malignant cells is usually helpful in ruling out PTE, except in the rare coexistence of PTE and pleural cancer.

The electrocardiogram is often normal or nonspecific (e.g., sinus tachycardia) in mild to moderate PTE; in massive PTE, generally with substernal pain and shock, the electrocardiogram is likely to show the classic pattern of acute cor pulmonale; S_I, Q_{III}, T_{III}, and inverted T-waves over the right precordium. A subtle clue is sudden or transient right axis shift, which requires early and frequent electrocardiograms to detect.

Most commonly, the chest radiographic findings in PTE are normal. The classic "Hampton's hump"—an infiltrate with the configuration of a truncated cone with its base at the visceral pleura and a convex apex or hump pointing toward the hilum—is rare. The principal evidence of embolism on the chest radiograph is often the lack of abnormalities in a patient who is ill. Oligemia (the Westermark sign), or a localized lack of normal pulmonary vascular shadows, is an indication of PTE without infarction. A normal preembolic control film for comparison may be most helpful. The central pulmonary artery may be enlarged—the so-called knuckle sign. The lung volume may be reduced, especially with an elevated hemidiaphragm. This is particularly common with the atelectasis that accompanies infarction. Enlarged heart with a right-sided configuration, distended superior vena cava and azygous vein, and distended, rapidly tapering pulmonary arteries are often seen late, especially with severe and chronic involvement. Infarction produces infiltrates on the chest film with segmental and patchy rather than lobar distribution; they are much more frequent in the lower lung (90%) than in the upper lung (10%). The infiltrate is generally alveolar in character and tends to be in contact with a visceral pleural surface and accompanied by some volume loss. Platelike or discoid atelectasis is commonly seen at the bases (Figs. 11-1 to 11-3).

The perfusion scan is obtained by the injection of radioactive particles (generally human serum albumin labeled with a gamma emitter, usually technetium 99m) into a peripheral vein; these particles embolize to the lung and lodge in the pulmonary arterioles and capillaries in proportion to the active blood flow. Any anatomic or physiologic abnormality of this perfusion will give a "positive" or "cold" area, that is, lack of radioactivity pattern. The ventilation scan utilizes the inhalation of a bolus of a radioactive gas, usually xenon 133. The classic abnormal vascularity pattern is one of normal ventilation and decreased perfusion. The perfusion scan can be almost diagnostic alone if done early while the chest radiograph is still normal or without infiltrates.

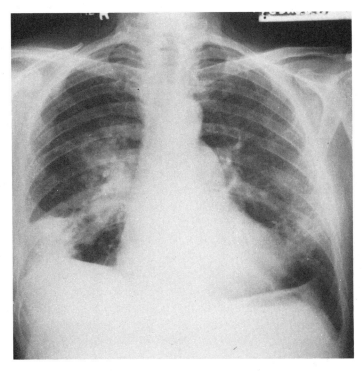

FIG. 11-1. Pulmonary thromboembolism, bilateral. **R;** Recent; **L;** old. *(Courtesy Medical Illustration Service, Veterans Administration Hospital, Denver, Colorado.)*

Pulmonary angiography is the most accurate diagnostic test for PTE. It not only provides a picture of the pulmonary arterial anatomy but this test can also be extended to examine the pulmonary veins, left atrium and ventricle, and thoracic aorta. In addition, since the procedure usually includes right heart catheterization, the pulmonary artery pressure can also be obtained. Diagnostic angiographic findings of PTE are intra-arterial filling defects and sharp cutoffs of vessels.

Treatment

Treatment is approached under the following four headings: (1) prophylaxis in high-risk patients before evidence of PTE, (2) treatment after PTE is diagnosed to prevent more PTE, (3) thrombolytic therapy, and (4) thromboembolectomy.

High-risk patients should be identified and their predisposing conditions

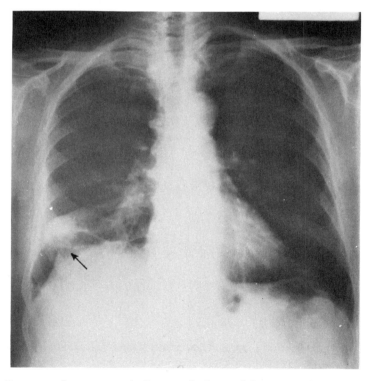

FIG. 11-2. Recent pulmonary embolism, right lower lobe. Note characteristic tenting of adjacent hemidiaphragm. *(Courtesy Medical Illustration Service, Veterans Administration Hospital, Denver, Colorado.)*

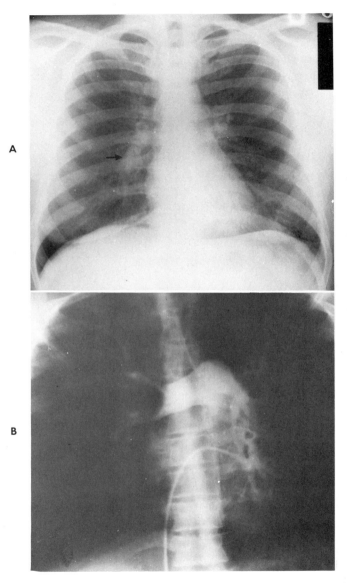

FIG. 11-3. Pulmonary embolism, "Westermark's sign." **A,** Decreased perfusion of right lung plus subtle "stuffing" of right pulmonary artery. **B,** Confirmation by angiogram. *(Courtesy Medical Illustration Service, Veterans Administration Hospital, Denver, Colorado.)*

treated vigorously to minimize the severity and duration of the disease. A low dosage of heparin (5000 u/8 hr) appears to have little risk and may be highly preventive. Use of well fitted elastic stockings with active and passive early postoperative leg movements is safe and probably helpful.

Treatment after PTE is diagnosed should include general cardiopulmonary support—oxygen, cardiotonic drugs, and intensive care monitoring. Aqueous heparin should be immediately initiated with a bolus of 5000 U intravenously and continued at the rate of 1000 to 1500 U/hr by continuous infusion. The exact amount of heparin given should be adjusted to elevate and maintain the activated partial thromboplastin time at 1½ to 2 times normal baseline levels. This should be continued for about 10 days, with conversion to adequate oral anticoagulation (e.g., warfarin) until the period of risk has passed (e.g., after a cast has been removed and full ambulation established) or empirically, from 6 weeks to even 6 months. If the patient cannot tolerate this anticoagulation regimen (i.e., develops serious bleeding), inferior vena cava interruption procedures and antiplatelet cohesive drugs (e.g., sulfinpyrazone [Anturane]) should be considered; many authorities believe that these procedures are seldom indicated, and hence they are still controversial.

Direct attack on the PTE by thrombolytic therapy is still experimental. Surgical thrombolectomy is considered only when the PTE has been massive, as manifested by syncope, shock, and severe hypoxemia, since the surgical mortality approximates 50%.

PULMONARY HYPERTENSION

The pulmonary arterial vascular system has a normal pressure range of up to 25 mm Hg during systole and 15 mm Hg during diastole. With exercise and the accompanying increase in cardiac output, the normal level may rise as high as 40/25 mm Hg. Sustained elevated levels of pressure can develop in the pulmonary system and are classified as *primary* (cause unknown) and *secondary* pulmonary hypertension. Currently, pulmonary artery pressure cannot be measured noninvasively; the medical profession still depends on right heart catheterization for accurate measurement.

Primary pulmonary hypertension

The cause of primary pulmonary hypertension is entirely unknown, and its incidence is low, especially when compared with systemic essential hypertension. Young adult females are characteristically the most frequently afflicted, although it may occur at all ages; a few familial cases have been reported. Patients with mild to moderate degrees of primary pulmonary hypertension are usually asymptomatic. When symptoms first appear, they indicate already severe disease and consist of exertional dyspnea, easy fatigability, syncope, and occasionally an anginal syndrome indistinguishable on history from the anginal pain of coronary artery disease. The examination at this time usually reveals a quiet precordium (low cardiac output) and the findings of right ventricular enlargement, namely, a sustained cardiac thrust or lift along the lower left sternal border. The second heart sound is often finely split and may have an accentuated pulmonic component. The electrocardiogram displays varying manifestations of right ventricular enlargement (see Chapter 10), while the chest film reveals prominent, enlarged central pulmonary arteries that taper (disappear) rapidly toward the periphery. The cardiac silhouette is only slightly to moderately enlarged until frank heart failure ensues.

No specific treatment for primary pulmonary hypertension is known, but long-term anticoagulation and isoproterenol have been tried. Recent reports on the efficacy of oral hydralazine and diazoxide for primary pulmonary hypertension have been encouraging. The prognosis, after the development of symptoms, is one of progressive disability and death, usually within 1 to 5 years.

Secondary pulmonary hypertension

The accompanying outline lists and classifies the major causes of secondary pulmonary hypertension. Since the cross-sectional area of the pulmonary vascular bed is large, with a reverse factor of several fold, the classic pulmonary diseases—Group A—are usually moderately severe to severe and therefore obvious before they cause pulmonary hypertension. Pulmonary function tests are usually diagnostic in questionable or atypical cases. Expiratory flow rates detected with simple spirometry are well below 50% of the predicted rates in COPD. Occasionally, early diffuse interstitial lung disease reveals little or no change on the chest film. In these cases, total lung capacity, vital capacity, and diffusing capacity are markedly decreased in comparison with normal or near normal values in primary pulmonary hypertension. Alveolar hypoventilation is easily recognized by an elevated $Paco_2$ and should not cause confusion because the $Paco_2$ is low in primary pulmonary hypertension.

Pulmonary vascular diseases of known cause—Groups B and C—may at times be very difficult to diagnose without the aid of a pulmonary perfusion scan and/or angiogram. When an angiogram is being done, a complete right heart catheterization should also be performed. Elevated capillary wedge pressures will indicate pulmonary venous disease, Group C, or left heart disease, Group D. The venous phase of a pulmonary angiogram or a left heart catheterization may be needed to evaluate and localize the cause of an ele-

CLASSIFICATION OF SECONDARY PULMONARY HYPERTENSION

A. *Classic pulmonary disease*
1. COPD—chronic bronchitis, emphysema, and chronic, severe bronchial asthma
2. Restrictive lung diseases
   a. Interstitial diseases (e.g., U.I.P., D.I.P., silicosis)
   b. Chest wall deformities (e.g., kyphoscoliosis, thoracoplasty, fibrothorax)
3. Alveolar hypoventilation
   a. Primary—idiopathic
   b. Obesity—pickwickian
   c. Neuromuscular—following poliomyelitis
   d. Cryptic upper airways obstruction in children

B. *Pulmonary arterial disease*
1. Pulmonary thromboembolism
2. Intravenous drug abuse (e.g., amphetamines, "blue velvet")
3. Collagenoses (e.g., scleroderma, periarteritis)
4. Nonthrombotic occlusion (e.g., tumor, schistosomiasis)

C. *Pulmonary venous disease*
1. Idiopathic veno-occlusive disease
2. Anomolous pulmonary venous return
3. Fibrosing mediastinitis

D. *Heart diseases*
1. Chronic left ventricular dysfunction (e.g., cardiomyopathy, constrictive pericarditis)
2. Mitral valve disease, especially stenosis
3. Left to right shunts (e.g., ASD, VSD, PDA)
4. Left atrial myxoma
5. Cor triatriatum

vated capillary wedge pressure. If mitral stenosis is a possibility, a cardiac ultrasound (echocardiogram) examination should be performed early, as a safe noninvasive test. Finally, left to right cardiac shunts, such as atrial and ventricular septal defects and patent ductus arteriosus are usually recognizable by finding hypervolemic lung fields on the chest film. Left to right cardiac shunts are a category of heart disease that causes pulmonary hypertension in which the capillary wedge pressure may be normal. However, an increase in the oxygen saturation (oxygen step-up) on the right side of the heart during a right heart catheterization is easy to detect and diagnostic of left to right cardiac shunts.

Treatment

Therapy for secondary pulmonary hypertension should first be directed toward the causative disease. In COPD every effort should be made to control bronchospasm and inflammation. Cessation of smoking is mandatory. Some reactive forms of airways obstruction, especially chronic bronchial asthma, and still active stages of interstitial lung disease such as sarcoidosis and desquamative interstitial pneumonia may respond to corticosteroid therapy. Recurrent PTE requires long-term anticoagulation. Some forms of primary hypoventilation may benefit from respiratory center stimulation with the hormone progesterone. Most of the cardiac diseases listed in the chart (i.e., Group D, 2 to 5) can be corrected with open heart surgery if they are diagnosed before the myocardium or pulmonary arteries have undergone irreversible changes (i.e., Eisenmenger's reaction). Finally, even if a definitive cure is not available, long-term nasal oxygen therapy may be beneficial in correcting hypoxemia and erythremia. This is particularly well documented in the "blue bloater" or type "B" COPD.

SUGGESTED READINGS
Pulmonary thromboembolism

Barnes, R.W., Wu, K.K., and Hoak, J.C.: Fallibility of the clinical diagnosis of venous thrombosis, J.A.M.A. **234**:605, 1975.

Breckenridge, R.T., and Ratnoff, O.D.: Pulmonary embolism and unexpected death in supposedly normal persons, N. Engl. J. Med. **270**:298, 1964.

Bynum, L.J., Wilson, J.E., III, Crotty, C.M., et al.: Noninvasive diagnosis of deep venous thrombosis by phleborheography, Ann. Intern. Med. **89**:162, 1978.

Cooperative study: urokinase pulmonary embolism trial. A national cooperative study, Circulation **47**:(Suppl. II), 1973.

Dalen, J.E., Banas, J.S., Jr., Brooks, H.L., et al.: Resolution rate of acute pulmonary embolism in man, N. Engl. J. Med. **280**:1194, 1969.

Fleischner, F.G.: Roentgenology of the pulmonary infarct, Semin. Roentgenol. **2**:61, 1967.

Gallus, A.S., Hirsh, J., Tuttle, R.J., et al.: Small subcutaneous doses of heparin in prevention of venous thrombosis, N. Engl. J. Med. **288**:545, 1973.

Gardner, A.M.N.: Inferior vena caval interruption in the prevention of fatal pulmonary embolism, Am. Heart J. **95**:679, 1978.

Hirsh, J.: Venous thromboembolism: diagnosis, treatment, prevention, Hosp. Pract. **10**:53, August, 1975.

McNeil, B.J.: A diagnostic strategy using ventilation-perfusion studies in patients suspect for pulmonary embolism, J. Nucl. Med. **17**:613, 1976.

Mobin-Uddin, K., McLean, R., and Jude, J.R.: A new catheter technique of interruption of inferior vena cava for prevention of pulmonary embolism, Am. Surg. **35**:889, 1969.

Moser, K.M., and Miale, A., Jr.: Interpretive pitfalls in lung photoscanning, Am. J. Med. **44**:366, 1968.

Novelline, R.A., Baltarowich, O.H., Athanasoulis, C.A., et al.: The clinical course of patients with suspected pulmonary embolism and a negative pulmonary arteriogram, Radiology **126**:561, 1978.

Robin, E.D.: Overdiagnosis and overtreatment of pulmonary embolism: the emperor may have no clothes, Ann. Intern. Med. **87**:775, 1977.

Szucs, M.M., Jr., Brooks, H.L., Grossman, W., et al.: Diagnostic sensitivity of laboratory findings in acute pulmonary embolism, Ann. Intern. Med. **74**:161, 1971.

Winebright, J.W., Gerdes, A.J., and Nelp, W.B.: Restoration of blood flow after pulmonary embolism, Arch. Intern. Med. **125**:241, 1970.

Wenger, N.K., Stein, P.D., and Willis, P.W., III: Massive acute pulmonary embolism: the deceivingly nonspecific manifestation, J.A.M.A. **220**:843, 1972.

Pulmonary hypertension

Blount, S.G., Jr.: Primary pulmonary hypertension, Mod. Concepts Cardiovasc. Dis. **36**:67, 1967.

Fraser, R.G., and Pare, J.A.P.: Diagnosis of diseases of the chest, Philadelphia, 1970, W.B. Saunders Co., pp. 832-852.

Neff, T.A., and Petty, T.L.: Long-term continuous oxygen therapy in chronic airway obstruction: mortality in relationship to cor pulmonale, hypoxia, and hypercapnia, Ann. Intern. Med. **72**:621, 1970.

Reeves, J.T.: Hope in primary pulmonary hypertension? N. Engl. J. Med. **302**:112, 1980.

Robertson, C.H., Jr., Reynolds, R.C., and Wilson, J.E., III: Pulmonary hypertension and foreign body granulomas in intravenous drug abusers: documentation by cardiac catheterization and lung biopsy, Am. J. Med. **61**:657, 1976.

Shettigar, U.R., Hultgren, H.N., Specter, M., et al.: Primary pulmonary hypertension: favorable effect of isoproterenol, N. Engl. J. Med. **295**:1414, 1976.

Sutton, F.D., Weil, J.V., Pierson, D.J., et al.: Long-term treatment of the pickwickian syndrome with sublingual progesterone, Clin. Res. **22**:512A, 1974.

Williams, M.H., Jr., Adler, J.J., and Colp, C.: Pulmonary function studies as an aid in the differential diagnosis of pulmonary hypertension, Am. J. Med. **47**:378, 1969.

Chapter 12

HYPERSENSITIVITY PNEUMONITIS (EXTRINSIC ALLERGIC ALVEOLITIS)

Robert B. Dreisin

Since the inhalation of organic dusts was first implicated in the production of pulmonary diseases in 1713, a wide variety of offending agents and their environmental sources have been identified. These are listed in Table 12-1. In the majority of clinically recognized instances the antigenic material is a fungal spore, although heterologous serum proteins and bacterial enzymes have also been implicated. The source of exposure is usually related to a specific occupation or hobby; however, in some instances the environmental source may be as apparently innocuous as a contaminated heating system or air conditioner. In addition, cases have been reported in which a patient has been exposed to antigenic material transported into the home on the clothes of an occupationally exposed spouse.

Whether or not any particular foreign material may act as an antigenic substance and elicit a pathologic host response depends on a multitude of factors including particle size, concentration of the dust, periodicity of exposure, and underlying immunologic reactivity of the patient. Most of the particles responsible for the production of hypersensitivity pneumonitis are extremely small, facilitating deposition within alveoli and terminal airways.

To understand fully the clinical and pathophysiologic features of these diseases, an understanding of hypersensitivity reactions in general is necessary.

Type I

Type I hypersensitivity reactions are those underlying allergic eczema, allergic rhinitis (hay fever), and asthma in the 10% of the population who are atopic. Type I hypersensitivity has also been termed *immediate hypersensitivity* because the reactions produced are seen within minutes following exposure to the offending antigen.

The antibody mediating immediate hypersensitivity reactions has been

126

TABLE 12-1. Classification of hypersensitivity reactions*

	Reaction	Pulmonary pathology	Skin test	Examples
Type I	Antigen + IgE bound to mast cell	Release of mediators of anaphylaxis with bronchoconstriction	Immediate wheal and flare	Bronchial asthma, allergic rhinitis, eczema
Type II	Cytotoxic antibody attacks cellular or tissue component and activates complement	Cellular and tissue inflammation	None	Goodpasture's syndrome, transfusion reactions
Type III	Antigenic-antibody complexes deposit locally	"Innocent bystander" interstitial inflammation with granuloma formation	Arthus (erythema, induration) at 4-6 hr.	Hypersensitivity pneumonitis (extrinsic allergic alveolitis), serum sickness
Type IV	Sensitized T-lymphocytes and macrophages attack antigen	Granuloma formation with or without caseation necrosis	Delayed (24-48 hr)	Tuberculosis, ? sarcoidosis, ? Wegener's granulomatosis

*Classification of Gell and Coombs.

identified as immunoglobulin E (IgE). Although it is true that the majority of atopic patients, those suffering from immediate hypersensitivity diseases, have elevated levels of IgE in their blood, these diseases are in fact mediated not by circulating IgE but rather by immunoglobulin bound to the surface of the mast cell. When an antigen combines with bound IgE, the level of cAMP within the mast cell is lowered. The mast cell subsequently loses its granules, releasing the mediators of immediate hypersensitivity: histamine, SRS-A, and a substance that attracts eosinophils known as eosinophil chemotactic factor (ECF-A). These and other mediators are probably responsible for most of the symptoms seen in atopic patients. If antigen is introduced into the skin of such a patient, an immediate wheal and flare reaction is seen. If the antigen-antibody interaction occurs at the nasal mucosa, allergic rhinitis is the clinical outcome. If the reaction occurs within the tracheobronchial tree of a sensitized patient, bronchoconstriction and wheezing result. This reaction is blocked by the prior inhalation of disodium cromoglycate, which specifically inhibits the degranulation of mast cells. The symptoms are alleviated by the administration of drugs such as isoproterenol and theophylline compounds, which increase intracellular cAMP concentration. The reaction is not blocked by prior or concurrent administration of corticosteroids. Type I reactions may be important in the initiation phase of *acute* allergic alveolitis (see below).

Type II

Type II hypersensitivity reactions are those mediated by circulating antibodies directed against endogenous cellular or tissue antigens. Type II cytotoxic antibodies directed against the pulmonary and glomerular basement membranes have been implicated in the development of Goodpasture's syndrome (see Chapter 30). Because the initiating antigen is endogenous, skin testing is not feasible. Type II reactions have not been implicated in extrinsic allergic alveolitis.

Type III

In the Type III (Arthus) reaction, both antigen and antibody are free. As the two react, complement is fixed and the resulting antigen-antibody complement complex may initiate an inflammatory reaction at the site of deposition. If the offending antigen is known, the antibodies responsible may be measured in an affected patient's serum by classic gel precipitation techniques. They are therefore known as precipitating antibodies, or precipitins. If a patient has circulating precipitins, a skin test with the corresponding antigen will elicit a local reaction consisting of erythema and induration. This reaction begins approximately 4 hours after challenge, reaches a peak at 6 hours, and fades by 24 hours. The reaction is termed an *intermediate hypersensitivity response,* although it has sometimes been erroneously termed a delayed response. This reaction, in contrast to the Type I response, may be blocked or alleviated by the prior administration of corticosteroids. Mounting experimental evidence indicates that Type III reactions are generally preceded by overt or occult Type I reactions elicited by the same antigen; it is possible that the increased vascular permeability engendered by the Type I response is necessary for the deposition of antigen-antibody complement complexes within tissues. The clinical counterpart of the preceding Type I reaction is frequently inapparent.

It appears that Type III reactions are responsible for most of the clinical manifestations of acute allergic alveolitis. The great majority of affected patients do have precipitating and complement-fixing antibodies in their blood that will react with the offending antigen and give rise to a classic intermediate (Arthus-type) skin response to it. The demonstration of immune complexes in early lesions further supports this concept. Type III responses cannot explain all the features of allergic alveolitis.

Type IV

In contrast to the first three types of hypersensitivity reactions, Type IV hypersensitivity is mediated by T-lymphocytes rather than by specific antibodies. In patients with previously sensitized T-lymphocytes, skin testing with the appropriate antigen produces a local reaction consisting of erythema and induration that reaches its maximum at 24 to 48 hours; it is thus properly termed a *delayed hypersensitivity response*. The Type IV response is responsible for classic tuberculin hypersensitivity and may play a role in other pulmonary diseases such as sarcoidosis and Wegener's granulomatosis. Type IV reactions now appear to account for many features of allergic alveolitis as well. Peripheral blood T-lymphocytes as well as the T-lymphocytes obtained by bronchoalveolar lavage of these patients recognize and react to the offending antigen. These reactive cells are better predictors of *disease* than even precipitating antibodies, which are found in many persons who have been exposed to the antigen but who have no evidence of illness. An impairment in the ability of a class of T-lymphocytes known as *suppressor cells* to prevent these responses may also be very important in the evolution of the disease.

Clinical features: Farmer's lung

Although many specific hypersensitivity pneumonitis reactions have been described (Table 12-2), the clinical features produced by each depend more

TABLE 12-2. Antigens, their source and the disease entities that can produce hypersensitivity pneumonitis

Disease	Source of antigen	Precipitins
Air-conditioner and humidifier lung	Fungi in air conditioners and humidifiers	Thermophilic actinomycetes
Aspergillosis	Ubiquitous	*Aspergillus fumigatus, A. flavus, A. niger, A. nidulans*
Bagassosis (sugarcane workers)	Moldy bagasse	*Thermoactinomyces vulgaris*
Bird fancier's lung	Pigeon, parrot, hen droppings	Serum protein and droppings
Byssinosis	Cotton, flax, hemp workers	Unknown
Farmer's lung	Moldy hay	*Micropolyspora faeni, T. vulgaris*
Malt worker's lung	Moldy barley, malt dust	*A. clavatus, A. fumigatus*
Maple-bark pneumonitis	Moldy maple bark	*Cryptostroma corticale*
Mushroom worker's lung	Mushroom compost	*M. faeni, T. vulgaris*
"New Guinea" lung	Moldy thatch dust	Thatch of huts
Pituitary snuff-taker's lung	Heterologous pituitary powder	Heterologous antigen of pituitary snuff
Sequoiosis	Moldy redwood sawdust	*Graphium Aurea basidium pullalans*
Sisal worker's lung	Unknown	Unknown
Smallpox handler's lung	Not yet demonstrated	Not yet demonstrated
Suberosis	Moldy oak bark, cork dust	Unknown
Wheat weevil disease	Infested wheat flour	*Sitophilus granarius*

on the intensity and duration of antigenic exposure than on the nature of the specific eliciting antigen. The following discussion of the clinical and pathophysiologic features of farmer's lung disease in general applies to the other diseases listed in Table 12-2 as well.

Farmer's lung is a form of hypersensitivity pneumonitis elicited by the inhalation of the spores of a group of fungi known as the thermatophilic actinomycetes, particularly *Micropolyspora faeni*. These fungi are known as *thermatophilic* because they grow best at elevated temperatures, between 40° C and 60° C. These temperatures are readily achieved by the growth of bacteria and fungi in the moldy vegetable matter found in barns and silos. Because of the enclosed spaces in which such fungi grow and the small size of their spores (less than 4 μm), an exposed farmer may retain within his tracheobronchial tree as many as 750,000 spores/min. Depending primarily on the intensity and duration of this antigenic challenge, two types of clinical response may be seen.

Acute response. The classic form of farmer's lung disease is seen in patients intermittently exposed to high concentrations of fungal spores. After working in a contaminated silo, an affected patient will usually remain asymptomatic for 4 to 6 hours. At this point, however, symptoms will develop that are both respiratory and systemic. These consist of a persistent nonproductive cough, dyspnea, malaise, anorexia, chills, and fever up to 104° F to 106° F. Chest pain is absent, and hemoptysis is rare. The symptoms will generally subside over the ensuing 12 to 48 hours, but frequently become so severe that hospitalization is required. Physical examination at this time may reveal fever and cyanosis as well as fine crepitant rales heard throughout the chest. Wheezing is not heard unless the patient is atopic. The development of leukocytosis parallels the fever curve; counts between 15,000 and 25,000 are common. Clubbing, signs of pulmonary hypertension, and cor pulmonale are not observed. The chest radiograph is usually normal but may demonstrate diffuse nodular infiltrates that may be alveolar or interstitial in appearance and that clear rapidly (Fig. 12-1).

Whether or not the disease is correctly diagnosed following its first manifestations, patients frequently return to the site of exposure, sometimes wearing protective facial masks. Because of the small size of the spores, such measures are ineffectual, and the typical patient experiences many episodes of the disease and spontaneous remission. During this period progressive weight loss is common, and generalized fatigue may be incapacitating.

Chronic form. The chronic form of hypersensitivity pneumonitis may be extremely difficult to diagnose. This form is generally seen in patients exposed to low concentrations of spores over a prolonged period. Acute reactions are mild and may not be recognized. Cough and dyspnea develop in-

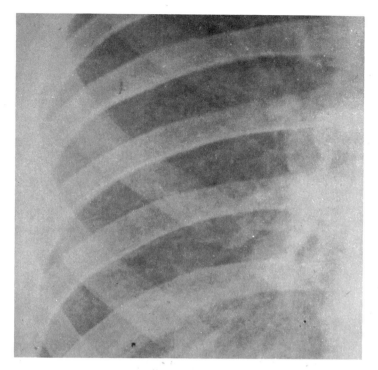

FIG. 12-1. Extrinsic allergic alveolitis. Note fine "soft" nodulation. *(Courtesy Medical Illustration Service, Veterans Administration Hospital, Denver, Colorado.)*

sidiously and are generally not related to specific episodes of antigenic challenge. Physical examination of such patients is variable and may show either the hyperexpansion, diminished breath sounds, hyperresonance, and rhonchi of COPD or the "Velcro" rales of diffuse interstitial fibrosis. Leukocytosis is absent. The chest radiograph usually demonstrates hyperexpansion with a generalized increase in interstitial markings, but may easily be mistaken for the picture of simple COPD.

Pulmonary function

Since the pulmonary abnormalities in the acute form of farmer's lung disease are completely reversible, results of pulmonary function testing depend on the stage of the episode at which the patient is tested. This is best considered in terms of the serial changes seen following a natural or aerosol-delivered antigenic challenge. The classic response is seen in Fig. 12-2, *A*. For 4 hours following challenge the patient remains asymptomatic. At this time, coincident with the development of fever and leukocytosis, both the FVC and

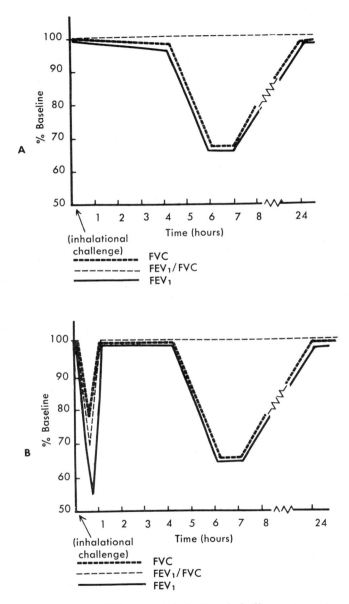

FIG. 12-2. Serial spirometry following inhalational challenge in patients with hypersensitivity pneumonitis. **A,** Classic response. **B,** "Dual response" in an atopic patient. *(Courtesy Medical Illustration Service, Veterans Administration Hospital, Denver, Colorado.)*

the FEV_1 fall dramatically, although the FEV_1/FVC ratio remains constant. The residual volume may be elevated, suggesting that some air trapping has occurred. These abnormalities gradually revert to normal by the next day.

In atopic patients a "dual response" is seen. In this situation, depicted in Fig. 12-2, *B*, inhalational challenge is immediately followed by a fall of the FVC and a disproportionately large fall in the FEV_1, with an accompanying fall in the FEV_1/FVC ratio. During this time the patient may experience wheezing. The spirogram classically returns to baseline levels within 1 hour but is followed at 4 to 6 hours by a response identical to that seen in Fig. 12-2, *A*.

Pulmonary function testing in individuals with chronic forms of hypersensitivity pneumonitis is quite variable, with degrees of both restrictive and obstructive diseases. Lung volumes are usually diminished, although ratio of residual volume to total lung capacity may be elevated. The diffusion capacity for carbon monoxide (D_{LCO}) is depressed.

Pathologic features

Lung biopsy of patients with the more acute forms of hypersensitivity pneumonitis demonstrates marked interstitial infiltration consisting of plasma cells, lymphocytes, and clumps of epithelial cells with scattered granulomas. Many foamy macrophages are seen within alveoli and terminal airways, and a terminal bronchiolitis may be present. In the chronic form of the disease, nonspecific peribronchial fibrosis with some degree of centrilobular emphysema is seen. These bronchial and bronchiolar changes may be responsible for the air trapping mentioned above. In neither instance does hilar or mediastinal adenopathy develop. Immunofluorescent staining of very early lesions may demonstrate a granular deposition of antigen-antibody complement complexes at the alveolar basement membrane.

Diagnosis

In the acute forms of hypersensitivity pneumonitis the diagnosis is usually apparent to both the patient and the physician. In the chronic forms the diagnosis may be much more elusive and will be missed unless the physician obtains a meticulous history of possible sources of antigenic exposure. In either instance a suspected diagnosis may be confirmed by three immunologic procedures.

1. An inhalational challenge with suspected antigens may be performed and, in afflicted patients, will elicit a response such as seen in Fig. 12-2. Inhalational challenge is rarely necessary, however, and should be performed only by personnel familiar with the disease and capable of treating the potentially severe pulmonary reactions that may ensue.

2. Because more than 70% of patients' sera will contain precipitating antibodies, agar gel precipitation tests may be performed. Generally, a standard Ouchterlony double diffusion test is sufficient, although more sophisticated techniques are currently being employed in specialized laboratories. The results must be interpreted in the light of other clinical data, as many exposed but healthy persons will also have precipitating antibodies.
3. Skin testing with the suspected antigen may elicit either a Type III (Arthus) response or a dual response consisting of a Type I response followed in several hours by the Arthus reaction. Generally, delayed hypersensitivity skin reactions are not seen in these patients, although they have been observed in some animal models of the disease.

In patients in whom the diagnosis remains uncertain an open lung biopsy is recommended. With the advent of the fiberoptic bronchoscope, transbronchial biopsy under fluoroscopic control has proven safe, but the widely scattered granulomatous lesions characteristic of hypersensitivity pneumonitis may easily be missed.

Treatment

The only effective treatment for hypersensitivity pneumonitis is complete avoidance of the offending antigen, since once the patient's immunologic abnormalities have become established, even small, intermittent antigenic challenges may produce relentlessly progressive disease. In the acute case, supportive care consisting of adequate hydration, bed rest, and oxygen administration is generally sufficient. Occasionally, however, pulmonary involvement in this disease may be so extensive as to be life threatening; endotracheal intubation with or without mechanical ventilation may then be necessary. Corticosteroids may dramatically abort the acute attack, with improvement seen as early as 1 or 2 hours following their administration.

Treatment of the more chronic forms of the disease is less successful. Patients whose lungs have progressed to a state of CLE emphysema with interstitial fibrosis, even if they avoid further antigenic exposure, rarely improve even with corticosteroid therapy. At a somewhat earlier state, when both cellular and fibrotic infiltrates are seen, the prognosis is somewhat brighter. Chronic ambulant corticosteroid therapy is rarely indicated, however, and will not halt the disease process unless the offending antigen is eliminated from the patient's environment.

SUGGESTED READINGS

Fink, J.N., Banaszak, E.F., Thiede, W.H., et al.: Interstitial pneumonitis due to hypersensitivity to an organism contaminating a heating system, Ann. Intern. Med. **74**:80, 1971.

Fink, J.N., Hensley, G.T., and Barboriak, J.J.: An animal model of a hypersensitivity pneumonitis, J. Allergy **46**:156, 1970.

Fink, J.N., Sosman, A.J., Barboriak, J.J., et al.: Pigeon breeder's disease: a clinical study of a hypersensitivity pneumonitis, Ann. Intern. Med. **68**:1205, 1968.

Fink, J.N., Sosman, A.J., Salvaggio, J.E., et al.: Precipitins and the diagnosis of a hypersensitivity pneumonitis, J. Allergy Clin. Immunol. **48**:179, 1971.

Gell, P.G.H., and Coombs, R.R.A.: Clinical aspects of immunology, Oxford, 1963, Blackwell Scientific Publications, Ltd.

Liebow, A.A., and Carrington, C.B.: Hypersensitivity reactions involving the lung, Trans. Coll. Physicians **34**:47, 1966.

Moore, V.L., and Fink, J.N.: Immunologic studies in hypersensitivity pneumonitis—quantitative precipitins and complement-fixing antibodies in symptomatic and asymptomatic pigeon breeders, J. Lab. Clin. Med. **85**:540, 1975.

Pepys, J.: Pulmonary hypersensitivity reactions to inhaled organic dusts, Trans. Med. Soc. London **85**:49, 1969.

Ramazzini, B.: DeMortis Artificum Diatriba, 1700, the Latin text of 1713, revised, with translation and notes by W.C. Wright, Chicago, 1940, The University of Chicago Press.

Salvaggio, J., Kawai, T., and Harris, J.: Cell-mediated (type IV) hypersensitivity pneumonitis, Chest **63**:51S, 1973.

Schuyler, M.R., Thigpen, T.P., and Salvaggio, J.E.: Local pulmonary immunity in pigeon breeder's disease, Ann. Intern. Med. **88**:355, 1978.

Sweet, L.C., Anderson, J.A., Callies, Q.C., et al.: Hypersensitivity pneumonitis related to a home furnace humidifier, J. Allergy Clin. Immunol. **48**:171, 1971.

Chapter 13

PULMONARY TUBERCULOSIS

John A. Sbarbaro *and* Paul T. Davidson

Infection with *Mycobacterium tuberculosis* involves a lifelong relationship between the host (human) and tubercle bacilli, in which dormant organisms remain alive in the host for years. These bacilli are held in check primarily by the host's immunologic defense system, but they remain capable of "reactivating" and causing a progressive and potentially life-threatening disease—tuberculosis. The diseased host may then serve as a nidus for the spread of infection to other individuals.

Etiology

Mycobacteria are nonmobile, nonsporulating, weakly gram-positive rods classified in the order Actinomycetales. The bacilli do not have a waxy capsule, but a high lipid content contributes to their acid-fast staining characteristic. The two mammalian bacilli, *M. tuberculosis* and *M. bovis*, are obligate aerobes; they do not grow under anaerobic condition but grow in proportion to the oxygen tension of the environment. The organisms are recognized by their characteristic colonial morphology, lack of pigmentation, and slow or delayed catalase activity. *M. tuberculosis* produces a positive reaction to the niacin test, an important way of differentiating it from other mycobacteria. *M. bovis*, which yields a negative niacin test, has for all practical purposes been eliminated as an important pathogen in many parts of the world by pasteurization of milk and cattle tuberculin testing control programs. *M. tuberculosis* organisms that have become isoniazid (INH) resistant lose their catalase activity.

Transmission and pathogenesis

M. tuberculosis is usually spread as or on an airborne "droplet nucleus." These particles, produced and disseminated as persons with pulmonary tuberculosis talk or cough, are small enough (1 to 10 μm) to remain airborne for extended periods. When inhaled, they can pass through the mucociliary airway defenses into the alveoli. Based on volume distribution of air within the lungs, the lower lung fields are the major site of initial bacillary implantation.

Once secure within the alveoli of a susceptible host, the bacilli multiply slowly, at a rate of about 1 multiplication every 24 hours. During the ensuing 3 to 10 weeks, while the host is developing a cellular immune response, these bacilli may be transported through lymphatic channels, first to the regional hilar lymph nodes and then into the bloodstream by way of the thoracic duct. They may also get into the bloodstream from the intestinal tract or pulmonary capillary system. In these ways, organisms are seeded throughout the host's entire body *before* the arrival of specifically reactive T-lymphocytes in sufficient numbers to control the infective process. Without an adequate immunologic response, the result of hematogenous spread is "miliary" tuberculosis (readily visible in the lung fields), "disseminated" tuberculosis (Fig. 13-1), or both.

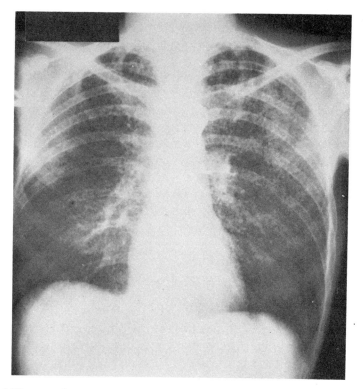

FIG. 13-1. Miliary tuberculosis, advanced. This appearance can be simulated by many other conditions. *(Courtesy Medical Illustration Service, Veterans Administration Hospital, Denver, Colorado.)*

Usually, this infective process is eventually brought under control by macrophages brought to the site of infection by the specifically reactive T-lymphocytes. The macrophages phagocytize the bacilli, but many organisms remain viable and continue to multiply within the phagocyte. In most cases this host defense process proves adequate in controlling further spread of the infection, and the host/parasite relationship settles into a state of equilibrium; some organisms are slowly destroyed as lesions heal, but significant numbers of bacilli retain their viability in a dormant condition.

About 5% of hosts are incapable of containing the initial infective process; an additional 5% of those who do pass successfully through the initial challenge phase later lose their capability of controlling the infection, and the dormant bacilli again begin to multiply. In both these circumstances progressive inflammation and tissue necrosis occur, primarily as the result of the cellular immune response process rather than from toxins produced by the bacteria. Because *M. tuberculosis* is an absolute aerobe, progression of tuberculous infection into active disease occurs most commonly in the lungs where contact with molecular oxygen is most likely. Progressive tissue destruction resulting in masses of caseous necrosis, cavity formation, compression of surrounding structures, and erosion of blood vessels with subsequent hemorrhage may lead to the host's ultimate death. The total number of organisms harbored by the host during these developments may reach hundreds of millions; the appearance of drug-resistant mutants is an inevitable result.

Some tissues of the body do not provide an optimum environment for the survival of tubercle bacilli, for example, muscle. However, in addition to the lungs, the kidneys and the ends of the long bones also appear to provide ideal conditions for tubercle growth for reasons that are not entirely clear but may be related to high tissue oxygen tensions. It is in these organs that one should look for progression of the initial infection, or, in later years, reactivation or awakening of dormant bacilli with progressive growth and subsequent tuberculous disease. The longer it takes for the host to bring the initial infective process under control, the larger the final bacillary population burden within the host and therefore the greater the opportunity for a dormant bacillus to reactivate. For example, the initial infective process results in hematogenous spread to the lungs. If immunologic control is achieved before further bacillary growth can cause macroscopic destruction (normal chest radiograph), the chance of later reactivation of the disease is estimated at 27 persons out of 100,000/so infected. But if the infection produces macroscopic damage before control is achieved ("old apical scar," "Simon foci," "fibrotic lesion"), the chance of late progressive disease increases to 2 persons out of 100/yr so diseased.

Clinical manifestations

Patients usually have chronic generalized constitutional complaints such as fatigue, anorexia, low-grade fever (usually in the afternoon), weight loss, and irregular menses in women. A chronic cough, sputum production, or hemoptysis suggests pulmonary disease. Some patients have acute symptoms such as fever and chills, pleuritic pain, myalgia, sweating (especially at night), and even pulmonary hemorrhage when first seen. However, it is not unusual to find patients, even those with progressive and extensive disease, who are asymptomatic.

Cough, at first quite mild, slowly progressive over weeks and months, and productive of mucoid or mucopurulent sputum, may be associated with a dull, recurring chest pain or a feeling of tightness in the chest. Dyspnea, on the other hand, is uncommon.

Pleural effusion may occur at any time after the initial infection; it is caused by the release of bacilli-laden caseous material into the pleural space, causing an inflammatory reaction and the exudation of a clear, protein-rich fluid.

Except for the findings characteristically associated with pleural effusion, the physical examination in tuberculosis is nonspecific and nondiagnostic. Apical rales and the physical signs of cavitation are quite unreliable. A normocytic, normochromic anemia and an elevated erythrocyte sedimentation rate with an associated normal white count are common findings; a monocytosis (8% to 15%) may be observed.

Diagnosis

Although isolation of *M. tuberculosis* by culture is necessary to confirm a progressive disease process, a number of factors contribute to the diagnosis of active tuberculosis.

History. A history of exposure to tuberculosis identifies an individual at definite risk. On the average, over 25% of household contacts exposed to contagious tuberculosis are found to have acquired the infection.

Tuberculin test. Infection with mycobacterial organisms results in delayed (white cell–mediated) hypersensitivity to certain products of the organisms produced during cellular growth. These by-product antigens have been extracted and refined into a product called *purified protein derivative* (PPD). Each production batch of tuberculin may differ markedly from other production batches. Products produced for general clinical use therefore must now be stabilized with Tween (PPD-T), standardized in human beings, and compared with reactions produced with the U.S. Standard PPD-S.

The most commonly used concentration of PPD-T is 5 tuberculin units (TU) (biologic equivalent), sometimes called *intermediate strength*. Injection of these materials (0.1 ml) into the skin produces a localized reaction in sensitized persons. Tuberculin and PPD-T are administered intracutaneously, usually on the volar surface of the forearm by either the Mantoux method or multiple puncture techniques. The reaction to injected tuberculin and PPD-T in sensitized individuals consists of an area of induration (usually with surrounding erythema that should be disregarded) that appears in 48 to 72 hours and varies in size and intensity according to the dosage of tuberculin and the sensitivity of the individual.

A positive tuberculin test usually develops 2 to 10 weeks after initial infection with *M. tuberculosis.* Although an induration measuring 10 mm or greater is considered indicative of infection with *M. tuberculosis,* 5 mm of induration is equally diagnostic in the presence of known exposure to *M. tuberculosis.* The PPD-T skin test is subject to variation. For instance, differences in interpreter readings of up to 15 mm have occurred among 4 trained readers.

Individual host response to the injected antigen may vary according to the host's immunologic condition at the time of the test. Viral infections, cancer, sarcoidosis, immunosuppressive drugs, overwhelming infection, and corticosteroid therapy adversely affect the test. Unexplained specific anergy to tuberculin exists in up to 5% of individuals who, although infected, do not react to tuberculin despite evidence of immunologic competence.

Because infection with mycobacteria other than *M. tuberculosis* is widespread, especially in warmer climates (see Chapter 15), sensitivity to mycobacterial antigens, some shared commonly with *M. tuberculosis,* is also widespread. Existing tuberculin products are not specific enough to identify only individuals infected with *M. tuberculosis;* they also detect sensitivity to these shared mycobacterial antigens. Epidemiologic studies have demonstrated that most tuberculin reactions of individuals infected with *M. tuberculosis* are larger than 10 mm of induration; however, this does not mean that reactions smaller than 10 mm of induration cannot indicate infection with *M. tuberculosis.* Rather, the larger reactions reflect only the likelihood that the sensitivity arises from infection with the mycobacteria from which the tuberculin was made. Organisms with antigens similar to *M. tuberculosis* will also elicit larger skin reactions. Stronger concentrations of tuberculins (100 to 250 TU) identify lower degrees of sensitivity to mycobacterial antigens, and positive skin reactions only to these products are more probably reflections of infection with atypical mycobacteria rather than with *M. tuberculosis.*

Multiple puncture devices, primarily valuable for screening purposes, have highly concentrated tuberculin on prongs that are designed to ensure intradermal placement of the test material. Because of their dependence on uncontrolled quantities of concentrated tuberculin, these devices are standardized for sensitivity but not specificity. A positive reaction indicates sensitivity to mycobacterial antigens and not necessarily infection with *M. tuberculosis*. A diagnostic Mantoux test should follow all positive multiple puncture tests except those causing blistering (and thereby indicating significant sensitivity to antigens from *M. tuberculosis*).

As individuals age, sensitivity to tuberculin may wane. A single tuberculin test properly interpreted as negative may anamnestically recall delayed white cell sensitivity 1 week later, with subsequent tests interpreted as positive. This phenomenon has frequently led to confusion and misdiagnosis of recent infection. The problem can be avoided by retesting 1 week later individuals over age 50 who had weak or negative reactions to the initial test. Recall phenomenon is 1% among persons aged 20, over 7% among persons aged 50, and up to 18% among individuals aged 80 or older.

Sputum smear and culture

Smear. Examination of a stained sputum obtained from a single sputum specimen may provide the first bacteriologic evidence of the presence of mycobacteria. Since over 10,000 bacteria/ml of specimen are required to produce a positive smear, its presence suggests that the patient source may be highly contagious. Positive sputum smears are almost always found in conjunction with cavitary tuberculous disease. In addition to the Ziehl-Neelsen technique, smears can now be quickly screened by low-power microscopy using fluorescent auramine/rhodamine. Centrifuging the specimen before staining increases the opportunity for detecting bacteria.

Culture. Tubercle bacilli can be cultured on synthetic media; however, because of their slow growth, other bacteria, if present, may quickly overgrow the media, suppressing the multiplication of tubercle bacilli needed for diagnostic identification. Although specimens obtained through biopsy are unlikely to be contaminated with other microorganisms and can be transferred directly to culture media, other specimens obtained from sputum, saliva, and even urine require decontamination. This "decontamination process" uses sodium hydroxide to kill nonmycobacteria. Although tubercle bacilli are somewhat resistant to this decontamination process, a significant number of tubercle bacilli may also be killed; excess decontamination may thus result in false-negative sputum cultures, especially in inexperienced laboratories. Clinicians must remain alert to this confusing possibility.

Newer media (such as 7H10 or 7H11) permit the identification of bacilli within 3 to 4 weeks; egg media (Löwenstein-Jensen) requires a longer time (up to 6 weeks). Most mycobacteria will grow in these media. Further differential testing is required for final identification. *M. tuberculosis* is niacin positive, catalase positive, and nonchromogenic. (See Chapter 15 for information regarding the other mycobacteria.)

Chest radiography

Because of its ability to identify macroscopic changes in physical structure, the chest radiograph has been most valuable in the diagnosis of pulmonary tuberculosis (Figs. 13-1 to 13-6). Lesions large enough to be visible are usually associated with large populations of viable tubercle bacilli. For example, during the initial stages of infection, a small peripheral inflammation, associated with hilar node involvement, results from unchecked multiplication of organisms. This early *primary complex* usually resolves into a calcified *Ghon complex* harboring only a few viable bacilli. Similarly, the initial hematogenous spread, when unchecked, is followed by progressive bacillary growth, especially in tissues with a high oxygen content such as the upper regions of the lungs. *Simon foci, apical scar,* and *old fibrotic lesion* are terms used to describe the residuals of this early progressive growth. Their presence signifies the likelihood that a large, albeit dormant, bacillary population remains viable within the host.

Treatment principles

With the availability of effective drugs, the treatment of tuberculosis—pulmonary or extrapulmonary—can be accomplished primarily in an ambulatory care setting. Only patients with significant signs or symptoms of disease now require inpatient care, although the hospital may serve as a site for isolation, patient education, and the monitoring of initial drug toxicity in selected cases.

Since reliable evidence now indicates that effective chemotherapy actually taken by the patient controls infectiousness within 2 to 4 weeks (even in the presence of persisting positive cultures and/or smears), the patient may be permitted to resume a normal life-style during the early phases of therapy. However, because of the potential risk to other persons, the treatment of tuberculosis imposes on the physician a responsibility to ensure adequate treatment of the patient. Numerous studies have demonstrated that 30% to 35% of patients do not follow their physician's instructions and therefore are best treated by the direct professional administration of drugs. Direct administration of medication is difficult on a daily basis but can be achieved if the drugs are given intermittently in higher dosages. All patients should be watched carefully for signs of drug toxicity.

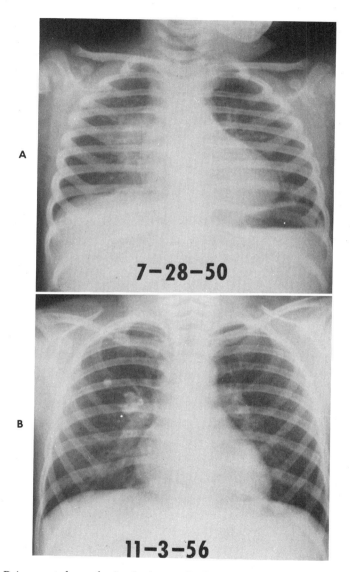

FIG. 13-2. Primary tuberculosis. **A,** Acute. **B,** Late. Parenchymal and hilar calcifications 6 years later. *(Courtesy Medical Illustration Service, Veterans Administration Hospital, Denver, Colorado.)*

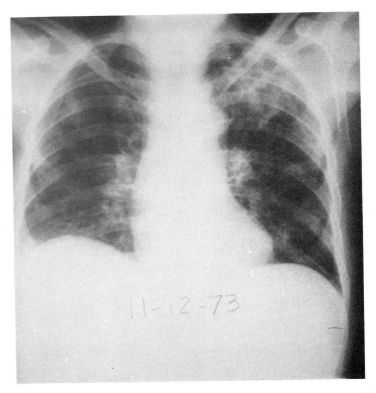

FIG. 13-3. Acute pneumonic pulmonary tuberculosis in all lobes, especially left upper lobe, with small right pleural effusion. *(Courtesy Medical Illustration Service, Veterans Administration Hospital, Denver, Colorado.)*

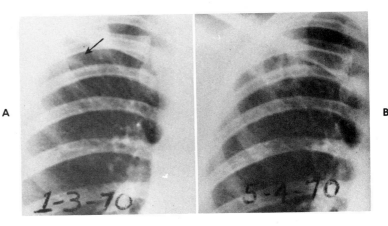

FIG. 13-4. Early pulmonary tuberculosis. **A,** Small "soft" infiltrate in first right anterior interspace beneath clavicle. **B,** Progression to 3 cm cavity in 4 months. *(Courtesy Medical Illustration Service, Denver General Hospital, Denver, Colorado.)*

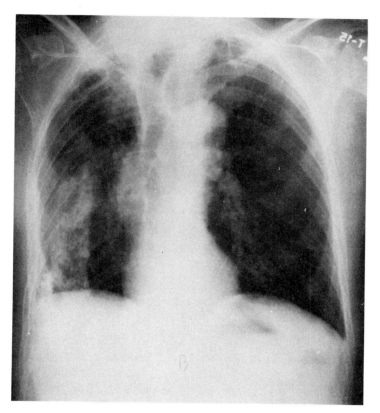

FIG. 13-5. Calcific pleural thickening, right, secondary to old tuberculous empyema. *(Courtesy Medical Illustration Service, Veterans Administration Hospital, Denver, Colorado.)*

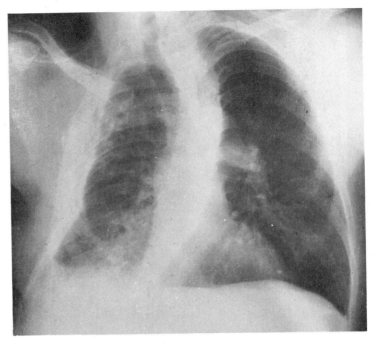

FIG. 13-6. Right fibrothorax: marked pleural thickening secondary to tuberculous empyema in childhood, with resultant scoliosis. *(Courtesy Medical Illustration Service, Colorado General Hospital, Denver, Colorado.)*

PRINCIPLE: *Chemotherapy is effective because of its action on the metabolic processes of the tubercle bacillus.*

Drug	Metabolic site of action	Daily dosage	Twice weekly dosage
Rifampin (Rm)	RNA synthesis	10-20 mg/kg up to 600 mg orally	600 mg*
Isoniazid (INH)†	DNA synthesis	5-10 mg/kg	15 mg/kg
Ethambutol (EMB)	RNA synthesis	15-25 mg/kg	50 mg/kg
Streptomycin (SM)	Protein synthesis	15-20 mg/kg	25-30 mg/kg
Pyrazinamide (PZA)	?	15-30 mg/kg up to 2 gm	70 mg/kg

Rifampin (Rm) and INH are considered bactericidal agents. Streptomycin (SM) also has bactericidal activity in neutral or slightly alkaline pH, but apparently is effective only against extracellular organisms. Pyrazinamide (PZA) requires an acid medium for its bactericidal activity and therefore is effective on mycobacteria within macrophages. When combined, SM and PZA are thought to act as a single bactericidal drug. Ethambutol (EMB)

---

*Hypersensitivity reactions are frequent if more than 600 mg is given.
†Vitamin B$_6$ (pyridoxine) should be given with INH to reduce the risk of peripheral neuritis.

in a daily dosage of 15 to 25 mg/kg is primarily a bacteriostatic agent. Other drugs such as kanamycin, viomycin, capreomycin, thiacetazone, ethionamide, cycloserine, and para-aminosalicylic acid (PAS) are also effective in varying degrees against *M. tuberculosis* and are employed in carefully planned retreatment regimens.

PRINCIPLE: *The number and type of drugs needed to control bacillary growth is related to the number of organisms involved in the disease process and the stage of their metabolic activity.*

Two important phases of an effective chemotherapeutic regimen have been identified as a result of 30 years of clinical experience and basic research.

Phase I consists of initial intensive chemotherapy directed toward the rapid destruction of large multiplying populations of tubercle bacilli. Bacterial resistance to individual drugs occurs by natural mutation (e.g., 1 of every 10^5 to 10^6 bacilli is resistant to INH, SM, and EMB; the number for Rm is 10^7. Therefore 1 of every 10^{12} bacilli would be resistant to both INH and Rm); large bacillary populations require 2 or 3 drugs to ensure the elimination of all actively metabolizing organisms and to avoid the risk of permitting the overgrowth of resistant mutants. Measurable reduction of organisms occurs about 14 days after the initiation of appropriate therapy and coincides with marked diminution of infectiousness, permitting discontinuation of pulmonary isolation.

This intensive phase of daily treatment should be continued for a total of 4 to 8 weeks, depending on the severity of the disease process. A regimen of 2 or 3 bactericidal drugs (INH, RM, and the SM/PZA combination) is the first choice for this chemotherapeutic phase.

Phase II consists of maintenance chemotherapy directed toward the elimination of the majority of the remaining bacilli (or at least the majority of dormant bacilli likely to return to an active stage of growth). This phase of treatment depends on the effect of a drug on relatively dormant organisms during their brief spurts of metabolic activity. Recent experience suggests that although this phase of treatment may be as short as 4 to 4½ months (total treatment of 6 months) if bactericidal drugs (Rm, INH) are used without lapses, relapse rates after this short a regimen range from 2% to 7% or more.

When treatment with bactericidal regimens including Rm is extended to a total therapy duration of 9 months (continuation phase treatment administered either daily or twice weekly), relapse rates fall to below 1%. If it is not possible to use this bactericidal combination throughout therapy and bacteriostatic agents such as EMB are substituted into the treatment regimen, this phase of therapy should be extended to a total of 18 months.

Although single drug (INH) maintenance therapy has been used and has apparently been effective, this maintenance phase of active treatment should incorporate two drugs (on the presumption that the host's immune system is incapable of containing the rather large bacillary population.

Nonmetabolizing (dormant) bacilli are unaffected by chemotherapy. This explains the necessity for continuing treatment for extended periods. During this period of therapy, it is reasonable to hypothesize that dormant bacilli again begin to metabolize from time to time; the continued presence of drugs ensures their elimination. Those bacilli remaining after cessation of treatment are held in check by the host's immune system. They remain a threat, however, should the immune system be compromised at some later date.

A directly administered, intermittent, twice weekly, high-dosage regimen using INH and Rm has been shown to be most effective during this second phase of treatment and has the advantage of ensuring patient compliance while reducing the potential for drug toxicity. Intermittent high-dosage combinations of INH and Sm and INH and EMB have also been proved effective, but again, treatment duration must be prolonged if Rm is removed from the regimen.

PRINCIPLE: *Under no circumstances, either in Phase I or Phase II, should a single drug be added to a* failing *regimen (implying both a potentially large bacillary population and the risk of emergence of resistance to the single new drug), but there is no problem in substituting one effective drug for another in a regimen successfully controlling the infection.*

A history of previous treatment should always raise the possibility of drug resistance, and susceptibility testing is required before combining new drugs with drugs used in the earlier treatment of the patient.

All antituberculosis drugs, in addition to their metabolic effect on tubercle bacilli, have the potential for adverse metabolic action on the host.

Transient elevated levels of serum glutamic pyruvic transaminase (SGOT and SGPT) may be observed in 10% to 20% of patients treated with INH; they do not require a change in either treatment regimen or dosage. The risk of severe hepatotoxicity, clinically manifested as jaundice, increases with age (0.3% below age 34 to 2.3% above age 50) and is reversible if medication is promptly discontinued. Peripheral neuritis may occur when INH is used in dosages greater than 5 mg/kg/day and can be prevented by the simultaneous administration of pyridoxine.

SM, capreomycin, and kanamycin may lead to damage of vestibular function (dizziness and imbalance), loss of high-tone hearing, and aggravation of renal impairment. Careful clinical monitoring is necessary.

Rm, when used daily, may lead to significant liver dysfunction (2% to 4% with jaundice), especially in individuals with preexisting liver damage. Minor side effects such as gastrointestinal intolerance and cutaneous reactions, usually pruritic, may also result. When used intermittently (never in dosages above 600 mg), Rm may result in the development of Rm-dependent antibodies, associated with flulike reactions characterized by fever, chills, headaches, malaise, and, rarely, severe problems such as thrombocytopenia and purpura.

When EMB is used in a dosage of 15 mg/kg/day, the risk of visual toxicity (optic neuritis, decrease in visual acuity and fields), is virtually nil; a risk does appear with increasing *daily* dosage (3% with dosages under 30 mg/kg to 20% in dosages greater than 35 mg/kg).

Preventive therapy is frequently offered to tuberculin reactors, contacts, and persons with residual radiographic lung changes suggestive of an earlier encounter with tuberculosis, provided the existence of active disease has been carefully excluded. A single drug (INH—5 mg/kg for adults, 10 mg/kg for children) is given daily for 12 months. The principle is again to eliminate the more active bacilli of the dormant population, thereby reducing the opportunity for later disease reactivation. Because the number of living bacilli in such cases must be small, the use of this one bactericidal drug is considered and has proved to be safe and effective.

Recent close contacts with infectious tuberculosis and persons with residual evidence of a tuberculous disease process (positive tuberculin test associated with apical lung stranding) should always be considered candidates for preventive treatment. Persons with a positive tuberculin test in the absence of other evidence of tuberculous disease should be considered for treatment if under 35 years of age. However, the risk of INH hepatotoxicity increases after 35 years of age, offsetting the risk of dormant bacilli reactivating to progressive disease. Unless complicating problems such as silicosis, diabetes, treatment with adrenocorticoids or immunosuppressive drugs, hematologic or reticuloendothelial disease such as leukemia or Hodgkin's disease, renal transplantation, ileal bypass surgery for obesity, or gastrectomy are present, preventive treatment is best withheld.

Summary

Because of its lifelong relationship to the host, tuberculosis holds a unique place in the practice of medicine. The chart on p. 150 reflects this interrelationship and serves as a constant reminder to physicians of their responsibility, both to the patient and to society, to consider recurrence of the disease process. This classification is of particular value for public health statistics and should be used when reporting a case to the health department. The reporting of all cases of tuberculosis is mandatory. And as with other chronic diseases, the diagnosis should become a permanent part of the patient's diagnosis or "problem" list and be considered actively throughout that individual's life.

CLASSIFICATION OF TUBERCULOSIS (1981)

A. *Tuberculosis exposure, no evidence of infection*

B. *Tuberculous infection, no disease*
1. Chemotherapy status (tuberculin positive, negative bacteriologic and radiologic studies; must be *considered* for preventive therapy)

C. *Tuberculosis, current disease*
1. Location of disease
2. Bacteriologic status
3. Chemotherapy status
4. Radiologic findings
5. Tuberculin skin test reaction

D. *Tuberculosis, no current disease*
1. Chemotherapy status

E. *Tuberculosis suspect, diagnosis pending*
1. Chemotherapy status

SUGGESTED READINGS

Bates, J.H.: Diagnosis of tuberculosis, Chest **76** (Suppl):757, 1979.

Comstock, G.W.: Untreated inactive pulmonary tuberculosis: risk of reactivation, Public Health Rep. **77**:461, 1962.

Comstock, G.W., and Edwards, P.Q.: The competing risks of tuberculosis and hepatitis for adult tuberculin reactors, Am. Rev. Respir. Dis. **111**:573, 1975.

Fox, W.: The chemotherapy of pulmonary tuberculosis: a review, Chest **76** (Suppl):785, 1979.

Fox, W., and Mitchison, D.A.: short-course chemotherapy for pulmonary tuberculosis, Am. Rev. Respir. Dis. **111**:325, 1975.

Iseman, M.D.: Tuberculosis. In D.H. Simmons, editor: Current pulmonology, Boston, 1979, Houghton Mifflin Co.

Johnston, R.F., and Wildrick, K.H.: The impact of chemotherapy on the care of patients with tuberculosis, Am. Rev. Respir. Dis. **109**:636, 1974.

Kopanoff, D.E., Snider, D.E., and Caras, G.J.: Isoniazid-related hepatitis. A U.S. Public Health Service Cooperative Surveillance Study, Am. Rev. Respir. Dis. **117**:991, 1978.

Stead, W.W.: The pathogenesis of pulmonary tuberculosis among older persons, Am. Rev. Respir. Dis. **91**:811, 1965.

Stead, W.W., and Dutt, A.A., Eds.: Tuberculosis clinics in chest medicine, vol. 1, no. 2, Philadelphia, 1980, W.B. Saunders Co.

Thompson, N.J., Glassroth, J.L., Snider, D.E., et al.: The booster phenomenon in serial tuberculin testing, Am. Rev. Respir. Dis. **119**:587, 1979.

Chapter 14

EXTRAPULMONARY TUBERCULOSIS

Michael D. Iseman

Over the past decade the number of cases of pulmonary tuberculosis in the United States had steadily declined; however, the incidence of extrapulmonary tuberculosis (XPTB) has remained stable at roughly 4,000 cases per year. The proportion of XPTB has thus risen to comprise roughly 14% of all new cases of tuberculosis in the United States.

Pathogenesis

In the great majority of cases, with the exceptions noted below, XPTB is a consequence of lymphohematogenous dissemination that occurs during the initial invasion or primary pulmonary infection. During this primary process a bacillemia deposits the mycobacteria in a variety of organs or spaces throughout the body. The microbes characteristically travel back from these primary foci to the lymph nodes draining the area, constituting a "primary complex." This invasion is usually clinically silent, and the microbes initially elicit little, if any, tissue response. However, with the appearance of delayed hypersensitivity (signaled by the appearance of tuberculin skin test reactivity) and the related, but not identical, phenomenon of cell-mediated immunity, a granulomatous inflammatory reaction occurs in which many of the organisms are eliminated. Nonetheless, some viable microbes usually persist and months or years later may undergo recrudescence, resulting in overt disease. A common feature of the sites in which mycobacteria most successfully hibernate is high oxygen tension. Mycobacteria are obligate aerobes and prosper in sites with a rich oxygen supply, including the lung apices, renal cortex, bone growth plates, and meninges.

Forms of XPTB not due to lymphohematogenous dissemination include (1) cervical lymphadenitis due to infection of pharyngeal lymphatic tissue, (2) pleural or chest wall tuberculosis due to immediate spread from a subpleural caseous focus, (3) ileocecal or perirectal disease that develops from invasion of the intestinal tract by organisms swallowed along with the respiratory secretions in a patient with active pulmonary disease, and (4) pericardial disease produced by a fistulous tract between an infected mediastinal lymph node and the pericardial sac.

Epidemiology

The proportion of extrapulmonary to pulmonary tuberculosis varies widely in different areas. In general, the higher the incidence of all tuberculous disease, the lower the percentage of XPTB. Although the majority of XPTB occurs among whites—reflecting the preponderance of whites in the United States—annual case rates of XPTB have become considerably higher among nonwhites: whites, 1.3; blacks, 6.5; others (primarily Orientals), 16.2 (cases per 100,000 per year). Among whites with XPTB, the percentage of Hispanics is quite high. Of 3674 cases the U.S. Public Health Service (USPHS) reported in whites, 836, or 34%, occurred in patients also noted to be Hispanic. The mean age of patients with various forms of XPTB was close to 43 years. Exceptions to this were meningeal tuberculosis, which usually occurs in younger patients (mean age 29.7 years) and miliary tuberculosis, which shows a predilection for the elderly (mean age 50.4 years). Bovine tubercle bacilli, usually entering the body by way of the gastrointestinal tract, commonly caused XPTB in the past; the elimination of bovine tuberculosis in North America is a major reason for reduced incidence of XPTB.

The common anatomic sites of XPTB are listed in Table 14-1. The relative proportion of each form of disease was remarkably consistent in the various regions surveyed by the USPHS and strikingly similar to experience with XPTB in Canada.

Only 18% of the XPTB patients surveyed by the USPHS were found to have concomitant active pulmonary disease. However, among XPTB patients in whom a chest radiograph was reported, 77% revealed abnormalities consistent with *previous* pulmonary tuberculosis.

TABLE 14-1. Frequency of extrapulmonary tuberculosis by organ site

Organ site	Annual case rate*	% XPTB†
Pleurae	0.54	26.5
Lymph nodes	0.45	21.3
Genitourinary tract	0.37	17.9
Disseminated (miliary)	0.22	10.6
Skeletal (bone/joint)	0.19	8.8
CNS	0.10	4.7
Abdomen	0.08	3.8
Pericardium	0.02	0.9
Endocrine glands	0.004	0.02

*Per 100,000 per year, 1969-1973.
†Total is less than 100% because very rare sites are excluded.

Tuberculin test in XPTB

Of those patients in the USPHS survey for whom a tuberculin skin test was reported, 124 of 865 (14%) had negative or doubtful reactions. This figure is comparable to the incidence of nonreactivity in several series of patients with pulmonary tuberculosis.

The message thus is clear: *the lack of a positive skin test does not allow the physician to exclude active tuberculous—including extrapulmonary—disease.*

General features of XPTB

General manifestations including weight loss, fatigue, malaise, fever, and diaphoresis may or may not be present in patients with XPTB. XPTB has a tendency to be mild in relation to the extent and severity of the tuberculous process. "Cold" abscesses and draining sinuses are common with bone or joint disease.

MILIARY TUBERCULOSIS

Miliary tuberculosis appears to occur in two general settings: (1) rapid spread in a young, immunologically naive subject shortly after the primary infection and (2) late or delayed dissemination in a host infected years before whose immunity has been compromised by a withering process (yet undefined) associated with aging or by specific immunologic alterations associated with various diseases (e.g., Hodgkin's and other lymphoproliferative diseases, leukemia, and some solid tumors) or immunosuppressive therapy. Although miliary tuberculosis tends to involve the extremes of age groups, the disease may attack patients of any age. Recent reviews have identified an increase in the average age of patients with miliary tuberculosis, a disparately high incidence among blacks, and a striking tendency for the disease to appear with subtle, cryptic manifestations. Patients may offer a variety of complaints including weakness, fatigue, anorexia, weight loss, fever, chills, sweats, headache, and abdominal pain; most of these symptoms are nonspecific and not particularly helpful in making the diagnosis. However, as pointed out by Sahn and Neff, the presence of headache or abdominal pain in such patients appears to be significantly associated with associated meningeal or peritoneal disease, respectively.

The term *miliary* refers to the millet seed size of the diffuse, finely nodular shadows usually seen on the chest radiograph. However, it is important to realize that symptoms may precede or follow the radiographic discovery of miliary TB; the film may also reveal extremely subtle abnormalities that defy recognition, even in retrospect, or unusual abnormalities including pleural effusions, hilar adenopathy, localized parenchymal lesions, and even noncardiogenic pulmonary edema (ARDS). Classic miliary changes alone were seen in only 50%, 66%, and 85% of patients in 3 recent series. In the USPHS survey of XPTB, among those cases of miliary tuberculosis for whom subsites of disease were reported, 248 of 574 (43%) patients were designated as "miliary nonpulmonary"; presumably these patients did not have radiologically detectable involvement of the lungs. *The presence of a normal chest radiograph or one with atypical findings should not exclude consideration of miliary tuberculosis in an otherwise suggestive clinical setting.*

The intermediate strength tuberculin skin test will be negative or doubtful in roughly 50% of patients with proven miliary TB. If pulmonary radiographic abnormalities are present and miliary TB is suspected, several diagnostic procedures may be helpful, including examination of sputum obtained by induction, by gastric aspiration, by transtracheal aspiration, or by fiberoptic bronchoscopy with bronchial lavage and transbronchial biopsy if necessary. Rarely, open lung biopsy may be indicated. Investigation of other organ systems or body spaces should be based on the presence of demonstrable abnormalities therein. Choice of which organ or body space to investigate first should be based upon consideration of the procedure's relative risk, the probability of a positive yield, and special therapeutic implications of finding tuberculous involvement of that area, for example, the indication for a course of steroids with tuberculous meningitis, pericarditis, or peritonitis. It should be stressed that the fluid extracted from body cavities involved with tuberculosis (cerebrospinal, pleural, pericardial, or peritoneal) usually yields highly characteristic if not diagnostic features. Bone marrow biopsy and culture is a safe, albeit painful, means of pursuing the diagnosis in patients with hematologic abnormalities. Lumbar puncture should be performed in patients with headache or altered mental status. In the presence of substantially increased intracranial pressure or focal neurologic findings suggestive of a mass lesion, a CAT scan of the brain should be obtained to exclude a tuberculoma. Liver biopsy will demonstrate abnormalities in many patients with miliary tuberculoses. However, the histologic findings may prove relatively nonspecific; early tuberculous granulomas in the liver do not undergo caseation, and many disorders (both infectious and noninfectious) may produce noncaseating granulomas of the liver.

Tuberculous *meningitis* may occur with or without the miliary disease. The onset is usually insidious with headache, behavioral changes, and progressive obtundation developing over several weeks. Focal neurologic abnormalities, including prominent cranial nerve involvement and seizures, usually signal the second phase of tuberculous meningitis. Coma is a late and ominous phase of this disease. Cerebrospinal fluid typically shows increased pressure, elevated protein, lowered glucose, and increased cells, mostly lymphocytes. When the fluid is allowed to stand, it forms a pellicle within which organisms can often be found. Treatment is usually effective but delay in starting therapy frequently results in substantial residual neurologic deficits.

Cerebral tuberculoma is usually indistinguishable from other forms of benign brain tumor.

Skin tuberculosis comes in numerous forms; these include lupus vulgaris, scrofuloderma, lupus miliaris disseminatus, tuberculosis verrucosa cutis, and erythema induratum.

The *eye* may be involved in at least two ways: *conjunctivitis,* in a very severe untreated pulmonary case, and *uveitis.*

Cervical lymph node tuberculosis—scrofula, the "king's evil"—produces matted, very firm masses fixed to the underlying structures and sometimes to the overlying skin, ultimately producing spontaneous drainage if untreated. Careful microbiology will frequently today identify the cause as scotochromogenic mycobacteria other than *M. tuberculosis.*

Tuberculous *laryngitis* used to be a dreaded complication of advanced pulmonary disease. Symptoms are hoarseness, cough, and, in advanced cases, severe dysphagia. Laryngoscopy will reveal redness, edema, and ultimately ulceration of the true cords, the arytenoids, and adjacent tissues. *Otitis media* was another rare complication of advanced lung disease.

Pleural tuberculosis is discussed in Chapter 19.

Endobronchial tuberculosis usually derives from a bathing of the bronchi in highly infected sputum; it may also arise from ulceration of an infected peribronchial node. Cough, dyspnea, wheezing, and hemoptysis are the most common symptoms. Complete bronchial obstruction with resultant atelectasis may occur. Diagnosis is made by bronchoscopy. The disease is suspected when symptoms are greater than radiographic involvement would indicate. Rarely, endobronchial tuberculosis may exist without chest radiographic abnormality.

Tuberculosis *pericardial* involvement begins with a serofibrinous effusion; however, cardiac tamponade is uncommon. Constrictive pericarditis supervenes some 2 to 5 years later in some patients. Pericardial decortication may then be needed to correct the mechanical problem despite chemotherapy.

Mediastinal tuberculous lymphadenopathy is common among infants and children with primary tuberculosis but is an unusual finding in adults. Although common among children of all races, when tuberculous hilar adenopathy is seen in adults, it occurs essentially among nonwhites. The temptation to treat hilar adenopathy presumptively in a nonwhite adult as sarcoidosis should be influenced by this knowledge. The definitive means of establishing the diagnosis in such cases is by finding the organisms or characteristic histologic features in the hilar nodes. Mediastinoscopy is usually the procedure of choice to obtain this tissue.

Intestinal tuberculosis* is most commonly located in the terminal ileum, cecum, or rectum. Rectal tuberculosis usually appears as ischiorectal abscess or fistula. Involvement in the ileocecal region may cause diarrhea or constipation, vague distress, or low-grade constitutional symptoms; diagnosis is confirmed by following the progress of barium through the area—a so-called motor meal.

Tuberculous *peritonitis* is difficult to diagnose because symptoms and signs are not very specific. Pain, abdominal masses, a "doughy" feel, and vague constitutional symptoms may be present. Diagnosis can be confirmed by peritoneal biopsy (Cope needle), peritoneoscopy, or laparotomy.

Genitourinary tuberculosis* comes in many forms. Renal tuberculosis begins with papillary ulceration that ruptures into the kidney pelvis and spreads to ureter and bladder. Symptoms are absent or mild early on; painless hematuria is a common early sign. Involvement of the ureter may cause ureteral obstruction and resultant renal destruction. Involvement of the *bladder* is apt to produce intense frequency of urination and pain. Involvement of the *prostate, seminal vesicles,* and *epididymis* may occur in men, and extension to the *ovaries, fallopian tubes,* and *uterus* may occur in women.

Skeletal tuberculosis takes many forms. Thoracolumbar spine involvement produces classic Pott's disease or kyphoscoliosis with "cold" psoas abscesses and frequent burrowing of secretions and draining sinuses. Pain is usually mild in relation to the extent and severity of the process but may result from nerve root irritation or vertebral body collapse. Other frequent sites are the hips and knees; tenosynovitis may occur. Diagnosis is suggested by the radiologic appearance—areas of boney rarefaction adjacent to areas of increased density—but can only be confirmed by obtaining secretions or tissue for careful microbiologic study.

Disseminated *lymphohematogenous* tuberculosis is a strange and fortunately uncommon manifestation of XPTB. Involvement of lymph nodes, especially the mesenteric nodes, plus at times the liver and the bone marrow, is characteristic. Symptoms are general, often mild, but with unexplained exacerbations; low-grade fever, weight loss, anorexia, and vague pains are the

---

*Transient intestinal or ureteral obstruction has occurred during the first few weeks of antituberculosis therapy, due to a Herzheimer type of reaction—temporary inflammatory swelling—in usually unsuspected lesions in these tubular organs.

most common. This rare form of XPTB should be suspected in any tuberculin-positive chronically ill patient with no clear-cut diagnostic findings.

• • •

The treatment of XPTB does not differ appreciably from that of pulmonary tuberculosis (see Chapter 13). Some physicians prefer to treat XPTB for a longer time and with perhaps more antituberculous agents. Controlled studies are few. Corticosteroid therapy may be indicated in various forms of the disease to relieve obstruction of some passage, tube, or airway (e.g., meningeal, pericardial, peritoneal).

SUGGESTED READINGS

Amerosa, J.K., Smith, R.P., Cohen, J.R., et al.: Tuberculous mediastinal lymphadenitis in the adult, Radiology **126**:365, 1978.

Ashby, M., and Grant, H.: Tuberculous meningitis treated with cortisone, Lancet **1**:65, 1955.

Baydur, A.: The spectrum of extrapulmonary tuberculosis, West. J. Med. **126**(4):253, 1977.

Bentz, R.R., Dimcheff, D.G., Nemiroff, M.J., et al.: The incidence of urine cultures positive for *Mycobacterium tuberculosis* in a general tuberculosis patient population, Am. Rev. Respir. Dis. **111**:647, 1975.

Berger, H.W., and Mejia, E.: Tuberculous pleurisy, Chest **3**:88, 1973.

Berney, S., Goldstein, M., and Bishko, F.: Clinical and diagnostic features of tuberculous arthritis, Am. J. Med. **53**:36, 1972.

Brownrigg, G.M.: Tuberculous peritonitis and salpingitis (letter), N. Engl. J. Med. **282**:1209, 1970.

Byrd, R.B., Bopp, R.K., Gracey, D.R., et al.: The role of surgery in tuberculous lymphadenitis in adults, Am. Rev. Respir. Dis. **103**:816, 1971.

Cameron, E.W.J.: Tuberculosis and mediastinoscopy, Thorax **33**:117, 1978.

Campbell, I.A., and Dyson, A.J.: Lymph node tuberculosis: a comparison of various methods of treatment, Tubercle **58**:171, 1977.

Christensen, W.I.: Genitourinary tuberculosis: review of 102 cases, Medicine **53**:377, 1974.

Cromartie, R.S., III: Tuberculous peritonitis, Surg. Gynecol. Obstet. **144**:876, 1977.

Emond, R.T.D., and McKendrick, G.D.W.: Tuberculosis as the cause of transient aseptic meningitis, Lancet **2**:234, 1973.

Extrapulmonary tuberculosis in the United States, DHEW pub. no. (CDC) 78-8360, Washington, DC, 1978, Department of Health, Education and Welfare.

Gelb, A.F., Leffler, C., and Brewin, A., et al.: Miliary tuberculosis, Am. Rev. Respir. Dis. **108**:1327, 1973.

Gooi, H.C., and Smith, J.M.: Tuberculous pericarditis in Birmingham, Thorax **33**(1):94, 1978.

Grieco, M.H., and Chmel, H.: Acute disseminated tuberculosis as a diagnostic problem. A clinical study based on 28 cases, Am. Rev. Respir. Dis. **109**:554, 1974.

Gryzbowski, S., Enarson, D.A., Ashley, M.J., et al.: Extrapulmonary tuberculosis in Canada: some epidemiological, clinical, and bacteriological features (Abstract), Am. Rev. Respir. Dis. (II), **119**:402, 1979.

Hermans, P.E., Goldstein, N.P., and Wellman, W.E.: Mollaret's meningitis and differential diagnosis of recurrent meningitis, Am. J. Med. **52**:128, 1972.

Huseby, J.S., and Hudson, L.D.: Miliary tuberculosis and adult respiratory distress syndrome, Ann. Intern. Med. **85**:609, 1976.

Levine, H., Metzger, W., Lacera, D., et al.: Diagnosis of tuberculous pleurisy by culture of pleural biopsy specimen, Arch. Intern. Med. **126**:269, 1970.

Liu, C.I., Fields, W.R., and Shaw, C.I.: Tuberculous mediastinal lymphadenopathy in adults, Radiology **126**:369, 1978.

Marcq, M., and Sharma, O.P.: Tuberculosis of the spine: a reminder, Chest **63**:403, 1973.

Matthay, R.A., Neff, T.A., and Iseman, M.D.: Tuberculous pleural effusions developing during chemotherapy for pulmonary tuberculosis, Am. Rev. Respir. Dis. **109**:469, 1974.

Mayers, M.M., Kaufman, D.M., and Miller, M.H.: Recent cases of intracranial tuberculomas, Neurology **28**(3):256, 1978.

Munt, P.W.: Miliary tuberculosis in the chemotherapy era: with a clinical review in 69 American adults, Medicine **51**:139, 1972.

Price, H.I., and Danziger, A.: Computer tomography in cranial tuberculosis, Am. J. Roentgenol. **130**(4):769, 1978.

Rooney, J.J., Crocco, J.A., and Lyons, H.A.: Tuberculous pericarditis, Ann. Intern. Med. **72**:73, 1970.

Sahn, S.A., and Neff, T.A.: Miliary tuberculosis, Am. J. Med. **56**:495, 1974.

Scerbo, J., Keltz, H., and Stone, D.J.: A prospective study of closed pleural biopsies, J.A.M.A. **218**:377, 1971.

Sporer, A., and Auerbach, O.: Tuberculosis of prostate, Urology **11**(4):362, 1978.

Steiner, P., and Portugaleza, C.: Tuberculous meningitis in children, Am. Rev. Respir. Dis. **107**:22, 1973.

Wechsler, H., Westfall, M., and Lattimer, J.K.: The earliest signs and symptoms in 127 male patients with genitourinary tuberculosis, J. Urol. **83**:801, 1960.

Chapter 15

DISEASES CAUSED BY OPPORTUNISTIC MYCOBACTERIA

Paul T. Davidson *and* Enrique Fernandez

It is now clear that mycobacteria other than *M. tuberculosis* (MOTT) can cause significant disease in humans. Although still relatively uncommon, diseases caused by these mycobacteria make up an ever-increasing percentage of the total number of patients with mycobacterial infections, particularly in a developed country such as the United States. This is largely the result of a steadily declining incidence of *M. tuberculosis* infections and an apparent stable incidence of infection with other mycobacteria. Disease caused by MOTT is clinically similar to tuberculosis but is often more difficult to treat.

Classification and identification

As a group, the mycobacteria other than *M. tuberculosis, M. bovis,* and *M. leprae* have also been designated as *atypical mycobacteria, unclassified mycobacteria,* and *anonymous mycobacteria.* In recent years a more precise classification into species has been developed, using the morphologic, biochemical and other properties of the microorganisms. This should result in less confusion regarding terminology and allow the clinician to designate disease caused by a specific species. For the purposes of this chapter, the general designation for this group of microorganisms is opportunistic mycobacteria. Most of them are saphrophytes and only cause disease in humans under opportunistic conditions; thus the name.

In 1959 Runyon proposed a tentative classification based largely on morphologic characteristics that has been very helpful and widely used. Table 15-1 lists the four Runyon groups and the associated species. Only certain species have been linked to disease in humans. The Group I photochromogens are nonpigmented when grown in the dark but rapidly develop a carotenoid pigmentation after exposure to light. The Group II scotochromogens are pigmented even when grown in the dark. Nonpigmentation is a charac-

TABLE 15-1. Identification of mycobacteria isolated from humans

Species and Runyon group	Relative clinical significance in humans	Optimal growth temperature (°C)	Growth rate	Pigmentation in dark	Pigmentation in light	Niacin test	Nitrate reduction	Catalase > 45 mm foam[1]	Aryl-Sulfatase—3 days	Tellurite reduction
M. tuberculosis	++++	37	S	−	−	+	+	−[2]	−	−
M. bovis	++++	37	S	−	−	−	−	−	−	−
M. ulcerans	++++	30	S	−	−	−	−	+	−	−
OPPORTUNISTIC MYCOBACTERIA										
Group I										
M. kansasii	+++	37	S	−	+	−	+	+	−	−
M. marinum	+++	30	S	−	+	F	−	−	−	−
M. simiae	++	37	S	−	+	+	−	+	−	?
Group II										
M. scrofulaceum	++	37	S	+	+[4]	−	−	+	−	−
M. gordoneae	0	37	S	+	+[4]	−	−	+	−	−
M. flavescens	0	37	S	+	+[4]	−	+	+	−	F
M. szulgai	+++	37	S	+[3]	+[3]	−	+	+	F	−
Group III										
M. avium-intra-cellulare	+++	37	S	−	−	−	−	−	−	−
M. xenopi	++	42	S	+[4]	−	−	−	−	M	−
M. gastri	0	37	S	−	−	−	−	−	−	−
M. terrae com-plex	0	37	S	−	−	−	+	+	−	−
M. triviale	0	37	S	−	−	−	+	+	F	+
Group IV										
M. fortuitum	+	37	R	−	−	−	+	+	+	M
M. chelonei	+	37	R	−	−	V	−	+	+	F
M. smegmatis	0	37	R	−	−	−	+	+	−	+
M. phlei	0	37	R	+	−	−	+	+	−	M
M. vaccae	0	37	R	V	+	−	+	+	−	M

KEY: S = slow growth (10-30 days); R = rapid growth (3-7 days); V = variable; + = positive; − = negative or <16% of strains +; M = 50-84% of strains +; F = 16-49% of strains +.
1. Catalase >45 mm foam = 5+ (violent bubbling) on plate test; catalase <45 mm = 3+ (intermediate bubbling) on plate test.
2. INH-resistant strains of M. tuberculosis are often catalase negative.
3. M. szulgai is scotochromogenic when grown at 37° C, but photochromogenic when grown at 25° C.
4. Pigment may intensify after prolonged incubation or exposure to light.

teristic of the Group III nonphotochromogens. Group IV consists of rapid growing organisms that are generally nonpigmented but are characterized by their ability to show significant growth within a few days of culturing. Table 15-1 lists the opportunistic mycobacteria and some of the methods by which the various species are differentiated. Additional information is available in standard texts.

Epidemiology

The opportunistic mycobacteria have a worldwide distribution. Soil is their most common source. Water, house dust, and milk also have been implicated. Certain strains are commonly found in association with animals, particularly chickens and swine.

The means by which infection is transmitted to humans are poorly understood. The lung is the most likely portal of entry in most instances. Infection as distinguished from disease is quite common in humans, since the organisms are ubiquitous in the environment. Most people have been exposed, particularly those living in certain climates. The organisms are obviously of low virulence because disease is uncommon. Skin test data using specific antigens suggest that infection among persons living in the southeastern United States is particularly common. The incidence of disease is very low, however, for the number infected.

Direct transmission from person to person has not been documented. The public health restrictions used in patients with *M. tuberculosis* disease are therefore not applicable to the diseases discussed in this chapter.

Estimates are that the opportunistic mycobacteria cause up to 10% of all new mycobacterial infection cases diagnosed each year. In the United States this is presently some 2500 to 3000 new cases each year. Disease usually occurs sporadically. Mini-epidemics have been observed in environments where the mycobacteria could multiply freely in a closed reservoir such as a swimming pool or water storage tank. Outbreaks have also been observed in animals.

Clinical presentation

Despite the fact that the opportunistic mycobacteria are generally saprophytic, some strains may cause disease in humans. The pathophysiology of these diseases is similar to that of diseases caused by *M. tuberculosis*. Because these organisms are generally less virulent in humans than *M. tuberculosis*, the disease process tends to be more indolent and progress more slowly. Alteration of host factors probably has significant influence, since many of the patients have underlying chronic diseases and some have received immunosuppressive medications.

Any organ of the body can be diseased with these organisms. Disseminated infection occurs, although rarely, and is usually fatal. The most commonly affected organ is the lung, which will be the major concern of this discussion.

Certain strains of mycobacteria are exclusively saprophytic; others have rarely been implicated in disease. The relative clinical importance of the strains is shown in Table 15-1. *M. kansasii* and *M. avium-intracellulare* strains are by far the most common causes of disease in humans.

Diagnosis

Because the opportunistic mycobacteria are ubiquitous in the environment, a few colonies are commonly isolated from the sputum of normal people. Generally, such an isolation has no clinical significance and should be ignored. The following criteria should be applied in making a definitive diagnosis of disease caused by a strain of opportunistic mycobacteria: (1) the organism should be isolated repeatedly from the same source in large numbers, (2) the patient should have clinical evidence of disease compatible with the diagnosis, and (3) all other potential causative agents should be excluded. The clinical presentations of disease caused by the various opportunistic mycobacteria are similar in many ways. However, certain aspects are distinct and the approach to treatment and its expected results are definitely different.

M. kansasii has two unique characteristics differentiating it from most of the other opportunistic mycobacteria: (1) it is not as commonly found in the environment and (2) it usually shows good in vitro susceptibility to several antituberculosis drugs.

The disease is more common in males than in females and may occur at any age. Underlying chronic lung diseases such as COPD and pulmonary fibrosis are common. A history of antecedent spontaneous pneumothorax is frequent. Presenting symptoms are usually mild and may persist for many months. They consist of cough, expectoration, and dyspnea; fever, chills, and hemoptysis may occur but are less common.

The appearance on chest radiography is nondiagnostic. The disease looks and acts like *M. tuberculosis* infection. Bilateral involvement is common.

Progression of disease with *M. kansasii* is unpredictable. However, without treatment the disease nearly always gradually worsens. Over many months or years, the disease will gradually destroy more lung tissue, sometimes an entire lung.

M. avium-intracellulare is a widely distributed and commonly found saprophyte. Disease caused by these organisms appears to occur more commonly in rural areas of low altitude, high humidity, and soil of high organic content. All strains of *M. avium-intracellulare* are characteristically resistant in vitro to most of the antituberculosis drugs.

The disease is more common in males than in females and may occur at any age. Pulmonary disease in children is rare and is usually associated with disseminated infection. Underlying lung disease, especially COPD, is very common. The symptoms and chest radiography are indistinguishable from those of *M. tuberculosis* infections. The onset may be in association with an acute pneumonia of viral or bacterial origin.

Since the virulence of the organism for the host is unpredictable, progression of disease is also unpredictable. In some cases, the major medical problem is the underlying lung disease, the progress of which has a profound influence on the overall outcome. Some patients will remain clinically stable for many years with active infection and no treatment. Unfortunately, the majority of patients with extensive involvement will ultimately show progression of disease without treatment. Progression can be extensive. An entire lung can eventually be destroyed.

Pulmonary disease caused by *M. scrofulaceum, M. fortuitum, M. chelonei, M. simiae, M. szulgai,* and *M. xenopi* is rare. The clinical presentation and course are similar to those described for *M. kansasii* and *M. avium-intracellulare.* Because of the generally saprophytic nature of these organisms, host resistance and the presence of other lung diseases play an important role.

M. scrofulaceum is usually scotochromogenic. It causes lymph node disease more commonly than pulmonary infection.

The rapid growing mycobacterial strains *M. fortuitum* and *M. chelonei* are being reported more frequently as pathogens in humans. Skin and tissue abscesses occur and are usually secondary to injury. Pulmonary disease is rare. Bronchiectasis and rheumatoid arthritis are commonly associated. Significant underlying disease is usually present.

M. simiae, originally isolated from monkeys, has been associated with disease in humans and animals. The organisms often grow poorly in the laboratory, are photochromogenic and niacin positive, and are highly resistant to antituberculosis drugs.

M. szulgai, a recently discovered scotochromogenic mycobacterium, has been isolated thus far only from human disease, most of it pulmonary. Drug susceptibility patterns are similar to those of *M. kansasii,* and response to therapy is consequently good.

Originally isolated from a toad, *M. xenopi* is a nonchromogenic mycobacterium that grows optimally at a temperature of 42° C to 45° C and may cause pulmonary disease. The significance and incidence of this organism as a cause of disease are yet to be determined.

Treatment

It is essential to obtain reliable documentation that the cause of the disease is in fact a strain of opportunistic mycobacteria before treatment is begun. When the sputum smear is positive for acid-fast bacilli, the most likely diagnosis is infection with *M. tuberculosis.* Treatment for this disease should be initiated immediately. Waiting for culture confirmation before starting therapy is usually not warranted, especially when the patient is clinically ill. When culture results are available, a definitive diagnosis is possible. If one of the opportunistic mycobacterial species other than *M. tuberculosis* is isolated, the clinician must reassess the situation and make appropriate therapeutic changes.

The approach to therapy and the expected response differ according to the species involved. For this reason, treatment of each infection will be discussed separately.

M. kansasii is usually susceptible in vitro to rifampin, ethionamide, cycloserine, and sometimes ethambutol. Some susceptibility to higher concentrations of isoniazid, capreomycin, kanamycin, viomycin, and streptomycin may also be present. Disease frequently responds to the usual initial treatment regimen of two or three drugs used in treating *M. tuberculosis* infection in spite of the susceptibility findings. A regimen containing three drugs is recommended. Because *M. kansasii* is always initially susceptible to rifampin, it should be included in any initial treatment regimen. At the present time, the best initial regimen is a combination of rifampin, isoniazid, and ethambutol. All three drugs are continued until sputum cultures have been negative for 1 year. Two drugs are continued for a second year. Such a regimen has proven successful in better than 95% of cases.

Strains of *M. avium-intracellulare* vary in susceptibility but frequently are highly resistant to all the antituberculosis drugs. Occasionally they may be susceptible to cycloserine, rifampin, or ethionamide and less commonly to other drugs. The in vitro drug resistance suggests that response to drug therapy should be limited. This is generally the case when two or three-drug regimens are used. Occasionally a patient will respond successfully to a standard regimen despite in vitro resistance to all the drugs used, but overall results are disappointing with this approach.

Some years ago at National Jewish Hospital in Denver a five- or six-drug regimen was tried in *M. avium-intracellulare* infections. It was a surprise to discover that this method worked in approximately 75% of patients. The plan is to use as many drugs as possible that the patient has not had before, up to six in number, always including those drugs that demonstrate some degree of in vitro susceptibility. The regimen is continued until the patient's cultures have been consistently negative for at least 1 year or until drug toxicity intervenes. Three or four drugs are continued for the second year following culture conversion.

The major limiting factor of this aggressive approach is the frequent occurrence of drug toxicity. Individual drugs frequently must be discontinued or dosages altered. Careful consideration must be given to the potential benefit versus the potential toxicity of treatment. It is essential to hospitalize the patient during the introduction of the regimen and until side effects have been initially stabilized. Following discharge, the patient should be seen frequently while on five or six drugs by a physician experienced in the use of the drugs. Evidence of clinical response may be delayed for 3 to 6 months. If the patient's sputum cultures have not been consistently negative after 6 months, the drug therapy should be discontinued. Evidence of radiologic improvement is unreliable as a means of following the clinical status. Regular monitoring of the sputum culture status is the only reliable guide.

Since antituberculosis chemotherapy of these infections has limited efficacy, resection of localized disease in subjects who can undergo operation should be given early and serious consideration. A multidrug regimen should be given for several weeks before surgery and continued for many months afterward.

The treatment of disease caused by the less commonly encountered mycobacteria should be individualized. *M. szulgai* and *M. xenopi* tend to have a good degree of drug susceptibility. *M. fortuitum, M. chelonei,* and *M. simiae* are usually highly drug resistant in vitro and respond poorly to multiple antituberculous drug treatment. Recent evidence indicates that amakacin and doxycycline may be effective in treating patients with disease caused by *M. fortuitum* or *M. chelonei.*

SUGGESTED READINGS
General

Chapman, J.S.: The Atypical mycobacteria and human mycobacteriosis. New York City, 1977, Plenum Medical Book Company.
Lester, W.: Unclassified mycobacterial diseases, Annu. Rev. Med. **17**:351, 1966.
Wolinsky, E.: Nontuberculous mycobacteria and associated diseases, Am. Rev. Respir. Dis. **119**:107, 1979.

Epidemiology

Edwards, L.B., and Palmer, C.E.: Epidemiological studies of tuberculin sensitivity. I. Preliminary results with purified protein derivatives prepared from atypical acid-fast organisms, Am. J. Hyg. **68**:213, 231, 1958.
Meissner, G., and Anz, W.: Sources of mycobacterium avium complex infection resulting in human diseases, Am. Rev. Respir. Dis. **116**:1057, 1977.
Wolinsky, E., and Rynearson, T.K.: Mycobacteria in soil and their relation to disease-associated strains, Am. Rev. Respir. Dis. **97**:1032, 1968.

Specific species

Dalovisio, J.R., and Pankey, G.A.: *In vitro* susceptibility of Mycobacterium fortuitum and Mycobacterium chelonei to amikacin, J. Infect. Dis. **137**:318, 1978.
Davidson, P.T.: *Mycobacterium szulgai:* a new pathogen causing infection of the lung, Chest **69**:799, 1976.

Davidson, P.T.: Treatment and long-term follow-up of patients with atypical mycobacterial infection, Bull. Int. Union Tuberc., Vol. 51, Tome 1, pp. 257-261, 1976.

Dreisen, R.B., Scoggin, C., and Davidson, P.T.: The pathogenicity of *Mycobacterium fortuitum* and *Mycobacterium chelonei* in man: a report of seven cases, Tubercle **57:**49, 1976.

Johanson, W.G., Jr., and Nicholson, D.P.: Pulmonary disease due to *Mycobacterium kansasii:* an analysis of some factors affecting prognosis, Am. Rev. Respir. Dis. **99:**73, 1969.

Krasnow, I., and Gross, W.: *Mycobacterium simiae* infection in the United States: a case report and discussion of the organism, Am. Rev. Respir. Dis. **111:**357, 1975.

Marks, J., and Schwabacher, H.: Infection due to *Mycobacterium xenopei*, Br. Med. J. **5426:**32, 1965.

Rosenzweig, D.Y.: Pulmonary mycobacterial infection due to Mycobacterium intracellulare-avium complex, Chest **75:**115, 1979.

Yeager, H., Jr., and Raleigh, J.W.: Pulmonary disease due to *Mycobacterium intracellulare*, Am. Rev. Respir. Dis. **108:**547, 1973.

Laboratory

Kubica, G.P., Gross, W., Hawkins, J.E., et al.: Laboratory services for mycobacterial diseases, Am. Rev. Respir. Dis. **112:**773, 1975.

Vestal, A.L.: Procedures for the isolation and identification of mycobacteria, DHEW pub. no. (CDC) 75-8230, Washington, D.C., 1975, Department of Health, Education and Welfare.

Chapter 16

PULMONARY FUNGUS DISEASES

Darryl D. Bindschadler

Fungi that are pathogenic for humans are nonmotile yeasts or molds with rigid cell walls. Mycotic infections result from the organisms' direct invasion of tissue, which creates microabscesses acutely and a granulomatous inflammatory response chronically. Further spread from the initial site of infection occurs by hematogenous dissemination or by direct extension into adjacent tissues. A firm diagnosis of active infection in the individual case is made by isolation of the organism by smear, culture, or histologic demonstration. Serologic testing is most important as an epidemiologic tool. Appropriate diagnosis in a suspected case of mycotic infection thus requires careful collection of appropriate specimens and attention to laboratory demonstration of the organism.

HISTOPLASMOSIS

Histoplasmosis is caused by the dimorphic fungus *Histoplasma capsulatum*, commonly found in the mycelial saprophytic form in the soil of chicken houses, in caves inhabited by bats, and in bird droppings, especially those of starlings and blackbirds. In the United States the organism is most prevalent in the Ohio and Mississippi River valleys. It is known to have a worldwide distribution with an interesting variant in Africa caused by *H. duboisii*.

Infection results from the inhalation of spores from an environmental source and leads to several clinical states. Asymptomatic infection results in the incidental finding of multiple parenchymal and/or hilar calcifications in the chest radiograph. Acute symptomatic infection may mimic a viral upper respiratory infection with low-grade fever, generalized somatic symptoms, and dry cough that lasts from a few days to a few weeks. Soft scattered pulmonary infiltrates plus hilar and mediastinal lymphadenopathy are characteristic and usually resolve without residual structural damage or persistent clinical illness. A severe confluent pneumonia persisting for 2 to 3 months or progression to ARDS and death follows inhalation of a large number of organisms from a heavily contaminated source.

Chronic cavitary histoplasmosis is the most common form. Clinically and radiographically it resembles pulmonary tuberculosis. Progressive destruction of lung tissue and loss of pulmonary function is due to continuing active mycotic infection. Apical fibrocavitary changes, bullous emphysema, lower lobe fibrosis, volume loss due to continuous inflammation, and retraction are seen along with obstructive airways disease. Treatment with amphotericin B appears to slow progression of the chronic cavitary disease but does not significantly improve lung function. Spread to mediastinal structures can result in fibrous mediastinitis and superior vena caval obstruction. Treatment of compressing mediastinitis with antifungal agents is unsuccessful because cultures for *Histoplasma* are negative; any organisms demonstrated are either dormant or dead.

Hematogenous spread occurs frequently during the course of acute infection, as documented by the isolation of *H. capsulatum* from the patient's bone marrow or urine at the time of primary infection. Multiple splenic and adrenal calcifications and liver granulomas attest to earlier benign dissemination. Oral mucosal lesions, gastrointestinal ulceration, thrombocytopenic purpura, granulomatous hepatitis, endocarditis, peritonitis, and chronic meningitis are among the more common situations noted in patients with chronic active disseminated disease.

Histoplasmomas are healed primary pulmonary or lymph node foci of infection. Typically they have a fibrotic capsule and a caseous center that contains a calcified nodule. In adults, histoplasmomas are usually single and do not contain viable organisms. They often increase in size from less than 1 cm to 3 to 4 cm over a 10- to 25-year period. Subpleural location and concentric rings of calcification or multiple calcified centers further characterize them. Distinguishing them from neoplasia may be difficult, especially if they grow rapidly. The diagnosis of histoplasmoma cannot be reliably established by skin test or serologic results.

Histoplasmin skin test antigen is made from a culture filtrate of the mycelial form of the organism. A single dilution of 1:100 is used, and a positive test is at least 5 mm induration 48 hours after intradermal injection of 0.1 ml of the reagent. Although valuable epidemiologic information has been gained from skin testing, no one clinical situation has been further clarified by the skin test results. Furthermore, the serologic tests for histoplasmosis are often made positive by a skin test and are thus a source of confusion. A summary of available data regarding serologic tests indicates that they may suggest but can neither establish nor exclude the diagnosis of active infection.

Amphotericin B is the only currently available effective antibiotic for histoplasmosis. Initial treatment should be 1 mg intravenously to test for hypersensitivity; if negative, this should be followed by 10 mg intravenously and a daily increase of 10 mg until a daily dose of at least 0.5 mg/kg has been reached. At this point, 1.0 to 1.2 mg/kg may be given every other day. Each dose should be infused slowly over a 4- to 6-hour period. Blood urea nitrogen (BUN), serum potassium, and urinary sediment should be closely monitored to detect the nephrotoxic effect of the drug. A progressively rising BUN and/ or serum creatinine is an indication to temporarily decrease the drug dosage. Other untoward reactions include chills, fever, nausea and vomiting, local thrombophlebitis, and an occasional blood dyscrasia. Results of renal biopsy in patients with a rising BUN reveal glomerular basement membrane thick- ·ening, tubular degeneration, and nephrocalcinosis. A total of 1.5 to 2.5 gm amphotericin B has been found to be 100% effective in treating chronic pulmonary histoplasmosis. Frequent relapse of progressive disseminated disease makes any plan as to total dose or duration difficult to recommend at present. Indications for administration of the drug include continuing posi- tive cultures in individuals with chronic active pulmonary disease and all forms of disseminated disease including chronic meningitis. Acute pul- monary histoplasmosis seldom requires treatment with antifungal drugs.

Surgical therapy is reserved for resection of compressing nodes, relief of cardiac tamponade, and the occasional removal of cavities or lesions sus- picious for neoplasm that prove to be histoplasmomas.

COCCIDIOIDOMYCOSIS

Coccidioidomycosis, caused by the dimorphic fungus *Coccidioides im- mitis,* is also known as San Joaquin fever, valley fever, desert rheumatism, or "the bumps." Until recently the organism was believed to be endemic only to the lower Sonoran life zone. This area, which includes parts of New Mexico, Utah, California, Texas, and Arizona, has an arid to semiarid climate with hot summers, few winter freezes, sparse flora, low altitude, and alkaline soil. Several recent small epidemics have occurred among groups of archeology students who were digging for Indian artifacts outside of known endemic areas. Other infections are commonly acquired from fomites transported through or from an endemic location or are due to reactivation of dormant disease in former endemic area inhabitants. The current estimates of 100,000 people infected annually will undoubtedly increase as the influx of people to the sunbelt area of the United States continues. Infection is most likely to occur toward the end of the wet season in the desert when the subsoil is still damp and the surface soil is dry.

Sixty percent of those infected are asymptomatic or have mild upper respiratory infection symptomatology. The other 40% develop an influenza-like picture from 1 to 3 weeks after exposure with symptoms of cough, fever, pleuritic pain, weakness, myalgia, and arthralgia. A small percentage will develop erythema nodosum or erythema multiforme. The chest radiograph during primary infection shows small areas of infiltration, hilar adenopathy, or frank pneumonia with or without pleural effusion. Most of these findings will resolve, and full clinical recovery can be expected. Radiographic residuals include nodules that may calcify or cavities. Thin-walled cavities can be asymptomatic, can result in recurrent and sometimes severe hemoptysis, or can become secondarily infected. A small percentage of patients who appear to have inadequate cellular immune systems will progress to develop chronic pulmonary disease with persistent pneumonia, progressive cavitary changes, granulomatous disease indistinguishable from tuberculosis, bronchiectasis, empyema, or bronchopleural fistula.

Less than 1% of patients with coccidioidomycosis develop disseminated disease. Nonwhites (especially Filipinos, blacks, and American Indians), pregnant women, and immunosuppressed persons have a much higher risk of developing extrapulmonary sites of infection. Chronic meningitis, musculoskeletal involvement including bony abscesses with draining fistulae, genitourinary infection, visceral organ involvement, and skin lesions have been recognized as areas of dissemination. High complement fixing (CF) antibody titers, negative skin tests, and poor cell-mediated immune mechanisms characterize the immunologic findings in these patients.

Mycelial phase antigen, Coccidioidin, has been the standard reagent for skin testing, but the newer parasitic phase reagent, Spherulin, is just as specific and more sensitive. Skin tests are positive in almost every symptomatic patient by the end of the third week of illness. Negative skin tests correlate with a deficit in cellular immunity in the face of latent or overt dissemination. Elevated CF titers remain the most reliable serologic indicator of dissemination. Caution should be taken to have serial measurements performed by a reliable reference laboratory, since the CF test is difficult to perform with adequate reproducibility and reliability. Rising titers of CF antibody indicate continued or increased activity of infection and predict a bad prognosis, whereas falling titers correlate with improvement. Precipitating antibodies are detectable with a commercially available latex agglutination kit but have little if any practical application in the management of an individual patient.

Diagnosis can be made by demonstrating spherules in potassium hydroxide preparations of infected material, by culturing the fungus from sputum, purulent drainage, or cerebrospinal fluid, or by detecting the organism in histologic sections. The mycelial phase of the organism grows on artificial media, producing highly infectious arthrospores that pose a hazard to laboratory personnel.

Amphotericin B to a total dose of 30 mg/kg is recommended for treatment of progressive or persistent pulmonary disease (see Histoplasmosis for details). Disseminated disease with meningitis requires both intrathecal and intravenous therapy for prolonged periods to total doses up to 10 gm intravenous amphotericin B. Miconazole and transfer factor appear to offer limited help as alternatives or adjuncts to amphotericin B.

Surgical removal is necessary for enlarging cavities that despite chemotherapy cause recurrent or severe hemoptysis or may result in spread of infection to the pleura. Amphotericin B to a total dose of 1 gm given before and following surgery is part of the recommended therapeutic approach in these situations.

BLASTOMYCOSIS

Blastomycosis is caused by *Blastomyces dermatitidis*, a dimorphic fungus that enters the respiratory tract to cause infection. Blastomyces is presumed to reside in the soil, although it has been exceedingly difficult to culture from that source. Most patients appear with the disseminated stage of the disease, most commonly with pulmonary, skin, bone, and genitourinary involvement. Autopsy material has documented the presence of the organism in every body organ. The histologic demonstration of a yeast with its characteristic thick double wall and broad-based bud can be used for presumptive therapy. Confirmation is made by isolation of the fungus from pus, skin lesions, urine, or sputum or by biopsy of lung, prostate, or bone. Rarely, initial infections are asymptomatic or associated with mild respiratory symptoms that do not lead to physician contact. Symptoms and signs of pneumonia plus infiltration in the chest radiograph occur in 50% to 80% of patients. Cavity formation, hilar adenopathy, single or multilobar involvement, or consolidation can all be found. In patients with mild, self-limited primary infection the blastomycin skin test is usually positive. Otherwise, skin test and serologic data are unreliable and often misleading. All patients with active infection should be treated, preferably with intravenous amphotericin B to a total dose of 2 gm. About 90% of those treated with this regimen will become and remain disease free. An alternative, less successful, agent is 2-hydroxystilbamidine given intravenously in individual dosages of 225 mg daily to a total dose of 8 gm.

SOUTH AMERICAN BLASTOMYCOSIS

The dimorphic fungus *Paracoccidioides brasiliensis* causes this uncommonly encountered mycosis. Its geographic distribution is localized to specific areas of Latin and South America. Reported cases from other countries have always involved individuals with previous residence in the endemic area. Adult males are peculiarly disposed to this infection that typically involves mucocutaneous, lymphatic, or respiratory tissue. Pulmonary manifestations are widely variable and consist of patchy pneumonia and confluent infiltrates or nodules that involve basal and midlung areas with sparing of the apices. On culture plates as well as in histologic specimens the yeast phase of the organism has a characteristic "pilot wheel" morphology. Paracoccidioidomycosis is the only systemic fungal infection that can be successfully treated with sulfa drugs. Sulfadiazine in a daily dose of 4 to 6 gm for several months followed by 2 to 3 gm a day for 3 to 5 years (if there is initial improvement) is the suggested schedule. Intravenous amphotericin B to a total dose of 1 to 7 gm over a prolonged period is the alternative choice of therapy, but sulfa is often required as an adjunct if a cure is to be obtained.

ASPERGILLOSIS

Aspergillosis is caused by species of the ubiquitous mold *Aspergillus*. Infection caused by *Aspergillus fumigatus*, *A. flavus*, *A. niger*, and others result in (1) allergic aspergillosis, (2) invasive or disseminated infection, or (3) fungus ball. Bronchopulmonary aspergillosis is frequently a progressive disease with IgE-mediated asthma and IgG-mediated Type III parenchymal reactions. Common findings are repeated attacks of wheezing with fever, evanescent pulmonary infiltrates, bronchiolar plugging, repeated isolation of aspergilli from the sputum, eosinophilia, and a positive skin test to *Aspergillus* antigen. Serum IgG antibody levels to *Aspergillus* and total serum IgE are elevated. Central saccular bronchiectasis can often be identified in the middle or upper lung fields in the chest radiograph. Patients expectorate brown sputum plugs that contain the organisms. Colonization of the tracheobronchial tree without resulting disease occurs in patients with COPD. Colonization of lung tissue results in concentric rings of hyphae with surrounding fibrosing granulomatous inflammation or chronic nonspecific inflammatory elements. PAS or silver stains are used to demonstrate *Aspergillus* hyphae in histologic sections. Long-term therapy with oral corticosteroids plus standard antiasthma regimens are often required to control the disease process.

Disseminated aspergillosis results from vascular invasion and subsequent hemorrhagic infarction of lung, brain, kidney, heart, or liver of patients who are either primarily or secondarily immunosuppressed. Intravenous amphotericin B plus surgical excision has had limited success in controlling this stage of infection.

Fungus ball is associated with other diseases that have already produced cavities, cysts, or ectatic bronchi. Conglomerate masses of hyphae outlined by a crescent of air form the "ball." IgG antibody to the fungus is found in patients with radiographically visible aspergillomas. Surgical excision of the involved area is sometimes required for repeated episodes of hemoptysis. Other complications include bacterial lung abscess, bronchopleural fistula with fungal empyema, and spread of infection to thoracic vertebral bodies.

CRYPTOCOCCOSIS

Cryptococcosis is caused by *Cryptococcus neoformans*, a yeast that can be isolated from the excreta of pigeons and other birds. Following inhalation of the organism, multiform pulmonary lesions can develop, ranging from an asymptomatic solitary nodule to nonspecific pulmonic infiltrates, occasionally associated with pleural effusion, cavitation, and calcification. Cryptococcal pneumonia as well as bronchial colonization often occurs without subsequent spread to the CNS. Although most cases of pulmonary cryptococcosis resolve without specific therapy, some go on to develop progressive pneumonic spread while others remain clinically and radiographically stable for extended periods. Those patients who have repeated isolation of the yeast from their sputum should have their cerebrospinal fluid cultured and their CNS function monitored. Because of false-negative as well as false-positive sputum cultures, the diagnosis of pulmonary cryptococcal infection often requires lung biopsy.

Most patients who develop cryptococcosis have demonstrable cell-mediated immune defects. Whether these defects are a result of the infection or act as predisposing factors is currently not known. Repeated culture and radiographic monitoring of stable or regressive pulmonary lesions appear to be adequate unless host defense problems as seen with leukemia, lymphoma, corticosteroid, or immunosuppressive therapy coexist. At present, decisions as to when and how much amphotericin B to give in the face of inadequate host defense must be individualized.

CANDIDIASIS

Candida species commonly colonize the mouth and tracheobronchial tree in healthy subjects and are easily identified in sputum smears and cultures. *Candida* pneumonia occurs almost exclusively as a result of hematogenous dissemination from a distant site in immunocompromised patients. Radiographic findings are widely variable, ranging from finely nodular diffuse infiltrates to confluent areas suggestive of pulmonary edema. Lung biopsy remains the only reliable method of making a diagnosis of pulmonary candidiasis. Blood cultures, biopsy of suspicious skin lesions, and careful ophthalmologic examination for fluffy exudates in the anterior chamber of the eye are helpful in establishing a diagnosis. Amphotericin B with or without 5-fluorocytosine has been used successfully to treat pulmonary and disseminated infection; 5-fluorocytosine should not be used alone because of the risk of primary resistance or the emergence of resistance to that agent during treatment. Documentation of pulmonary infection should be followed promptly by the administration of antifungal therapy.

MUCORMYCOSIS

Mycoses due to organisms of the order Mucorales are most commonly due to the genera *Mucor*, *Absidia*, and *Rhizopus*. More than 75% of patients with pulmonary mucormycosis have leukemia or lymphoma, are neutropenic, and are being treated with corticosteroids. Diabetes mellitus, renal failure, burns, and immunosuppression for organ transplantation are other predisposing factors. Widely variable, nonspecific chest radiographic findings predominate with the pulmonary infarct syndrome an occasional finding. Demonstration of these fungi by sputum examination or culture should be confirmed by histologic examination of tissue obtained by fiberoptic bronchoscopy with brush biopsy, transbronchial lung biopsy, or open lung biopsy. Distinguishing the hyphae of *Mucor* from *Aspergillus* in tissue sections is difficult. Disseminated infection frequently originates in a pulmonary focus and results in CNS infarction and abscesses. Systemic amphotericin B and surgical removal of accessible foci along with control of chronic acidosis and reversal of immunosuppression are all necessary for successful treatment. It has been suggested that amphotericin B be started empirically in immunosuppressed individuals before the diagnosis is firmly established.

SPOROTRICHOSIS

Sporothrix schenckeii causes lymphocutaneous disease in 75% of reported cases. Pulmonary sporotrichosis is rare and generally occurs following inhalation of the organism and not secondary to hematogenous dissemination. The most common radiographic findings are upper lobe involvement with a smoldering process that may progress to thin-walled cavities, nodules, or fibrosis. Most cases are initially misdiagnosed as being due to tuberculosis, histoplasmosis, or coccidioidomycosis. Histologic confirmation is difficult because of the variability of appearance of the organism in tissue sections. Intravenous amphotericin B to a total dose of 1.5 to 2.5 gm is the treatment of choice.

ACTINOMYCOSIS AND NOCARDIOSIS

Actinomycosis and nocardiosis, until recently grouped with fungus infections, are due to higher bacteria, either aerobic or anaerobic *Actinomyces*. In addition to other characteristics that distinguish these organisms from fungi, their growth is inhibited by antibiotics and not by amphotericin B. Most human actinomycosis is caused by *Actinomyces israelii*, a facultative or anaerobic, filamentous, gram-positive bacterium. Pulmonary involvement follows aspiration of infected oral material from cervicofacial or dental infection and rarely is secondary to diaphragmatic penetration of abdominal infection. Normal tissue planes are regularly crossed by the infectious process, creating empyema, chest wall fistula, or mediastinitis.

The diagnosis of actinomycosis is rarely made by routine sputum examination and only becomes apparent when the organism is isolated from exudates obtained from an area of secondary spread. Suggestive radiographic findings include extension of pulmonary lesions through the chest wall, destruction of ribs or other adjacent bony structures, infiltrates that cross interlobar fissures, and vertebral erosion from posterior chest structures. Superior vena caval obstruction and tracheoesophageal fistula have also been described.

"Sulfur granules" are large aggregate masses of *Actinomyces* that are rarely seen today, partially because of the widespread use of antibiotics in earlier stages of infection. Similar conglomerates of other fungi are seen in other mycoses or with infection due to *Nocardia*, *Streptomyces*, or *Staphylococcus*.

Intravenous Penicillin G, 10 to 20 million U daily for 4 to 6 weeks, followed by oral phenoxymethyl penicillin, 2 to 4 gm daily for 6 to 12 months, will cure most severe infections. Occasional failures require alternative antibiotic schedules. Appropriate surgical excision or drainage can play an important role in successful treatment.

Nocardia species are soil-born, aerobic, partially acid-fast actinomycetes that enter the body through the respiratory tract. Most infections are opportunistic in patients with a predisposing condition such as lymphoreticular malignancy, long-term high-dose corticosteroid usage, pulmonary alveolar proteinosis, bronchiectasis, Cushing's disease, or dysglobulinemia or in transplant recipients. Bronchopneumonia progressing rapidly to consolidation, multiple widespread cavities, and early pleural involvement are radiographic clues to *Nocardiosis*. Dissemination occurs from the lung to the CNS, heart, or pericardium or to retroperitoneal or subcutaneous structures. Occasionally multiple organ miliary infection is found. No serologic or skin test methods are currently available to help with documentation of infection.

Sulfadiazine in doses to maintain plasma levels of 8 to 16 mg/100 ml and surgical drainage remain the best current recommendations for treatment.

Antibiotics often must be continued for many months beyond the minimal 6 weeks recommended because of the tendency for relapse or late appearance of abscesses in previously uninvolved areas. Infection due to other opportunistic organisms can complicate the course of illness. Mortality is estimated at 15% in patients without underlying disease and much higher in those receiving corticosteroids or immunosuppressive drugs.

SUGGESTED READINGS

Drutz, D.J., and Catanzaro, A.: Coccidioidomycosis, Am. Rev. Respir. Dis. **117:**559, 727, 1978.

Goodwin, R.A., Jr., and DesPrez, R.M.: Histoplasmosis, Am. Rev. Respir. Dis. **117:**929, 1978.

Hammerman, K.J., Powell, K.E., Christianson, C.S., et al.: Pulmonary cryptococcosis: clinical forms and treatment, Am. Rev. Respir. Dis. **108:**1116, 1973.

Mandell, G.L., Douglas, R.G., Jr., and Bennett, J.E., editors: Principles and practice of infectious disease, vol. 2, section F, New York City, 1979, John Wiley & Sons, Inc., pp. 1962-2080.

Medoff, G., and Kobayashi, G.S.: Strategies in the treatment of systemic fungal infections, N. Engl. J. Med. **302:**145, 1980.

Sarosi, G.A., Hammerman, K.J., Tosh, F.E., et al.: Clinical features of acute pulmonary blastomycosis, N. Engl. J. Med. **290:**540, 1974.

Weese, W.C., and Smith, I.M.: A study of 57 cases of actinomycosis over a 36-year period, Arch. Intern. Med. **135:**1562, 1975.

Chapter 17

BRONCHIECTASIS

Roger S. Mitchell

Definition

The term *bronchiectasis* means simply dilation of the bronchi, but in general usage it also implies the destruction of bronchial walls. *Saccular* bronchiectasis is the classic advanced form characterized by irregular dilatations and narrowings. The term *cystic* is used when the dilatations are especially large and numerous. *Tubular* bronchiectasis is simply the absence of normal bronchial tapering and is usually a manifestation of severe chronic bronchitis rather than of true bronchial wall destruction.

Etiology

The causes of bronchiectasis include repeated or prolonged episodes of pneumonitis, especially those complicating pertussis or influenza during childhood; this is particularly true when these illnesses have been neglected or inadequately treated and are slow to resolve. Bronchial obstruction caused by neoplasm or the inhalation of a foreign body may also result in bronchiectasis. When the bronchiectatic process involves most or all of the bronchial tree, whether in one or both lungs, it is believed to be genetic or developmental in origin.

Mucoviscidosis, Kartagener's syndrome (bronchiectasis with dextrocardia and paranasal sinusitis), and agammaglobulinemia are all examples of inherited or developmental diseases associated with bronchiectasis. The term *pseudobronchiectasis* is applied to cylindric bronchial widening, which may complicate a pneumonitis but which disappears after a few months. *Dry bronchiectasis* is true saccular bronchiectasis but without cough or expectoration; it is located especially in the upper lobes where good dependent drainage is available. A proximal form of bronchiectasis (with normal distal airways) complicates aspergillous mucus plugging.

Most cases of bronchiectasis are accompanied by severe chronic bronchitis, which is really the other extreme of a wide clinical spectrum of

177

bronchial disease. Advanced bronchiectasis is often accompanied by anastomoses between the bronchial and pulmonary vessels; these cause right-to-left shunts, with resulting hypoxemia, pulmonary hypertension, and cor pulmonale.

Clinical picture

The principal clinical feature of bronchiectasis is a chronic, loose cough, productive usually of large amounts of mucopurulent, often foul-smelling sputum. In advanced cases the sputum settles out into three layers: cloudy mucus on top, clear saliva in the middle, and cloudy purulent material on the bottom. It is frequently associated with chronic paranasal sinusitis. Hemoptysis, occasionally severe, sooner or later occurs in at least half of all cases. Frequent bronchopulmonary infections and, as the case advances, chronic malnutrition, sinusitis, clubbing, cor pulmonale, and right heart

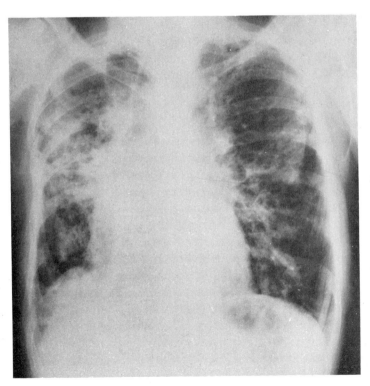

FIG. 17-1. Advanced bilateral bronchiectasis, right more than left. Note scattered small cavities, some with fluid levels. *(Courtesy Medical Illustration Service, Veterans Administration Hospital, Denver, Colorado.)*

failure are characteristic features of advanced untreated disease. Physical signs are variable; rales are present at times. The plain chest radiograph is not too helpful, except when recognizable dilations containing tiny air-fluid levels are present (Fig. 17-1).

Diagnosis

The diagnosis of bronchiectasis can often be made from the history alone. It is confirmed in patients being considered for surgery by bronchography, which should only be performed in these patients after the use of vigorous bronchial hygiene, postural drainage, and a course of antimicrobial therapy for at least 1 week. Bronchography should include every lung segment, but both lungs should not be studied at one time in patients with significantly impaired pulmonary function. The principal indication for bronchography is in patients with known or suspected bronchiectasis who are being considered for resection and who can tolerate the resection of at least one lobe or more. Occasionally, bronchography is used in patients who are candidates for pulmonary surgery to localize the lesion to be resected.

Iodized oil and iodine in water have been the standard contrast media for many years. Powdered tantalum appears to offer a reliable substitute without risk of iodine hypersensitivity.

Bronchoscopy in bronchiectasis often reveals a velvety deep red mucosa and pus welling up from the areas of involvement. Gram stains of sputum often show a variety of organisms, especially the fusospirochetal organisms. Cultures also reveal a variety of nonspecific organisms including the common mouth flora, anaerobic streptococci, and many others. Microscopic examination of the sputum may reveal necrotic elastic tissue, muscle fibers, and epithelial debris.

Treatment

The most important feature of the treatment of bronchiectasis is regular, daily, vigorous bronchial hygiene, with postural drainage, generally continued for the rest of the patient's life (see Chapter 10). Antimicrobial therapy for periods of 7 to 10 days may be helpful in the management of acute exacerbations of bronchiectasis. Prolonged, and especially multiple, antimicrobial drug therapy tends to eliminate the drug-susceptible organisms, allowing drug-resistant organisms to multiply in the irreversibly ulcerated bronchi, and thus should be avoided. Local treatment of an accompanying purulent sinusitis is also important. Successful resection of bronchiectactic segments or lobes depends on the unequivocal demonstration of irreversible involvement of localized areas plus freedom from involvement of all other parts of both lungs. Palliative surgery is seldom beneficial, except in patients with severe symptoms including recurrent hemoptysis, for example, a severe process in one portion with only mild changes elsewhere. Resection in bronchiectasis is always an elective procedure and should be postponed until all efforts at medical management have failed; results of surgical treatment so planned are highly successful.

Except for the congenital forms of the disease, bronchiectasis should be regarded as a preventable disease. A child who inhales a foreign body should have it immediately removed by bronchoscopy or surgery if necessary. Vigorous antimicrobial and other appropriate treatment for all forms of pneumonia will greatly reduce the frequency of complicating bronchiectasis. Timely vaccination against measles, pertussis, and other childhood diseases commonly complicated by pneumonia is also a preventive measure.

Complications and prognosis

Complications include chronic bronchitis, pneumonia with or without atelectasis, cor pulmonale, metastatic brain abscess, empyema, and amyloidosis.

The prognosis of severe untreated bronchiectasis is poor, generally with no more than 10 to 15 years of survival; death is generally a result of pneumonia, empyema, right heart failure, or exsanguinating hemorrhage. The outlook has been greatly improved by the appropriate use of antimicrobial therapy during periods of exacerbation.

SUGGESTED READINGS

Bass, H., Henderson, J.A.M., Heckscher, T., et al.: Regional structure and function in bronchiectasis: a correlative study using bronchography and ^{133}Xe, Am. Rev. Respir. Dis. **97**:598, 1968.

Baum, G.L., Racz, I., Bubis, J.J., et al.: Cystic disease of the lung: report of 88 cases, with an ethnologic relationship, Am. J. Med. **40**:578, 1966.

Fine, A., and Baum, G.L.: Long-term follow-up of bronchiectasis, Lancet **86**:505, 1966.

Fleshman, J.K., Wilson, J.F., and Cohen, J.J.: Bronchiectasis in Alaska native children, Arch. Environ. Health **17**:517, 1968.

Glauser, E.M., Cook, C.D., and Harris, G.B.: Bronchiectasis: a review of 187 cases in children with follow-up pulmonary function studies in 58, Acta Paediatr. Scand. Suppl. **165**:1, 1966.

Jaffe, H.J., and Katz, S.: Current ideas about bronchiectasis, Am. Family Phys. **7**:69, 1973.

Konietzko, J.F.J., Carton, R.W., and Leroy, E.P.: Causes of death in patients with bronchiectasis, Am. Rev. Respir. Dis. **100**:852, 1969.

Nadel, J.A., Wolfe, W.G., Graf, P.D., et al.: Powdered tantalum: a new contrast medium for roentgenographic examination of human airways, N. Engl. J. Med. **283**:281, 1970.

Phillips, F.J., Lalli, A., and Buhler, W.: Bronchographic studies as a guide to the surgical treatment of pulmonary tuberculosis, J. Thorac. Cardiovasc. Surg. **32**:820, 1956.

Sealy, W.C., Bradham, R.R., and Young, W.G., Jr.: The surgical treatment of multisegmental and localized bronchiectasis, Surg. Gynecol. Obstet. **123**:80, 1966.

Woolcock, A.J., and Blackburn, C.R.: Chronic lung disease in the territory of Papua and New Guinea: an epidemiological study, Ann. Med. **16**:11, 1967.

Chapter 18

LUNG ABSCESS

Roger S. Mitchell

Definition and etiology

A lung abscess is a circumscribed suppurative inflammation followed by central tissue necrosis, indistinguishable in its early stages from any localized pneumonitis. Only after it has communicated with a bronchus and started to drain will the characteristic air-fluid level be seen within the area of inflammation.

Single lung abscesses usually arise from suppurative inflammation behind a bronchial obstruction or after aspiration. The following may cause an obstruction: (1) aspirated foreign material such as food, blood, pieces of tonsil or teeth, or vomitus—the aspiration often occurs during surgery on the throat, teeth, or sinuses, or during unconsciousness resulting from alcoholism, oversedation, or an epileptic seizure, (2) benign or malignant tumors, or (3) inspissated bronchial mucus. Single lung abscess may also result from superinfection of a cavitated infarct or from metastasis of amebiasis from the liver, most commonly into the right lower lobe. A malignant tumor may cavitate because of tissue necrosis, that is, by outgrowing its blood supply.

Multiple lung abscesses may be a feature of hematogenous dissemination of *Staphylococcus, Klebsiella pneumoniae*, or other necrotizing organisms. Multiple abscesses may be caused by septic emboli arising from infected foci or septic phlebitis, especially in association with some coexistent chronic debilitating condition such as alcoholism, cirrhosis, congestive heart failure, or malnutrition. Lung abscesses also commonly occur in the clinical setting of immunosuppressive therapy, as in organ transplantation.

Single abscesses may be putrid or nonputrid. Multiple abscesses are almost always nonputrid. Putrid abscesses are virtually always associated with carious teeth, infected gums, and alcoholism and are usually located in the posterior segments of either the upper or lower lobes. Putrid abscesses are caused by many different organisms, especially anaerobic streptococci, *Bacteroides*, and fusospirochetes.

181

Pathology

During its early acute phase the pathology of lung abscess does not differ noticeably from that of ordinary pneumonia. As the pneumonia progresses, it fails to heal; ultimately, necrosis involving all elements of lung tissue occurs. As an abscess becomes chronic (present for 6 weeks or more), it may spread to and destroy adjacent tissue or it may empty and the wall lining its cavity may become partially covered with regenerated epithelium.

Clinical picture

The early symptoms, physical findings, and chest radiograph of lung abscess are similar to those of any acute severe bronchopneumonia: fever, chills, prostration, pleuritic pain, cough, and leukocytosis. When the abscess ruptures into a bronchus, the patient begins to cough up copious amounts of purulent, often foul-smelling and foul-tasting sputum. When the sputum is foul, it is generally the result of infection with mixed flora, especially the

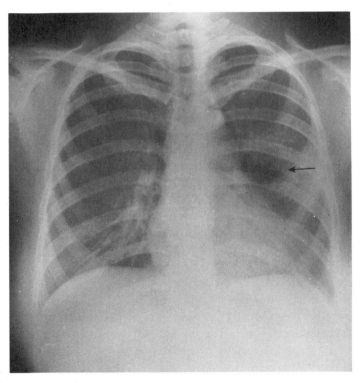

FIG. 18-1. Left lobar (lingular) pneumonia with abscess cavity (near left hilum). *(Courtesy Medical Illustration Service, Veterans Administration Hospital, Denver, Colorado.)*

fusospirochetes and anaerobic organisms. Rarely, a peripherally located abscess ruptures primarily into the pleura, causing an empyema. Multiple abscesses may or may not drain into a bronchus or the pleural space. The early use of inadequate antimicrobial therapy is likely to modify the course temporarily. Hemoptysis is a common feature, especially at the time of rupture into a bronchus. When a lung abscess has become chronic, severe debility, pulmonary osteoarthropathy (clubbing), and even secondary amyloidosis may occur.

The physical findings are those of pneumonia in the early stages; only after the development of a large air-containing cavity will the signs of cavitation (amphoric breath sounds and consonating rales) be found.

Diagnosis

The diagnosis of lung abscess usually presents no difficulty. The chest radiograph is typical (Figs. 18-1 and 18-2). The differential diagnosis should

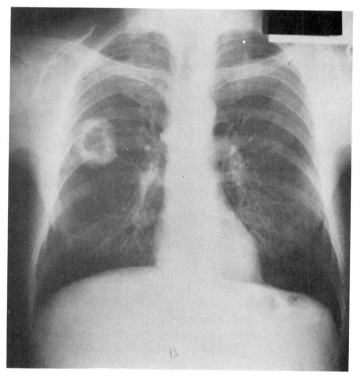

FIG. 18-2. Primary bronchogenic carcinoma: large, irregularly outlined right lung mass with thick-walled cavity. *(Courtesy Medical Illustration Service, Veterans Administration Hospital, Denver, Colorado.)*

include primary and metastatic neoplasms, tuberculosis, fungus diseases, actinomycosis, nocardiosis, bronchiectasis, pulmonary infarction, pneumonia, aseptic necrosis of a tumor or silicoma, and secondary infection of an emphysematous bulla or cyst. Precise identification is often difficult—the cultures are usually mixed and often include anaerobes; it is sometimes impossible to be sure of the responsible organism(s). Previous antibiotics will often have been given.

Treatment

Regardless of the organisms originally identified in the sputum, the initial treatment of lung abscess, especially the putrid variety, should be 2 to 6 million U crystalline penicillin G intravenously daily; 600,000 U procaine penicillin G intramuscularly every 6 hours for 4 weeks may be sufficient in milder cases. Penicillin by mouth may be effective in simple lung abscesses, especially after initial improvement has occurred. In the presence of serious penicillin hypersensitivity, clindamycin 600 mg 4 times daily, lincomycin 600 mg intramuscularly every 6 hours, or erythromycin 2 gm/day may also be used. Some observers are in favor of adding streptomycin 1 gm intramuscularly daily for at least the first 7 to 10 days or tetracycline 2 gm daily for 3 to 5 days, then 1 gm daily. The temptation to modify therapy in accordance with the sputum bacteriology and susceptibility tests should be resisted in patients who are doing well. Therapy should be continued for at least a week after complete symptomatic and radiographic control has been achieved.

If *Staphylococcus aureus* is found and believed to be the causative agent, the patient should receive intravenous methicillin, or an equivalent drug such as nafcillin, 8 to 16 gm daily, *if* penicillin resistant. Vancomycin, 500 mg intravenously every 6 hours, is an effective antistaphylococcus drug but has significant toxicity and probably should not be used. Antimicrobial treatment should be continued in such cases for at least 2 to 3 months, sometimes even longer.

If *Klebsiella* organisms are found and believed to be the causative agent, the initial therapy should include kanamycin, 15 mg/kg/day intramuscularly in 2 or 3 divided doses, the total dose being decreased if renal insufficiency is present or appears. Antibiotic susceptibility studies may allow the use of a less toxic antibiotic or suggest the need for a different aminoglycoside.

When *Pseudomonas* is clearly the causative organism, gentamycin or tobramycin should be used.

Penicillin is useful for most *Bacteroides* infections that are causally related to lung abscesses, although penicillin-resistant bacteroides have been identified in this setting and may require tetracycline, clindamycin, or chloramphenicol.

Bronchoscopy, if performed early, is helpful in removing any foreign matter that may be obstructing the bronchus and permits the application of suction to the orifice of the bronchus leading to the involved area of the lung in the hope of initiating or improving drainage of the abscess contents. The procedure may also detect a tumor if one is present.

Postural drainage may be helpful. Vigorous bronchial hygiene is often useful. Surgical drainage of an abscess through the chest wall is seldom if ever indicated today. Surgical extirpation should be postponed until it is clear that the abscess will not heal or if the possibility of an associated malignant tumor is high.

Lung abscess may often be prevented by following certain practices. Tonsillectomy, tooth extraction, and paranasal sinus operations should be performed under local rather than general anesthesia and under penicillin and/or other appropriate antibiotic coverage, especially in overtly infected cases. When any foreign material is inhaled during these procedures or under any circumstances, the inhaled material should be promptly removed by bronchoscopy; empiric therapy with corticosteroids and penicillin should be instituted. Prompt and appropriate antimicrobial management of acute bacterial pneumonias or any severe infection that could lead to a bacteremia and the maintenance of good oral hygiene should all reduce the risk of occurrence of lung abscess.

Complications and prognosis

The complications of lung abscess include pleural effusion; empyema; bloodstream dissemination, especially to the brain; fatal pulmonary hemorrhage; and, after a period of continued suppuration, the development of localized bronchiectasis, recurrent pneumonia in the surrounding lung, and amyloidosis.

The prognosis of lung abscess has improved in recent years, but a 15% to 20% mortality is still seen in single lung abscess and a 50% mortality occurs in the multiple, hematogenous abscesses. Advanced age, debility, and alcoholism and other chronic diseases are unfavorable accompanying features.

SUGGESTED READINGS

Bartlett, J.G., Garbach, S.L., Talley, F.P., et al.: Bacteriology and treatment of primary lung abscess, Am. Rev. Respir. Dis. **109**:510, 1974.

Bartlett, J.G., and Garbach, S.L.: Treatment of aspiration pneumonia and primary lung abscess, J.A.M.A. **234**:935, 1975.

Bigelow, D.B., and Mitchell, R.S.: Lung abscess. In Conn, H.F., and Conn, R.B., Jr., editors: Current diagnosis, Philadelphia, 1971, W.B. Saunders Co.

Brock, R.C.: Lung abscess, Baltimore, 1952, The Williams & Wilkins Co.

Flavell, G.: Lung abscess, Br. Med. J. **1:**1032, 1966.

Perlman, L.V., Lerner, E., and D'Esopo, N.: Clinical classification and analysis of 97 cases of lung abscess, Am. Rev. Respir. Dis. **99:**390, 1969.

Petty, T.L., and Mitchell, R.S.: Suppurative lung diseases, Med. Clin. N. Am. **51:**529, 1967.

Schweppe, H.I., Knowles, J.H., and Kane, L.: Lung abscess: an analysis of the Massachusetts General Hospital cases from 1943 through 1956, N. Engl. J. Med. **265:**1039, 1961.

Shafron, R.D., and Tate, C.F., Jr.: Lung abscesses: a five-year evaluation, Dis. Chest **53:**12, 1968.

Strieder, J.W.: Surgical management of pulmonary abscess and empyema, Am. J. Surg. **107:**683, 1964.

Chapter 19

PLEURAL EFFUSIONS

Steven A. Sahn

Pleural effusions are common findings in the practice of clinical medicine. A thorough knowledge of the physiology of fluid formation and the chemistry of the fluid in conjunction with the history and physical examination will enable the physician to determine the etiology of the effusion in a high percentage of cases. In most instances the diagnosis will be presumptive; only in malignancy, empyema, or lupus erythematosus will the diagnosis be definitive.

Physiology of formation of normal pleural fluid

The passage of fluid across the pleural membrane in healthy humans depends on the sum of opposing hydrostatic and osmotic pressures. Knowledge of the magnitude of these forces suggests that fluid is formed at the parietal pleural surface and absorbed at the surface of the visceral pleura (Fig. 19-1). Approximately 10 to 20 ml of low-protein fluid is found in each normal pleural space.

Conditions under which pleural fluid develops

Abnormal amounts of fluid may accumulate when one or more of the following changes occurs: (1) increase in hydrostatic pressure, (2) decrease in colloid osmotic pressure, (3) increase in capillary permeability, (4) increase in intrapleural negative pressure, and (5) decrease in lymphatic drainage. Increased hydrostatic pressure causes the pleural transudation that occurs in congestive heart failure, while increased capillary permeability causes inflammatory and neoplastic effusions. Decreased osmotic pressure is seen in severe hypoalbuminemia or with massive hypotonic fluid overload, while increased intrapleural negative pressure causes effusions that occur with major atelectasis. Impaired lymphatic drainage from mediastinal tumor involvement is the primary mechanism responsible for the formation of pleural fluid in malignancy. The ultimate fate of pleural fluid is also influenced by the absorptive capacity of the pleural lymphatics.

Clinical picture

The symptoms that cause a patient to see a physician are seldom caused by the effusion itself but by the underlying disease process. However, a large effusion may compress enough lung tissue to cause exertional dyspnea.

When a pleural effusion occurs, the lung is separated from the chest wall by a layer of fluid that interferes with sound transmission. The signs of a pleural effusion vary depending on the degree of lung compression and displacement and the amount of fluid present in the pleural space. Sounds are

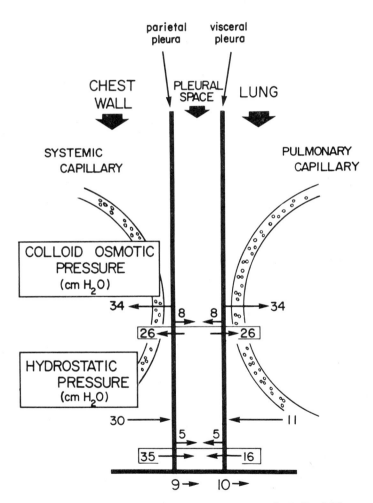

FIG. 19-1. Pleural fluid dynamics. *(Courtesy Division of Medical Photography, University of Colorado Medical Center, Denver, Colorado.)*

altered if bronchial obstruction or consolidation of the underlying lung tissue is present. These physical signs are summarized in Table 19-1.

Free pleural fluid has a characteristic appearance on the upright chest radiograph in the absence of pleural disease (Fig. 19-2). It has a ground glass density through which lung markings can frequently be seen near the medial

TABLE 19-1. Physical signs of pleural effusion

Amount of fluid (cc)	Expansion	Fremitus	Percussion	Breath sounds	Contralateral midsternal shift
<300	Normal	+	Normal	v	0
300-1000	↓	↓	f	↓ v	0
1000-2000	↓ ↓	↓ ↓	f	↓ ↓ bv	+
>2000	↓ ↓ ↓	0	f	0	++

KEY: ↓ = decreased; f = flat; v = vesicular; bv = bronchovesicular; 0 = absent; + = present.

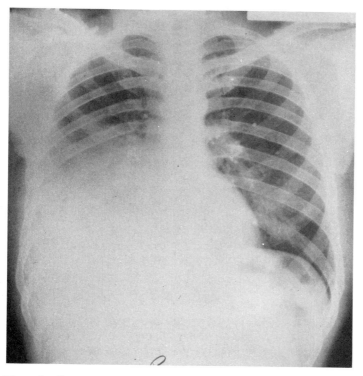

FIG. 19-2. Pleural effusion, right, recent. *(Courtesy Medical Illustration Service, Veterans Administration Hospital, Denver, Colorado.)*

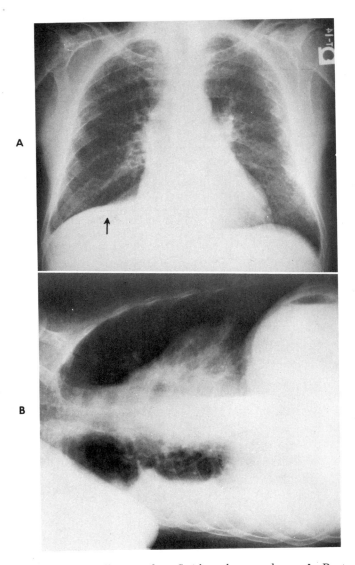

FIG. 19-3. Subpulmonic effusion: free fluid under one lung. **A,** Posteroanterior. **B,** Confirmed by ipsilateral decubitus film. *(Courtesy Medical Illustration Service, Veterans Administration Hospital, Denver, Colorado.)*

margin. The upper margin forms a meniscus (concave upward) at the lateral chest wall. Small effusions may reveal only a blunting of the costophrenic angle; effusions of approximately 300 cc or more in the adult are detectable on the upright chest radiograph. A lateral decubitus film, however, will demonstrate lesser amounts of free fluid. Occasionally, more than 300 cc of fluid will be situated between the bottom of the lung and diaphragm (subpulmonic effusion), which again is easily demonstrated in the lateral decubitus position (Fig. 19-3). Fluid may loculate in the pleural space, especially in the interlobar areas, and produce rounded densities or so-called *pseudotumors*.

Diagnosis

When the diagnosis of a pleural effusion is established radiographically and localized by physical examination, a diagnostic thoracentesis should be performed. In cases of obvious, uncomplicated congestive heart failure and other situations in which the clinical diagnosis is secure and the amount of pleural fluid is small, continued observation without thoracentesis is warranted. When the thoracentesis is performed, certain observations should be made and the fluid analyzed in a systematic manner. Fluid color, odor, and character should be noted. Results of the following tests should be noted depending on the clinical situation: red cell count; white cell count with differential; protein; sugar; lactic dehydrogenase (LDH); amylase; pH; Wright, Gram, and acid-fast bacilli (AFB) stains; aerobic, anaerobic, tuberculosis, and fungal cultures; and cytology.

Analysis of pleural fluid

Observation. Transudative fluids and some exudates are clear and straw colored. Additional hints from simple observation include a white, milky color suggesting chylothorax, a reddish tinge indicating blood, and an anchovy color found in an amebic liver abscess that ruptures into the pleural space. Elevated white cell counts and increased amounts of lipids make pleural fluid turbid. Pus aspirated from the pleural space confirms the diagnosis of empyema. Anaerobic empyemas have a characteristic foul odor. A very bloody viscous fluid suggests a malignant mesothelioma.

Leukocytes. If the patient's leukocyte count is greater than $1000/\mu l$ the fluid is likely exudative. Neutrophils generally predominate early in effusions associated with inflammation such as pneumonia, pulmonary infarction, pancreatitis, and subphrenic abscess. Lymphocytes are the predominant cell in transudative pleural effusions, but also are the predominant cell in chronic exudates (tuberculosis, lymphoma, carcinoma, uremic pleurisy, and rheumatoid pleurisy). Eosinophils (over 10%) in the pleural fluid suggest no specific diagnosis but offer certain helpful information. The presence of pleural fluid eosinophilia makes the diagnosis of tuberculosis unlikely. These cells are usually found in the presence of blood or air in the pleural space. When eosinophils are in abundance in parapneumonic effusions, it suggests that the fluid will not progress to an empyema. Pleural fluid eosinophilia may also be found in pulmonary infarction, polyarteritis nodosa, and parasitic and fungal diseases.

Erythrocytes. An erythrocyte count of 5000 to 10,000/μl causes pleural fluid to appear hemorrhagic. When a pleural fluid is grossly hemorrhagic in the absence of trauma, malignancy must be carefully ruled out. When the red cell count is greater than 100,000/μl, the diagnosis of malignancy, trauma, or pulmonary infarction should be strongly considered. It is quite rare to find a transudate or a tuberculous effusion that is grossly bloody. Congestive heart failure with a bloody effusion should raise the possibility of pulmonary infarction, although 10% of pleural effusions secondary to congestive heart failure alone may be serosanguinous.

Glucose. Pleural fluid glucose is helpful in the following situations: (1) rheumatoid pleural effusions almost always have a pleural fluid glucose less than 30 mg/100 ml and (2) other entities sometimes associated with low pleural fluid glucose (range 0 to 60 mg/100 ml) are empyema, carcinoma, tuberculosis, and rheumatoid and lupus pleurisy. The mechanism by which glucose is lowered in pleural effusions appears to be a combination of glycolysis by cellular elements in pleural fluid and pleural tissue and impairment of glucose diffusion into the pleural space secondary to damage of the pleural membrane. For the most accurate interpretation it is best to perform the thoracentesis in a patient who has fasted and to obtain both serum and pleural fluid glucose levels simultaneously.

Amylase. An elevated pleural fluid amylase, usually twice the serum amylase, suggests one of four possibilities: (1) acute pancreatitis, (2) pancreatic pseudocyst, (3) esophageal rupture, and (4) primary or metastatic carcinoma of the lung. High levels of pleural fluid amylase are probably caused by lymphatic passage or seepage of the enzyme across the diaphragm or by direct transdiaphragmatic communication.

Lipids. Examination of the supernatant of the centrifuged pleural fluid will determine if opalescent fluid is caused by empyema or lipid. The supernatant in empyema is clear, while in lipid pleural effusion the supernatant remains cloudy. Chylous effusions (caused by severing or obstructing the thoracic duct) contain chylomicrons and a high triglyceride concentration and stain positive with Sudan III stain. Chyliform effusions (long-standing, loculated effusions seen occasionally in tuberculosis, malignancy, trapped lung, or rheumatoid disease) contain a high colesterol concentration and do not stain positive with Sudan III.

pH. A low pleural fluid pH (under 7.30) has been found in empyema, esophageal rupture, rheumatoid pleurisy, tuberculosis, and carcinoma. Thus a pH less than 7.30 narrows the differential diagnosis of the exudative effusion. At present, its greatest use is in differentiating uncomplicated parapneumonic effusions from empyemas. If the pleural fluid pH in a parapneumonic effusion is greater than 7.30, the fluid will usually resolve spontaneously with antibiotic therapy without sequelae. However, if the pH is less than 7.30, the fluid is either an empyema, will progress to an empyema, or will behave like an empyema. Such fluid should be drained from the pleural space with a chest tube. Pleural fluid should be handled as an arterial blood sample and maintained anaerobically at 0° C until analyzed.

Cytology. In cases of documented carcinoma of the pleura, cytology is positive in only 50% to 60% of patients. Characteristics that suggest malignancy include cells that have large nuclei, a high nucleocytoplasmic ratio, and a clumping tendency. If the first specimen is negative and carcinoma is suspected, other fluid samples should be obtained that will yield fresher cells and a lower percentage of degenerative mesothelial cells. A low pleural fluid pH suggests that cytology should be positive.

AFB, Gram, and Wright stains. These stains should be performed on all pleural effusions. Smears of the effusion for acid-fast bacilli are positive in approximately 20% of patients with tuberculous pleurisy. If the Gram stain is positive in an uncentrifuged specimen, it suggests a bacterial count of at least approximately 10^5 organisms/cc. A Wright stain of the sediment enables more precise identification of cell types and frequently narrows the differential diagnosis.

Transudates versus exudates. In the differential diagnosis of a pleural effusion, it is extremely helpful to classify the fluid as either a *transudate* or an *exudate*. The differential diagnosis of a transudative pleural effusion is limited and can usually be discerned from the history and physical examination. The number of causes of exudative pleural effusions is much larger. They occur most commonly when inflammation or malignant disease of the pleura is present. If any one of the three following criteria is present, the fluid is usually an exudate: (1) a pleural fluid-to-serum total protein ratio of greater than 0.5, (2) a pleural fluid LDH of greater than 200 international units (IU), or (3) a pleural fluid-to-serum LDH ratio of greater than 0.6.

The etiologies of transudates and exudates are shown in the chart on p. 194.

ETIOLOGIES OF PLEURAL EFFUSIONS

A. *Transudates*
1. Congestive heart failure
2. Cirrhosis of the liver
3. Nephrotic syndrome
4. Atelectasis, early
5. Myxedema
6. Peritoneal dialysis

B. *Exudates*
1. Parapneumonic effusion
2. Pulmonary infarction
3. Neoplasm
4. Viral disease
5. Collagen disease (rheumatoid arthritis, lupus erythematosus)
6. Tuberculosis
7. Fungal disease
8. Parasitic disease
9. Rickettsial disease
10. Gastrointestinal disease (pancreatitis, subphrenic abscess)
11. Drug reaction (e.g., nitrofurantoin, methysergide)
12. Asbestosis
13. Meigs' syndrome
14. Postmyocardial infarction syndrome
15. Trapped lung
16. Lymphatic abnormality
17. Uremic pleurisy
18. Atelectasis, late
19. Chylothorax

Pleural biopsy and therapeutic thoracentesis

A pleural biopsy using a Cope or Abrams needle should be performed if an undiagnosed exudative pleural effusion is present. However, it is usually helpful only when lymphocytes predominate as in tuberculosis, carcinoma, or lymphoma. The biopsy should be performed with a sufficient amount of pleural fluid to protect against damage to the visceral pleura and underlying lung.

A therapeutic thoracentesis need only be performed when the effusion is large enough to cause severe dyspnea. Nasal oxygen should be given during and for several hours following therapeutic thoracentesis, since marked transient falls in Pao_2 may occur despite relief of dyspnea.

Parapneumonic effusions and empyemas

A parapneumonic effusion is any pleural effusion associated with a bacterial pneumonia or lung abscess. The fluid may be clear and sterile and resolve without further sequelae, or it may be frankly purulent, that is, an empyema.

When patients are carefully evaluated with lateral decubitus radiographs, the incidence of uncomplicated parapneumonic effusions is significantly greater than reported in the literature. *Streptococcus pneumoniae* probably causes parapneumonic effusions in up to 60% of patients and especially in those patients with positive blood cultures. *Staphylococcus aureus* pneumonias are frequently complicated by pleural effusions (90% in infants, 50% in adults). *Streptococcus pyogenes* pneumonias are not frequent but are almost always associated with massive pleural effusions.

The gram-negative pneumonias (*Klebsiella, E. Coli, Bacteroides,* and *Pseudomonas*) are associated with a high incidence of parapneumonic effusions.

Empyema, or pus in the pleural space, is today most commonly caused by bronchopulmonary infection. Empyema may be diagnosed from gross observation of the fluid, a positive Gram stain, a positive culture, or a low pleural fluid pH. Empyema fluid has a high leukocyte count (usually greater than 50,000/mm^3), a predominance of neutrophils, a high total protein concentration, and a low pleural fluid glucose. Currently, the most common organisms producing empyemas are anaerobes, *Staphylococcus aureus,* and enteric gram-negative bacilli.

An empyema should be suspected when the patient has pneumonia but remains febrile despite antibiotic therapy, develops a loculated pleural effusion, or develops an increased amount of pleural fluid. A diagnostic thoracentesis should be performed immediately in the latter two situations and when fluid is observed on a radiograph in the first situation.

The treatment of empyema consists of immediate and complete drainage of the pleural space, preferably by a chest tube, and the administration of appropriate antimicrobial agents selected on the basis of careful aerobic and anaerobic cultures. Antimicrobial treatment alone is seldom sufficient. In many cases this combination of tube drainage and antimicrobial therapy is adequate. However, if treatment is instituted late or drainage is not adequate, rib resection drainage with opening of all pockets by blunt dissection may be necessary. A late sequela of inadequately treated empyema is fibrothorax, or trapped lung, sometimes necessitating decortication.

SUGGESTED READINGS

Dodson, W.H., and Hollingworth, J.W.: Pleural effusion in rheumatoid arthritis: impaired transport of glucose, N. Engl. J. Med. **275**:1337, 1966.

Good, J.T., Jr., Taryle, D.A., Maulitz, R.M., et al.: The diagnostic value of pleural fluid pH, Chest **78**:55, 1980.

Griner, P.F.: Bloody pleural fluid following pulmonary infarction, J.A.M.A. **202**:947, 1967.

Light, R.W., MacGregor, M.I., Luchsinger, P.C., et al.: Pleural effusions: the diagnostic separation of transudates and exudates, Ann. Intern. Med. **77**:507, 1972.

Potts, D.E., Levin, D.C., and Sahn, S.A.: Pleural fluid pH in parapneumonic effusions, Chest **70**:328, 1976.

Sahn, S.A.: Evaluation of pleural effusions and pleural biopsy. In Petty, T.L., editor: Pulmonary diagnostic techniques, Philadelphia, 1975, Lea & Febiger, pp. 105-131.

Yam, L.T.: Diagnostic significance of lymphocytes in pleural effusions, Ann. Intern. Med. **66**:972, 1967.

Chapter 20

PNEUMOTHORAX AND PNEUMOMEDIASTINUM

Steven A. Sahn

Pneumothorax

SPONTANEOUS PNEUMOTHORAX

Definition

The term *pneumothorax* means that air has collected between the parietal and visceral pleurae, causing this area to become a real instead of a potential space. Air can enter the cavity by way of either the visceral or parietal pleura and may be the result of disease, trauma, or the deliberate introduction of air. A pneumothorax is described as *open* when air moves freely in and out of the pleural space during respiration, *closed* when no movement of air takes place, and *valvular* or *tension* when air enters during inspiration but is prevented from escaping during expiration. A tension pneumothorax may lead to cardiac and respiratory embarrassment.

Pathogenesis

Spontaneous pneumothorax is usually the result of rupture of an air-containing space at or just below the visceral pleura. This is usually a pleural bleb, most frequently located in the apex of the lung. The cause of such blebs and the immediate cause of bleb rupture are unknown. Rupture appears not to be related to exceptional effort or trauma, since the majority of patients are at rest when spontaneous pneumothorax occurs. Although blebs and bullae distend and even rupture with a decrease in atmospheric pressure, as during an airplane flight, this mechanism cannot be invoked in the majority of cases.

Many diseases have been associated with spontaneous pneumothorax (see the accompanying list).

196

DISEASES ASSOCIATED WITH SPONTANEOUS PNEUMOTHORAX

1. COPD
2. Status asthmaticus
3. Staphylococcal pneumonia with pneumatocele formation
4. Eosinophilic granuloma and other interstitial lung diseases
5. Pulmonary infarction
6. End-stage sarcoidosis
7. Marfan's syndrome
8. Primary or metastatic carcinoma of the lung
9. Endometriosis
10. Pneumoconiosis
11. Tuberculosis

Clinical features

Spontaneous pneumothorax usually occurs in young, thin males who are otherwise healthy. The onset is sudden, and unilateral pleuritic or non-pleuritic pain and dyspnea are the most common features. Dyspnea, which may be severe when the pneumothorax occurs, frequently disappears within 24 hours regardless of whether the collapsed lung undergoes partial reexpansion. The degree of dyspnea varies with the size of the pneumothorax and any preexisting lung pathology. Cough, when present, is nonproductive; the patient is rarely febrile. Signs of intravascular volume depletion occur when severe hemorrhage into the pleural space results from rupture of a pleural adhesion containing arteries under systemic pressure.

The physical signs depend on the degree of lung collapse and the presence or absence of an associated pleural effusion. A small pneumothorax usually is not detectable by physical examination. The most common physical signs are absence of breath sounds and fremitus. Decreased movement on the involved side and hyperresonance are noted in large pneumothoraces.

Radiographic appearances

The radiographic diagnosis of a pneumothorax can only be made with identification of the visceral pleural line (Fig. 20-1). The radiographic density of a collapsing lung changes little until the volume is greatly reduced, since blood flow to the lung diminishes in proportion to the amount of collapse. When pneumothorax is suspected and not visualized, an upright radiograph during expiration may be useful.

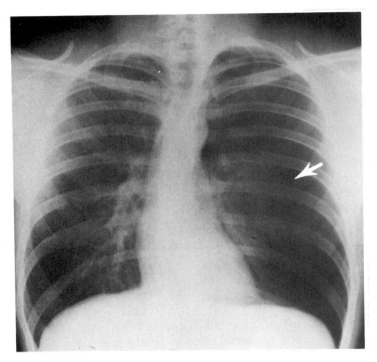

FIG. 20-1. Spontaneous pneumothorax, left. *(Courtesy Medical Illustration Service, Veterans Administration Hospital, Denver, Colorado.)*

Treatment

The management of an uncomplicated spontaneous pneumothorax depends on the degree of collapse. A small pneumothorax (less than 15% to 20%) causes little disability in the healthy patient. Bedrest is not essential, although activities should be limited. The reabsorption of air occurs spontaneously, usually within 30 days. It has been calculated that reabsorption of air from a sealed pneumothorax is 1.25% of the radiographic lung volume per day. A pneumothorax of less than 50% would take approximately 40 days to reexpand spontaneously if no air leak persisted. The economic consequences of such delayed healing are obvious, and many physicians resort to tube thoracostomy for rapid lung reexpansion.

In pneumothoraces larger than 20%, especially those accompanied by dyspnea, the air should be evacuated from the pleural cavity immediately. The usual method is the insertion of a chest tube connected to underwater seal drainage to permit one-way evacuation of air and to promote local pleural interadherence. The chest tube is usually left in place for 24 to 48 hours after reexpansion has occurred and the air leak has stopped.

TENSION PNEUMOTHORAX

Tension pneumothorax is a medical emergency and occurs when the air leak is valvular. When increasing positive pressure builds in the pleural space, it impairs venous return to the heart with a resultant fall in cardiac output, tachycardia, and shock. The radiographic features of a tension pneumothorax are those of marked contralateral mediastinal shift and ipsilateral hemidiaphragmatic depression.

When a tension pneumothorax is diagnosed, treatment must be immediate. The increased pleural pressure must be reduced promptly by inserting a large bore needle into the pleural space. If the diagnosis is correct, a rush of air will be heard, confirming that the pleural space contained air under high pressure. As soon as possible the needle should be replaced by a chest tube.

TRAUMATIC PNEUMOTHORAX

Pneumothorax complicating trauma may occur with or without radiographic evidence of rib fractures. When a fracture is present the likely cause of pneumothorax is laceration of the visceral pleura by rib fragments; hemothorax is a common accompaniment. When no fractures are visible radiographically the cause is usually either direct parenchymal laceration or rupture of a preexisting bleb. Rarely, pneumothorax develops on the side contralateral to the trauma, presumably as a result of a contrecoup transmission of forces.

Other causes of traumatic pneumothorax are thoracentesis, pleural biopsy, transthoracic needle biopsy, transbronchial biopsy, and bronchial brushing through the fiberoptic bronchoscope.

RECURRENT PNEUMOTHORAX

Twenty percent of cases of spontaneous pneumothorax recur, most within a year. A few cases become chronic (persisting for 3 months or longer) because of the development of a bronchopleural fistula. This occurs if adhesions prevent the lung from collapsing and closing the fistula, if the air leak is through a congenital cyst (its epithelial tissue does not readily seal over), or if multiple leaks are involved in emphysema. A further reason for persistence of pneumothorax, especially the therapeutic variety, is the development of a fibrous peel over the visceral pleura (i.e., trapped lung).

Recurrent pneumothorax may be treated by the instillation of a sclerosing agent into the pleural cavity, but this procedure is unpredictable and may impair pulmonary function. The treatment of choice is parietal pleurectomy or pleural abrasion, both requiring a thoracotomy. Parietal pleurectomy consists of stripping the parietal pleura from the chest wall and upper mediastinum, which promotes adherence of the visceral pleura. Another method of promoting pleural interadherence is simple scrubbing or irritation of the visceral pleura. Recurrence after these procedures is rare, and impairment of ventilatory function is remarkably slight. When recurrence of a pneumothorax is complicated by the development of a contralateral pneumothorax, one of these procedures is indicated with a minimum of delay on the side first affected. Other surgical procedures used effectively for this condition include removal of the leaking segment, if sufficiently localized, and oversewing the leaking area, if feasible.

In cases of chronic pneumothorax, decortication of the visceral pleural peel may be necessary. This procedure has been carried out after many years of collapse; its success depends on the patency and freedom from active disease of both airways and vasculature.

ARTIFICIAL PNEUMOTHORAX

Artificial pneumothorax was once a mainstay of treatment in pulmonary tuberculosis. The procedure has now been abandoned. The only use of artificial pneumothorax today is as a diagnostic procedure for the differentiation of a peripheral pulmonary lesion from one in the parietal pleura or chest wall.

Pneumomediastinum

Definition and etiology

Air in the mediastinal tissues is referred to as *mediastinal emphysema* or *pneumomediastinum*. Pneumomediastinum is seen most commonly in newborns, in whom the incidence has been reported from 0.4% to 1%. Pneumomediastinum may be spontaneous or result from penetrating or blunt chest trauma, esophageal perforation, tracheal or bronchial perforation, ruptured lung abscess, gas-forming intrathoracic infections, carcinoma of the lung, or maxillofacial trauma.

Pathogenesis

It has been postulated that spontaneous pneumomediastinum may result from a number of circumstances all having in common vigorous abdominal, diaphragmatic, and thoracic muscle contraction against a closed glottis. These events result in alveolar distension with elevation of intra-alveolar pressure. If the pressure in the alveolus exceeds the pressure in the pulmonary vessels, alveolar rupture occurs and air gains access to the perivascular space. The free air migrates along perivascular sheaths and eventually reaches the mediastinum.

Spontaneous decompression of the pneumomediastinum occurs as air moves through the fascial planes to the subcutaneous spaces of the neck and chest. Up to one third of cases of spontaneous pneumomediastinum also have an associated pneumothorax.

Clinical features

Spontaneous pneumomediastinum in adults, which by definition has no relation to underlying lung disease, frequently occurs with an antecedent history of vomiting, coughing, sneezing, defecation, weightlifting, or childbirth. Occurrence during diabetic ketoacidosis has been reported. Symptoms and signs depend largely on the amount of air in the mediastinal space. The diagnosis may be suspected by a history of abrupt onset of retrosternal pain. The pain is aggravated by respiration and sometimes by swallowing. The degree of dyspnea varies considerably. Physical examination commonly reveals air in subcutaneous tissues of the neck above the clavicles; it may spread over the thoracic wall later. Hamman's crunch may be detected on auscultation and is best heard over the left sternal border from the third to sixth intercostal space with the patient sitting upright or in the left lateral decubitus position; this sign consists of a crunching or clicking noise synchronous with the heartbeat and occurs in about 50% of patients. Rarely, when air does not freely escape from the mediastinum, impaired venous filling of the heart with associated tachycardia and hypotension may occur.

Air in the mediastinum is recognized as a translucency outlining the upper mediastinum and the heart borders. The lateral radiograph may show a substernal collection of air. Air is usually also evident in the subcutaneous tissues of the neck. It should not be confused with pneumopericardium.

Treatment

Most patients with pneumomediastinum respond to symptomatic management consisting of observation, rest, and analgesia. This course can be pursued safely when the possible causes of pneumomediastinum have been ruled out by careful history, physical examination, and chest film evaluation. In most cases spontaneous absorption of air occurs within 1 week. In the patient who develops significant cardiopulmonary compromise from mediastinal air, a decompression procedure may be performed by an incision into the tissues just above the suprasternal notch.

SUGGESTED READINGS

Adwers, J.R., Hodgson, P.E., and Lynch, R.: Spontaneous pneumomediastinum, J. Trauma **14:**414, 1974.

Bodey, G.P.: Medical mediastinal emphysema, Ann. Intern. Med. **54:**46, 1961.

George, R.B., Herbert, S.J., Shames, J.M., et al.: Pneumothorax complicating pulmonary emphysema, J.A.M.A. **234:**389, 1975.

Hyde, L.: Benign spontaneous pneumothorax, Ann. Intern. Med. **56:**746, 1962.

Lindskog, G.E., and Halasz, N.A.: Spontaneous pneumothorax: a consideration of pathogenesis and management with review of 72 hospitalized cases, Arch. Surg. **75:**693, 1957.

Macklin, C.C.: Transport of air along sheaths of pulmonic blood vessels from alveoli to mediastinum: clinical implications, Arch. Intern. Med. **64:**913, 1939.

Ruckley, C.V., and McCormick, R.J.M.: The management of spontaneous pneumothorax, Thorax **21:**139, 1966.

Chapter 21

PULMONARY NEOPLASMS

Charles W. Van Way III *and* Thomas A. Neff

Prevalence

The prevalence of lung cancer (strictly speaking, carcinoma of the bronchus) has increased progressively since the turn of the century. The peak incidence occurs in persons aged 60 to 70 years. In 1980 in the United States, 85,000 new cases were diagnosed in men and 32,000 in women. Lung cancer occurs at least twice as commonly in urban as in rural environments.

Etiology

Epidemiologic data and animal experiments suggest that carcinogenic substances inhaled over long periods play a major causative role. The most important factor is cigarette smoking.

Cigarette smoking. Lung cancer is at least 10 times more common among cigarette smokers than among nonsmokers. The more an individual smokes, the greater the risk. The relationship between cigarette smoking and lung cancer is strongest for oat cell carcinoma, very strong for squamous cell carcinoma, weak for adenocarcinoma, and practically nonexistent for bronchiolar-alveolar cell carcinoma. Pipe and cigar smoking appear to be minor risk factors. Various carcinogens, notably 3,4-benzpyrene and radioactive polonium 210, have been implicated as the offending agents in tobacco smoke. Important considerations are the *inhalation* of tobacco smoke and the *temperature* at which the tobacco is burned—cigarettes burn at a much hotter temperature than either cigars or pipes, presumably producing a different spectrum of polycyclic hydrocarbons and other substances.

Industrial exposure. *Asbestos*, a substance of worldwide distribution and extensive industrial use, is the most important industrial material with a relation to lung cancer. Workers exposed to asbestos develop carcinoma of the lung 10 to 50 times more often than the general population, but the increased risk is confined almost entirely to those asbestos workers who also smoke cigarettes. The smoke apparently acts as either a potentiator or a cocarcinogen. Asbestos also predisposes individuals to pleural and peritoneal mesothelioma. *Uranium* miners have an increased risk of lung cancer. The risk is greatly increased if the miners are also cigarette smokers. Refining of *nickel* ore, manufacture of *bichromates*, mining of *hematite*, and mining and industrial use of *arsenic* also appear to increase the risk of lung cancer.

Tuberculosis. Carcinoma of the lung occurs at the site of active or inactive pulmonary tuberculosis frequently enough to suggest more than a coincidental relationship (so-called *scar carcinoma*). Adenosquamous or epidermoid carcinoma is occasionally found in the region of a pulmonary scar, whether or not it is related to tuberculosis. When carcinoma appears concomitantly with tuberculosis, the latter diagnosis often serves to delay the diagnosis of carcinoma.

Classification

The classification and the approximate frequency of each histologic type of lung cancer are as follows: (1) squamous (epidermoid), 35%; (2) adenocarcinoma, 20%; (3) undifferentiated large cell and undifferentiated small cell (i.e., oat cell), 40%; (4) bronchiolar-alveolar cell, less than 5%; and (5) giant cell, mixed, and other, less than 1%. Some very recent series have reported that adenocarcinoma is now more frequent than squamous cell carcinoma. Approximately 40% of lung cancers arise in the main and lobar bronchi, while 60% have their site of origin in the segmental or more distal bronchi.

Clinical picture

The patient with bronchogenic carcinoma is generally past age 40. Only 3% of cases are diagnosed in patients before 40 years of age. At the time of radiologic diagnosis, symptoms may be absent or the patient may show one of the following symptom complexes.

Bronchopulmonary symptoms. Although symptoms may be of recent onset, more often the patient complains of long-standing chronic cough and expectoration that have become more severe. A change in the quantity or character of sputum production is also common. Other common symptoms and manifestations are vague nonpleuritic chest pain, dyspnea on exertion, localized wheeze sometimes aggravated by lateral recumbency, hemoptysis, and recurrent pneumonia, especially in the same segment or lobe. Less often, patients have general debility, anorexia, weight loss without any clearly localizing pulmonary symptoms, or symptoms and signs of a distant metastasis.

Extrapulmonary intrathoracic features. The most common sites of metastasis are the mediastinal lymph nodes. The presence of mediastinal involvement at the time of initial examination depends largely on the cell type and location and size of the primary lesion. Oat cell carcinomas have commonly involved the mediastinal nodes by the time the diagnosis is established. The superior vena cava may be obstructed by involved lymph nodes or by direct invasion, especially in undifferentiated carcinoma. Hilar lymph nodes on the left may involve the recurrent laryngeal nerve, producing vocal cord paralysis and hoarseness. Pericardial effusion or direct invasion of the heart may occur. Pleural effusion may be caused either by mediastinal node involvement or by pleural metastases and is a poor prognostic sign.

Superior sulcus tumor. Tumors of the superior pulmonary sulcus, the so-called *Pancoast tumors*, present a special problem. Generally slow-growing epidermoid carcinomas, they tend to produce symptoms locally and to metastasize late. They are located near the angle the first rib makes with the vertebral column, and as a result extend early into the chest wall, involving specifically the sympathetic chain, the stellate ganglion, and the lower roots of the brachial plexus. From this distribution comes the classic Pancoast picture of severe pain in the involved shoulder, arm, and upper chest, together with ipsilateral Horner's syndrome. The chest radiograph may show a mass in the apex, or the involvement may simulate apical pleural thickening. The apical lordotic film is often helpful. The management of this tumor is markedly different from that used in the other forms of lung cancer (see Surgical resection).

Metastatic disease. One third of all patients with bronchogenic carcinoma first present with evidence of metastasis. Regional lymph nodes, liver, adrenal glands, bone, brain, kidneys, and the contralateral lung are common early sites. Adenocarcinoma tends to show early hematogenous metasteses and is the most common histologic type to involve the pleura. Oat cell carcinomas metastasize early to brain and bone. Lymphogenous dissemination throughout both lungs may occur, causing severe dyspnea and cough, marked hypoxemia, weight loss, and rapid death.

Extrathoracic nonmetastatic manifestations. Neuromuscular manifestations occur in 5% to 15% of cases of bronchogenic carcinoma. These may simulate myasthenia or polymyositis. Other neurologic manifestations are peripheral neuropathy, subacute cerebellar degeneration, encephalopathy, and necrotizing myelopathy. Hypertrophic pulmonary osteoarthropathy occurs in 5% of patients. This lesion consists of periosteal thickening, new bone formation, swelling and pain in the joints, and clubbing—usually painful. It is most commonly seen in oat cell carcinoma. The reason for its occurrence in lung cancer and numerous other disease states is unknown.

Endocrine and metabolic manifestations. Endocrinopathies that have been associated with bronchogenic carcinoma include hyperthyroidism, the syndrome of inappropriate secretion of antidiuretic hormone (SIADH), secretion of an insulin analogue, and excessive production of gonadotrophin. Hypercalcemia is most commonly associated with squamous cell carcinomas. Cushing's syndrome is unusual and has been found only with oat cell carcinoma and bronchial carcinoid. SIADH has been associated with both squamous and oat cell carcinomas. One of these endocrinopathies is manifested in 5% to 10% of patients with bronchogenic carcinoma.

Vascular and hematologic manifestations. Migratory thrombophlebitis, often in unusual sites and resistant to treatment, is seen in lung cancer as in various other malignancies, but it is not common. Thrombocytosis, thrombocytopenic purpura, fibrinolysis, hemolysis, and red cell aplasia have also been described.

Diagnosis (Figs. 21-1 to 21-5)

Patients with lung cancer generally appear in one of two ways. They may be asymptomatic but have an abnormal chest radiograph taken for routine or non-lung-cancer symptoms, or they may see a physician about any of the symptoms or manifestations listed above. If the symptoms are due to lung cancer, 98% of these patients will have some abnormality on their chest radiograph. It is helpful to follow an orderly diagnostic routine, beginning with the chest radiograph, as shown in the flow diagram in Fig. 21-6. The differential diagnosis of the peripheral nodule includes granuloma, benign tumor, and primary or metastatic cancer (see Chapter 22). Central tumors or large peripheral masses are usually approached with early bronchoscopy. Even if the lesion cannot be seen directly, bronchial washings for cytology or transbronchial biopsy under fluoroscopic control may be diagnostic.

Pleural effusion in the patient with suspected carcinoma should be aspirated for cytologic examination. Needle pleural biopsy is sometimes diagnostic even when the cytologic findings are negative. If both pleural biopsy and cytologic examination of the pleural fluid are accomplished, the diagnosis of carcinomatous involvement will be established in 80% to 90% of patients. Pleural involvement contraindicates resection of the tumor.

A number of procedures have been advocated to detect mediastinal spread of tumor. The two best are mediastinoscopy and parasternal mediastinotomy (Chamberlain procedure). Although safer than thoracotomy, these procedures usually require general anesthesia and are associated with some risk. Either procedure may produce injury to the great vessels, pneumothorax, or wound infection, although the mortality for both is less than 1% and the complication rate less than 10%. They are usually done as a staging procedure in patients who are otherwise candidates for thoracotomy, al-

Text continued on p. 213.

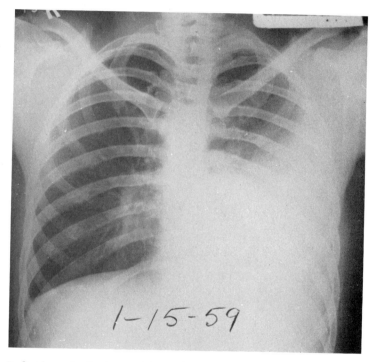

FIG. 21-1. Left pleural effusion, with mediastinal displacement *toward* the effusion, that is, underlying partial left lung atelectasis caused by completely occlusive bronchogenic carcinoma. *(Courtesy Medical Illustration Service, Veterans Administration Hospital, Denver, Colorado.)*

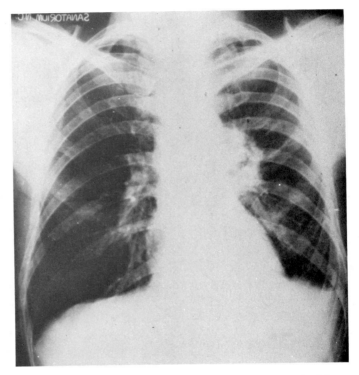

FIG. 21-2. Bronchogenic carcinoma: mass at left hilum and obliteration of left costophrenic angle. *(Courtesy Medical Illustration Service, Veterans Administration Hospital, Denver, Colorado.)*

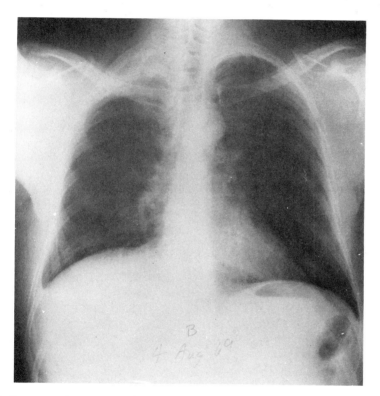

FIG. 21-3. Pancoast (superior sulcus) tumor: primary bronchogenic carcinoma, right apex, involving bone, pleura, brachial plexus, and cervical sympathetic nerves (producing Horner's syndrome). *(Courtesy Medical Illustration Service, Veterans Administration Hospital, Denver, Colorado.)*

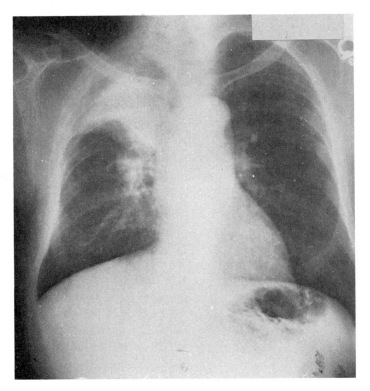

FIG. 21-4. Bronchogenic carcinoma, right upper lobe: **S** sign of Golden, lateral concavity caused by partial lobar collapse, medial convexity caused by mass in right upper lobe bronchus. *(Courtesy Medical Illustration Service, Veterans Administration Hospital, Denver, Colorado.)*

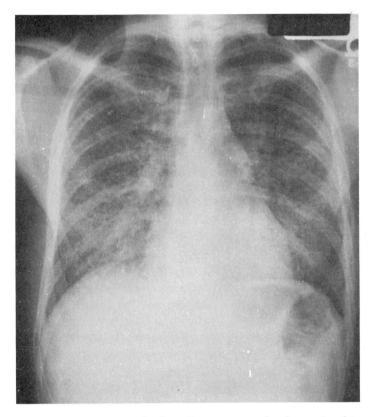

FIG. 21-5. Lymphogenous spread of malignancy to the lung: in this case, from stomach carcinoma. *(Courtesy Medical Illustration Service, Veterans Administration Hospital, Denver, Colorado.)*

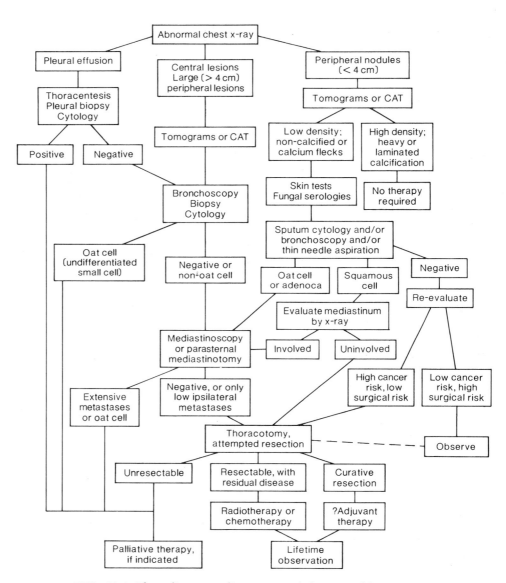

FIG. 21-6. Flow diagram: diagnosis and therapy of lung cancer.

though mediastinoscopy in particular is sometimes done to obtain tissue for diagnosis in a patient whose tumor is obviously unresectable. The decision to explore the mediastinum and the choice of procedure should be made in conjunction with the surgeon who will perform the thoracotomy. The choice of procedure generally depends on the location of the tumor. Both right and left paratracheal nodes are accessible to the mediastinoscope. However, left-sided tumors often spread to the periaortic nodes, which cannot be approached with the mediastinoscope. When these lesions are suspected, a parasternal mediastinotomy should be done.

The problem of when to do one of these procedures is complicated by the fact that mediastinal spread, although ominous, does not invariably contra-indicate resection. If the spread is confined to the low ipsilateral or para-aortic nodes and if radiotherapy is given after resection, the 5-year survival rate may reach the 10% to 20% range. In a healthy young patient without radiographic evidence of mediastinal involvement, one may elect to proceed directly to thoracotomy. Cell type is an important consideration. One should never consider operation for oat cell carcinoma with mediastinal involve-ment, but squamous cell or bronchiolar-alveolar carcinoma or adenocarci-noma, in that order, may be resected in the absence of distant metastases and other contraindications.

Other laboratory tests are of some value. The serum calcium, alkaline phosphatase, and platelet counts may suggest occult marrow involvement. The alkaline phosphatase is often elevated with liver or bone metastases. Hypercalcemia suggests either bone involvement or ectopic hormone pro-duction. Arterial blood gases and ventilation tests should always be part of the preoperative evaluation.

Screening for metastatic disease is best initiated by a thorough history and physical examination. Brain, bone, and liver radionuclide scans, CAT scans, and ultrasound studies are often used in an effort to detect clinically occult metastases. In general, these techniques are most productive if the patient has symptoms or signs suggestive of metastatic disease. The bone scan may be positive without clinical signs or symptoms, but it is also the most likely scan to give a false-positive result. The brain scan will be positive in about 5% of patients without clinical signs, the liver scan in about 5%, and the bone scan in 10% to 15%.

Gallium scanning is of some use in assessing whether a given lesion is malignant, although active granulomas will also be positive by this method. It is of less use in evaluating the mediastinum, missing about 50% of medias-tinal metastases.

The CAT scan has some usefulness in detecting mediastinal metastases, although other radiologic techniques, including the standard posteroanterior chest radiograph, 30-degree oblique tomograms, and xerotomography have been useful as well. Frontal tomograms are often used but rarely useful, and lateral tomograms are often useful but rarely used.

Long-term survivors with lung cancer are almost always those with a relatively localized, slow-growing process in whom successful resection has been carried out. About a third of long-term survivors have had disease beyond the primary lesion, usually in the hilar or interlobar nodes, and have had irradiation. The primary aim of diagnostic procedures is to identify such patients. The obvious corollary of this is to identify patients whose tumors cannot be resected successfully. It should be clear that all patients in the latter group are considered terminally ill. The decision to withhold surgery should be made only with proof, preferably histologic, that the situation is hopeless.

Treatment

Surgical resection. The techniques of surgical resection have remained relatively constant for the past 20 years. The basic principle is to carry out the most conservative resection that will remove the tumor and an adequate margin of uninvolved lung. Wedge and segmental resections, primarily used for small peripheral nodules, therefore carry a better prognosis than larger resections. For larger tumors, lobectomy or bilobectomy is performed if the tumor is favorably situated. But many tumors, most notably those of the left upper lobe, involve the pulmonary artery centrally and can be completely extirpated only with pneumonectomy.

Contraindications to resection are evidence of distant metastasis, mediastinal invasion, pleural involvement, and severe impairment of pulmonary or cardiac function. Age is not critical, given normal or near normal cardiac and pulmonary function. Of the pulmonary function tests, the MVV and the FEV_1 give the best indications of the patient's overall lung function. An MVV of less than 40 L/min or an FEV_1 of less than 1.0 L is associated with a greatly increased operative mortality. However, with modern techniques of ventilatory support, resection can be successfully performed in patients previously classified as prohibitive operative risks. The major pitfall is removal of too much lung tissue to permit survival, but this hazard is sometimes more apparent than real. If an area of lung is poorly ventilated and/or perfused, removal of that portion of lung will produce little respiratory compromise and, in fact, may even improve overall pulmonary function. Ventilation-perfusion radionuclide lung scans are very useful in evaluating borderline cases.

The risk of death after thoracotomy varies from less than 1% in a healthy patient undergoing wedge resection to 20% in a poor-risk patient undergoing pneumonectomy. An average risk for a lobar resection in an acceptable operative candidate is 5%.

The superior sulcus or Pancoast tumor requires special consideration. The accepted treatment is preoperative radiotherapy followed by an extensive en bloc resection of the upper chest wall with the involved upper lobe. Five-year survival rates of up to 35% have been reported by Paulson in a series of tumors that were relatively favorable. Because the superior sulcus tumor is often inaccessible to bronchoscopy, both the radiotherapy and the operation may have to be carried out without tissue diagnosis. By definition, superior sulcus tumors are small; a tumor larger than 3 cm is really just a large apical tumor and carries a much poorer prognosis than the classic small superior sulcus tumor.

Radiotherapy. Oat cell is the most radiosensitive histologic type of lung cancer; the rest are not very radiosensitive. A British Medical Research Council multicenter prospective study showed, however, that resection and radiotherapy individually were both poorly effective in oat cell cancer, with a 5-year survival rate of 0% to 4%, respectively. The problem is that although the tumor melts away under radiotherapy, it also grows back rapidly unless chemotherapy is given. Presently, radiotherapy *and* chemotherapy are regarded as a primary mode of therapy for oat cell cancer; the results are mildly encouraging.

In other types of lung cancer, radiotherapy is used postoperatively when positive nodes are found or when residual thoracic tumor is left behind after the resection. Except for the superior sulcus tumor, preoperative radiotherapy has been shown to be ineffective. Palliative radiotherapy should be used selectively. Indications include the following: severe hemoptysis, bronchial obstruction, recurrent effusion, superior vena caval obstruction, intractable pain (especially bone), and to relieve symptoms of CNS metastases. Although radiotherapy may temporarily relieve such symptoms, survival is lengthened in patients with unresectable lung cancer by 1 or 2 months at the most.

Chemotherapy. Multiple agent chemotherapy is beginning to show some real hope for oat cell carcinoma, especially when given to patients with limited disease. However, long-term, multiple drug regimens are toxic and must be used only by oncologic teams experienced in such therapy.

The role of chemotherapy for nonresectable tumors other than oat cell is still experimental and has not shown much promise to date. This therapy is best reserved for patients who wish to enter research protocols.

Immunotherapy. Preliminary studies with squamous cell carcinomas suggest that postresection intrapleural tuberculosis vaccine instillation prolongs life. However, the relationship between this attempt at immunoenhancement and a favorable clinical course remains unproved at present. Several long-term studies are in progress.

General. Both radiotherapy and chemotherapy, especially at low doses, are commonly used as part of the psychotherapy of fatal malignant disease. Judicious, humane care using family, social, and psychologic support must not be forgotten. Often, narcotics and oxygen are the best palliative drugs.

Results of treatment and prognosis

The overall prognosis in lung cancer is dismal. Of 100 average unselected patients with this disease, approximately 60 will have tumors that are obviously unresectable by clinical, laboratory, or radiologic evaluation. Of the remaining 40, 10 to 20 will have tumors that are unresectable because of mediastinal involvement at mediastinoscopy or mediastinotomy. Of the 20 to 25 patients undergoing thoracotomy and resection, approximately 5 will be alive 5 years later.

In highly selected favorable lesions the picture is better. The 5-year survival rate following resection for squamous cell carcinoma without mediastinal metastases is 30% to 40%. Even with mediastinal metastases that are not extensive, resection and postoperative radiotherapy will produce a 5-year survival rate of 15% to 20%. The survival rate for adenocarcinoma and large cell and undifferentiated carcinomas is 5% to 15%. Bronchiolar-alveolar carcinoma is an uncommon form of lung cancer with a bimodal distribution; 80% of patients have multifocal, often bilateral presentation, and their prognosis is dismal. In 20% the presentation is unifocal; the prognosis is about 50% for 5-year survival.

When primary, non-oat-cell cancer presents as a peripheral nodule, the picture is mildly encouraging. The overall 5-year survival rate for nodules 2.0 cm or less is 70%; for those 4.0 cm or less, 45% to 50%. Again, patients with squamous cell cancers have the most favorable prognosis.

BRONCHIAL ADENOMAS

Bronchial adenomas are relatively uncommon tumors of the lung occurring chiefly in young patients. They occur at a rate of approximately 1 per 50 cases of bronchogenic carcinoma. These tumors arise from the duct epithelium of the bronchial mucous glands and show some relationship to endocrine tumors. They are *usually benign* in behavior, but some show low-grade malignancy and may recur after resection. The most common type is the carcinoid, seen in 90% of cases; the remaining 10% are cylindromas, mucoepidermoid adenomas, and pleomorphic adenomas. Occasionally, a tumor is seen that resembles an oat cell carcinoma, but which is localized and noninvasive. The sex incidence of bronchial adenoma is equal, unlike bronchogenic carcinoma, which predominates in males. Because 80% to 90% of bronchial adenomas arise from either the main or lobar bronchi, they can be seen with the bronchoscope.

Clinical manifestations depend on the location of the tumor and on the degree of bronchial obstruction. Patients usually have symptoms referable to the tumor, although a small percentage of tumors are found by routine chest radiography. The most common early symptoms are cough and hemoptysis. Other symptoms include recurrent respiratory tract infections, fatigue, dyspnea, chest pain, and wheezing. The common radiologic findings are persistent segmental infiltrates or lobar atelectasis, peripheral nodule, or hilar mass. Rarely, the carcinoid variety is associated with either the carcinoid syndrome or Cushing's syndrome. On bronchoscopy the tumor appears as a reddish brown, shiny lesion that may bleed copiously when a biopsy is done. Treatment consists of surgical excision, which offers a favorable prognosis, particularly if the tumor is of the carcinoid variety, not locally invasive, and without lymph node metastases.

SUGGESTED READINGS

Ashraf, M.H., Milsom, P.L., and Walesby, R.K.: Selection by mediastinoscopy and long-term survival in bronchial carcinoma, Ann. Thorac. Surg. **30**:208, 1980.

Auerbach, O., Hammond, E.C., Kirman, D., et al.: Effects of cigarette smoking on dogs. II. Pulmonary neoplasm, Arch. Environ. Health (Chicago) **21**:754, 1970.

Donahue, J.K., Weichert, R.F., and Ochsner, J.L.: Bronchial adenoma, Ann. Surg. **167**:873, 1968.

Hammond, E.C., Auerbach, O., Kirman, D., et al.: Effects of cigarette smoking on dogs. I. Design of experiment, mortality, and findings in lung parenchyma, Arch. Environ. Health (Chicago) **21**:740, 1970.

Hansen, M., Hansen, H.H., and Dombernowsky, P.: Long-term survival in small cell carcinoma of the lung, J.A.M.A. **244**:247, 1980.

Hutchinson, C.M., and Mills, H.L.: The selection of patients with bronchogenic carcinoma for mediastinoscopy, J. Thorac. Cardiovasc. Surg. **71**:768, 1976.

Jackman, R.J., Good, C.A., Clagett, O.T., et al.: Survival rates in peripheral bronchogenic carcinomas up to four centimeters in diameter presenting as solitary pulmonary nodules, J. Thorac. Cardiovasc. Surg. **57**:1, 1969.

Karasik, A., Modan, M., Jacob, C.O., et al.: Increased risk of lung cancer in patients with chondromatous hamartoma, J. Thorac. Cardiovasc. Surg. **80**:217, 1980.

Kelly, R.J., Cowan, R.J., Ferree, C.B., et al.: Efficacy of radionuclide scanning in patients with lung cancer, J.A.M.A. **242**:2855, 1979.

Kirsh, M.M., Dickerman, R., Fayos, J., et al.: The value of chest wall resection in the treatment of superior sulcus tumors of the lung, Ann. Thorac. Surg. **15**:339, 1973.

Kirsh, M.M., Prior, M., Gago, O., et al.: The effect of histological cell type on the prognosis of patients with bronchogenic carcinoma, Ann. Thorac. Surg. **13**:303, 1972.

McKneally, M.F., Maver, C., and Kausel, H.W.: Regional immunotherapy of lung cancer with intrapleural BCG, Lancet **1**:377, 1976.

Martini, N., Flehinger, B.J., Zaman, M.B., et al.: Prospective study of 445 lung carcinomas with mediastinal lymph node metastases, J. Thorac. Cardiovasc. Surg. **80**:390, 1980.

Miller, A.B., Fox, W., and Tall, R.: Five-year follow-up of the Medical Research Council comparative trial of surgery and radiotherapy for the primary treatment of small-celled or oat-celled carcinoma of the bronchus, Lancet **2**:501, 1969.

Paulson, D.L.: Carcinoma of the lung, Curr. Probl. Surg. 1-64, Chicago, November 1967, Year Book Medical Publishers, Inc.

Pearson, F.G.: Use of mediastinoscopy in selection of patients for lung cancer operations, Ann. Thorac. Surg. **30**:205, 1980.

Richardson, J.V., Zenk, B.A., and Rossi, N.P.: Preoperative noninvasive mediastinal staging in bronchogenic carcinoma, Surgery **88**:382, 1980.

Saccomanno, G., Archer, V.E., Auerbach, O., et al.: Development of carcinoma of the lung as reflected in exfoliated cells, Cancer **33**:256, 1974.

Shields, T.W.: Bronchial carcinoma, Springfield, Ill., 1974, Charles C Thomas, Publisher.

Shields, T.W., Higgins, G.A., Jr., Lawton, R., et al.: Preoperative xray therapy as an adjuvant in the treatment of bronchogenic carcinoma, J. Thorac. Cardiovasc. Surg. **59**:49, 1970.

Shields, T.W., Humphrey, E.W., Matthews, M., et al.: Pathological stage grouping of patients with resected carcinoma of the lung, J. Thorac. Cardiovasc. Surg. **80**:400, 1980.

Chapter 22

THE SOLITARY PULMONARY NODULE

Thomas A. Neff *and* Charles W. Van Way III

Definition

The solitary pulmonary nodule (SPN) is defined in radiographic terms as an opacity on the chest film that is (1) single, (2) round to ovoid, (3) less than 6 cm (large nodules are usually called lung masses), (4) has distinct margins (i.e., surrounded by aerated lung parenchyma and therefore not abutting chest wall, diaphragm, or mediastinum), and (5) may or may not contain calcium obvious on the plain film. The vast majority of SPNs do not cause symptoms or signs. Rare symptoms associated with an SPN include hemoptysis, cough, clubbing, and endocrinopathy. Up to a third of patients have vague or nonspecific chest pain with no evidence of its having been caused by the SPN.

Management

The management of the SPN hinges on the physician's ability to separate each nodule into a malignant or a benign category. About one third of SPNs in patients who have undergone operation are malignant (bronchogenic carcinoma, solitary metastasis, or bronchial adenoma). However, by selection of patient populations, the malignant percentage has varied from as low as 3% to as high as 80%. The 3% occurred in the one series based upon a true population survey (Holin). The overwhelming number of benign SPNs are granulomas caused by tuberculosis, histoplasmosis, or coccidioidomycosis; however, hamartoma, cysts, and a host of rare benign neoplasms and other lesions have been reported.

The crux of patient management involves removing primary malignant tumors and adenomas after carefully excluding all evidence of extrathoracic metastases. Some 25% to 50% of patients with "localized" bronchogenic carcinoma (appearing as SPNs) will have 5-year cures; a few more may have their longevity improved by early surgical removal. With careful clinical

ABCs of SPN

No thoracotomy (observation)	Possible thoracotomy (continue work-up)
A. Age	A. Age
1. Under 35 years	1. Over 35 years
B. "Before" radiograph	B. "Before" radiograph
1. Shrinking	1. Growing
2. Volume doubled before 1 month or after 16 months	2. Volume doubled between 1 and 16 months
C. Calcium (tomograms)	C. Calcium (tomograms)
1. Present	1. Absent
2. High-density CAT scan	2. Low-density CAT scan
D. Smoking history	D. Smoking history
1. Nonsmoker	1. Smoker

selection, some patients with a "controlled" extrathoracic cancer (e.g., kidney, colon) will benefit from resection of a single or a small number of pulmonary metastatic nodules. Conversely, most patients with benign lesions do not need an operation. A simple mnemonic device to help one remember how to differentiate benign from malignant SPNs is the ABCs (see the accompanying chart).

Age. The chance of an SPN being a primary bronchogenic carcinoma in patients less than 35 years of age is about 1%.

"Before" chest radiographs (for growth rate). If available, previous chest films are extremely helpful because the growth rate of primary bronchogenic carcinoma is well known. If the nodule has not "doubled" in volume (note that the diameter of a tumor sphere must increase by only a factor of 1.26 to double in volume) within 16 months, the lesion assuredly is not malignant. SPNs that double in volume within 30 days, on the other hand, are almost always inflammatory.

Calcification. Definite calcification seen in an SPN almost always indicates a benign lesion (Figs. 22-1 to 22-4). Tomography of SPNs will often reveal or confirm calcium not seen or only suspected on plain films and is therefore useful. An exception is the fact that a fleck of calcium may sometimes be seen within a so-called *scar* carcinoma. Most recently, the great sensitivity of CAT scanning to determine density has been used to diagnose two thirds of all granulomas by their high density. The remaining one third of granulomas with low density must for the present be managed as possible carcinomas.

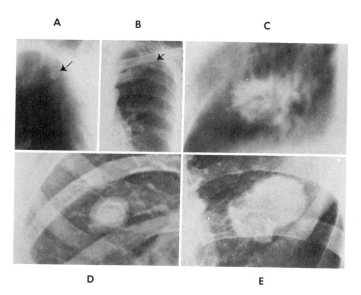

FIG. 22-1. Pulmonary nodules. **A,** Primary bronchogenic carcinoma, tiny nodule with spicular radiations on tomogram. **B,** Same patient: nodule is almost invisible on routine posteroanterior film. **C,** Right basal nodule with spicular radiations, very indicative of primary carcinoma. **D,** Concentric laminations, very indicative of a healed histoplasmosis. **E,** *Total* calcification, indicative of a healed granuloma (in this case, tuberculosis). *(Courtesy Medical Illustration Service, Veterans Administration Hospital, Denver, Colorado.)*

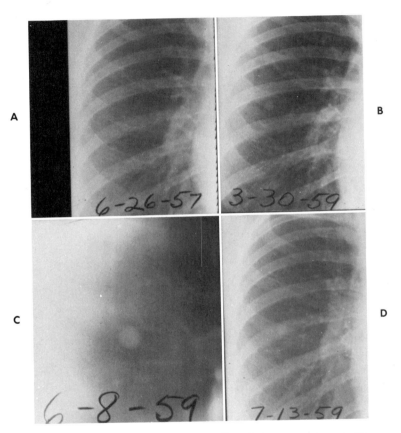

FIG. 22-2. Hamartoma. **A,** Clear film. **B,** Small nodule appearing at 40 years of age. Note smooth walls in 6/8/59 tomogram. **D,** Slight enlargement 3½ months after **B.** *(Courtesy Medical Illustration Service, Veterans Administration Hospital, Denver, Colorado.)*

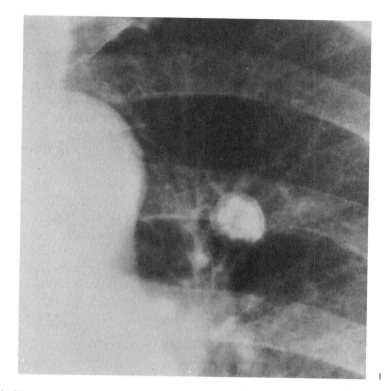

FIG. 22-3. Hamartoma nodule containing "popcorn" calcification. *(Courtesy Medical Illustration Service, Veterans Administration Hospital, Denver, Colorado.)*

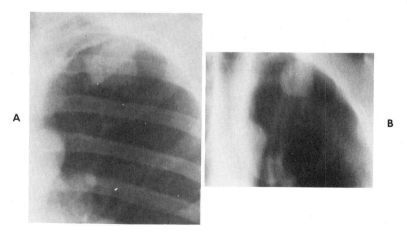

FIG. 22-4. Pulmonary nodule, 4 cm, smooth-walled nodule, left apex. It appeared to be a malignancy, but proved to be tuberculosis. **A,** Posteroanterior film. **B,** Tomogram. *(Courtesy Medical Illustration Service, Veterans Administration Hospital, Denver, Colorado.)*

Smoking history. Finally, the patient's smoking history is statistically very helpful. Oat cell, squamous cell, and undifferentiated bronchogenic carcinomas are all highly related to cigarette smoking history and rarely occur in nonsmokers. Adenocarcinoma, bronchial adenoma, and alveolar cell carcinoma are not closely related to smoking. Overall, nonsmoking patients with SPNs have about a 9:1 chance of having a benign disease. This low risk is not low enough to enable physicians to make an absolute decision on surgery versus observation, but is a reassuring statistic to the nonsmoker awaiting further evaluation.

Finally, a certain number of smoking patients over 35 years of age will have a noncalcified, low-density (as shown by CAT scan) SPN with no previous chest film available. If the patient is a good surgical risk, thoracotomy is often the best diagnostic and therapeutic procedure. Since larger lesions are more likely to have spread to the mediastinum, mediastinoscopy is recommended before thoracotomy in patients with nodules larger than 1.5 cm and, of course, in all patients with suspiciously enlarged mediastinum on plain chest film. In older, sicker, high-risk surgical patients, biopsy procedures such as bronchoscopy or percutaneous "skinny" needle aspiration can help the physician choose the best management plan.

SUGGESTED READINGS

Geddes, D.M.: The natural history of lung cancer: a review based on rates of tumor growth, Br. J. Dis. Chest **73**:1, 1979.

Holin, S.M., Dwork, R.E., Glaser, S., et al.: Solitary pulmonary nodules found in a community-wide chest roentgenographic survey, Am. Rev. Tuberc. **79**:427, 1959.

Jereb, M., and US-Krasovec, M.: Thin needle biopsy of chest lesions: time-saving potential, Chest **78**:288, 1980.

Lillington, G.A.: Solitary pulmonary nodules: benign or malignant? J. Respir. Dis. **1**:11, 1980.

Neff, T.A.: When the x-ray shows a "spot" on the lung, Med. Times **106**:65, 1978.

Siegelman, S.S., Zerhouni, E.A., Leo, F.P., et al.: CT of the solitary pulmonary nodule, Am. J. Roent. **135**:1, 1980.

Chapter 23

SLEEP APNEA

David W. Hudgel

There is rapidly growing awareness in the medical profession of the importance of respiratory abnormalities that can occur during sleep. Sleep apnea and arterial oxygen desaturation have been identified in some young, otherwise healthy individuals and in a greater number of older adults.[1] In addition, sleep apnea has been identified as the underlying disorder in many patients who have one or more of the following: pulmonary or systemic hypertension, secondary erythrocytosis, intellectual deterioration, mental depression, impotence, and daytime fatigue or somnolence. The purpose of this chapter is to review the etiology, clinical picture, diagnosis, complications, and treatment of sleep apnea.

Certain terms must first be defined:

apnea Interruption of normal ventilatory exchange for at least 10 seconds by one of of the following mechanisms:

   central apnea Complete or nearly complete cessation of abdominothoracic respiratory effort (Fig. 23-1).

   obstructive apnea Lack of ventilation exchange due to pharyngeal occlusion. During this type of apnea, abdominothoracic respiratory efforts continue (Fig. 23-2).

   mixed or complex apnea A combination of central and obstructive apneas within one apneic episode. Usually the central component precedes the obstruction.

Etiology

Little is known about the etiology or mechanism of sleep apnea. Whether the basic defect resides within the CNS is uncertain, but some evidence suggests this is so.[2] Patients with obstructive apnea have changes in ventilation timing for a few breaths before apnea. In addition, the arousal response to airway occlusion may be diminished in these patients. Whether these are primary or secondary events is unknown. Brain stem blood flow also seems to be decreased as compared to nonapneic individuals.[3] In obstructive apnea the mechanism of airway occlusion is pharyngeal muscle hypotonia.[4] For

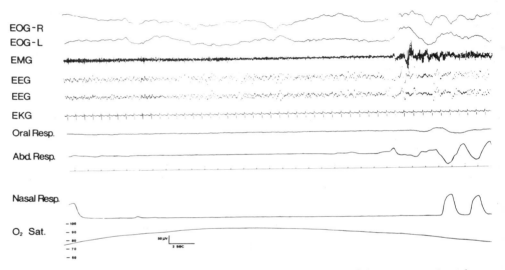

FIG. 23-1. Central apnea. Absent respiratory effort (abdominal respiration) without oral or nasal airflow. EOG-R and EOG-L, electro-occulogram; EMG, chin electromyogram; EEG, electroencephalogram; EKG, electrocardiogram; O_2Sat, arterial oxygen saturation as measured by ear oximeter. Because of circulation time from the lungs to the ear, there is a time lag in the decrease of the O_2Sat related to the apnea.

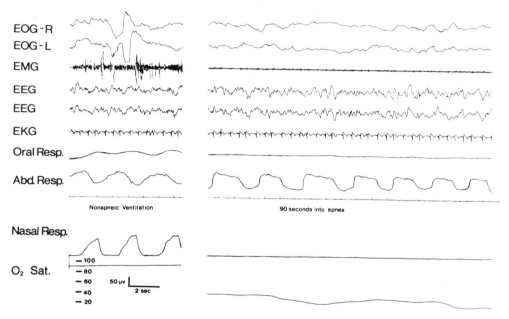

FIG. 23-2. Obstructive apnea. Left portion of figure shows normal sleep ventilation; right portion demonstrates absent nasal and oral flow but continual abdominal respirations, since O₂Sat is declining to extremely low levels. (See **Fig. 23-1** for key.)

unknown reasons the lateral and posterior pharyngeal muscles, as well as the genioglossus muscle, suddenly become hypotonic. With the next inspiration the negative intrathoracic pressure causes these hypotonic muscles to collapse inward, obstructing the airway. The muscle tone later returns, and ventilatory exchange resumes. The factor(s) leading to recovery of pharyngeal muscle tone are unknown. It is conceivable that decreased blood flow alters the acid-base or oxygenation status of the brain stem, resulting in dysfunction of the respiratory center or the neural controls of pharyngeal muscles.

The etiology of central apnea is not well understood. In animals, during certain stages of sleep, ventilation is nearly totally dependent on the input of peripheral receptors; the normal rhythmicity of the respiratory center appears to be absent during these times. If some disorder were to interfere with the activity or input of these receptors, central apnea might result. In patients with mixed apnea, treatment with tracheostomy resolves the obstruction, but the central component persists. However, after 3 to 4 weeks the central apnea also disappears. This suggests a mechanistic connection between the central and the obstructive apnea. Possibly, elimination of the obstructive component improves blood flow to the brain stem, which leads to improved function of the respiratory center and clearing of the central apnea.

Clinical picture

Patients with sleep apnea may have a variety of complaints relating to various organ systems. These complaints can occur individually or in combination. For instance, a middle-aged overweight man who snores, is mentally depressed, and has erythrocytosis may very likely have sleep apnea as the underlying disease process. In addition, patients with sleep apnea may have memory loss, intellectual deterioration, impotence, daytime somnolence, fatigue, and morning headaches.

The most important historical information, about which the patient is often unclear, concerns his or her snoring pattern. The patient's bed partner must be questioned regarding the presence and severity of snoring. In addition, the bed partner can often relate details of the patient's sleep breathing pattern, body position in which snoring occurs, and extent of restlessness. Typically, patients with obstructive sleep apnea snore extremely loudly and also have very restless sleep. Snoring and restlessness occur in the following way: Once the upper airway is obstructed, respiratory efforts by the thoracic and abdominal respiratory muscles increase. During this time the patient often flails around the bed, occasionally ending up on the floor. When the obstruction is finally broken, loud snoring or snorting occurs with the ensuing breaths. After a few normal breaths the cycle repeats. Patients with central sleep apnea may have mild snoring; bed partners may relate a history of intermittent pauses in respiration, but these patients do not have the dramatic restlessness mentioned above.

On physical examination several important aspects should be evaluated. One is body habitus. Overweight men with "bull" necks seem to be susceptible to sleep apnea. Metabolic and thyroid status, mandibular and maxillary anatomy, tonsillar, adenoid, and tongue size, nasal patency, tracheal position, pulmonary status, right ventricular activity, and general neurologic status (especially bulbar functions) are other areas on which the physician must focus. Patients with hypothyroidism, micrognathia, old mandibular fractures, tonsillar or adenoid hypertrophy, microglossia, and other upper airway–obstructing lesions may be predisposed to obstructive sleep apnea. Physical findings of pulmonary hypertension or right ventricular failure may indicate significant sleep hypoxemia. The neurologic examination may reveal cranial nerve or brain stem dysfunction or other entities possibly associated with breathing abnormalities during sleep.

Diagnosis

Definitive diagnosis of sleep apnea and type of apnea is best made in a specialized laboratory designed to evaluate sleep disorders. Unless the patient is extremely hypersomnolent, it is best to study him or her during normal sleeping hours rather than during a daytime nap. In this way the typical sleep pattern can be analyzed. In addition, sleep hypoxemia is often at its worst after several hours of sleep and during rapid eye movement (REM) sleep. Prolonged and REM sleep may not occur during a daytime nap; a more quantitative analysis can be made during a whole night's evaluation.

Sleep is categorized into light (Stages I & II), deep (Stages III & IV) and REM sleep by monitoring the electro-occulogram (EOG), the chin electromyogram (EMG), and the electroencephalogram (EEG). Electrocardiogram (ECG) is also usually recorded in order to identify cardiac arrhythmias that may occur in some apnea patients. To monitor the respiratory pattern, the patient's respiratory effort is recorded with an abdominothoracic strain gauge or an esophageal balloon. Nasal and oral airflow usually are traced with a thermistor or a capnograph. It is important to record both nasal and oral airflow simultaneously, since flow will often alternate between these two routes. Arterial oxygen saturation is followed by an ear oximeter. If this instrumentation disturbs the patient's usual sleep pattern and the suspected diagnosis is not confirmed, the evaluation should be repeated.

Central apnea is characterized by minimal or no strain gauge or esophageal pressure activity movement and no airflow (Fig. 23-1). Obstructive apnea is characterized by continued and increasing strain gauge or esophageal pressure amplitudes, but no airflow is present (Fig. 23-2). When ventilation resumes at the conclusion of the apneic episode, a short arousal (lightening of sleep) or awakening occurs. This repeated interruption of the sleep pattern often prevents the patient from reaching deep stages of sleep. The extent of arterial desaturation accompanying an apnea depends on the length and type of apnea. Obstructive apneas are accompanied by greater decreases in arterial oxygen saturation than central apneas. During obstruction, the patient is in effect performing the Müller maneuver and thereby pooling blood in major thoracic veins and altering the distribution of pulmonary blood flow.

Complications

Sleep apnea, primarily obstructive apnea, may be associated with many complications. As oxygen saturation decreases during apnea, pulmonary artery pressure increases. When this takes place repeatedly over months or years, at some point persistent pulmonary hypertension appears.[5] For unknown reasons, some of these patients also develop systemic hypertension that resolves with treatment of the apnea. Bradyarrhythmias or tachyarrhythmias may occur during apneic episodes. If these are ventricular in origin and considered dangerous, immediate treatment of the apnea with tracheostomy is indicated. Congestive right heart failure and secondary erythrocytosis can occur in the patient with sleep apnea who experiences repetitive hypoxemia.

The most bothersome complication is sleep deprivation.[6] Because each episode of apnea causes an arousal or awakening, the patient remains in the light stages of sleep and obtains very little or no deep, restful sleep. Patients do not awaken refreshed, but rather go through the day fatigued or fall asleep frequently, often at inappropriate and even dangerous times (e.g., while driving). These patients often have no warning of ensuing sleep, a characteristic that makes their behavior on the highway quite dangerous to themselves and others. Continuous sleep deprivation over time may lead to mental depression, memory loss, intellectual deterioration, behavioral changes, and impotence. These symptoms can destroy a patient's work, social, and family life. If the etiology of these problems goes unrecognized, the patient may be impaired and afunctional for life.

Other complications of sleep apnea are morning headaches, thought to be secondary to hypoxemia or CNS fluctuations in an acid-base balance that occur with apneas. Enuresis may also occur. Surprisingly, some apnea patients, especially those with central apnea, will have insomnia instead of hypersomnolence. This insomnia may result from repeated awakenings during the night or too much sleep during the day. Some patients will experience vivid hallucinations during daytime sleep episodes. Somnambulism has been reported infrequently.

Many patients with sleep apnea are obese.[7] Obese people who snore heavily and have daytime hypersomnolence fall into the category of obesity-hypoventilation or *Pickwickian syndrome,* so called after an obese character in Charles Dickens' *Pickwick Papers.* Obesity is thought to predispose individuals, especially but not exclusively men, to sleep apnea. The mechanism is not clear. Infiltration of adipose tissue into the pharyngeal muscles is one explanation, but this seems unlikely in view of the EMG studies mentioned above. It is clear that weight loss decreases apnea time, but it usually does not resolve the problem totally. It is important to note that some patients with apnea are not overweight; normal body habitus should not exclude the diagnosis of sleep apnea if other suggestive findings are present.

Treatment

Development of adequate treatment regimens for sleep apnea is just beginning. For instance, the primary treatment for obstructive apnea was tracheostomy until very recently. Now several pharmacologic agents appear to be helpful; the need for tracheostomy may be eliminated in most cases if these agents prove efficacious after further evaluation.

The presence of apnea does not necessarily indicate that treatment is necessary. To date, the natural history of apnea is unknown; it is not known whether treatment of uncomplicated apnea prevents complications. Therapy is therefore based on the presence of one or more of the following complications: (1) potentially life-threatening cardiac arrhythmias during sleep, (2) evidence of chronic cardiovascular effects (e.g., pulmonary hypertension with or without systemic hypertension, right ventricular hypertrophy, congestive right heart failure, or erythrocytosis), and (3) interference with daytime functioning (e.g., hypersomnolence, depression, memory loss, intellectual impairment).

Presently, tricyclic antidepressants appear to be quite helpful in sleep apnea.[8] Secondary amine compounds, such as protriptyline, have less sedating side effects than the tertiary amine products such as amitriptyline. Protriptyline decreases the frequency and duration of both central and obstructive apneas. The mechanism of action is unknown. These agents decrease the amount of REM sleep and thereby diminish the most prolonged apneas, but protriptyline also suppresses apneas in other sleep stages. One must be alert for cardiac rhythm disturbances and other major side effects such as glaucoma, gastrointestinal ileus, urinary retention, and interference with antihypertensive agents such as guanethidine, methyldopa and clonidine. Most patients can usually tolerate minor side effects such as dry mouth, mild tremor, and anxiety. If these effects do not unduly bother the patient, treatment should continue, since an uncomfortable tracheostomy may be the only alternative. The most effective dose for sleep apnea is unknown; 20 mg protriptyline at bedtime is usually well tolerated and produces a blood level greater than 70 ng/100 cc 24 hours after administration. This blood level of protriptyline is above the minimal therapeutic level for treatment of depression. Whether this is the most effective dose, schedule of administration, or blood level for treatment of sleep apnea remains to be seen. Tolerance has been reported with protriptyline, but in this study blood levels were not recorded.[8] It is possible that drug clearance increases or that a higher blood level is required after a period of therapy.

Medroxyprogesterone is a respiratory stimulant and has been used in sleep apnea.[9] It appears to be most effective in Pickwickian-type patients, since its primary effect is on daytime ventilation and alertness. It also decreases the extent of sleep hypoxemia, possibly because it improves chemical ventilatory drives. However, medroxyprogesterone does not eliminate apneas or change the sleep pattern in the majority of patients.[10]

Acetazolamide may prove to be a helpful agent in sleep apnea, but it has not yet been objectively evaluated. By producing a metabolic acidosis, this drug stimulates ventilation and thus may decrease the amount of sleep hypoxemia in patients with sleep apnea.

Tracheostomy effectively eliminates obstructive apnea.[7,11] Continued normal ventilation is ensured when the site of obstruction in the pharynx is bypassed. Complications clear quickly. The tracheostomy tube can be plugged when the patient is awake for normal cough and voice functioning. Of course, the patient must consider this procedure's hygienic and aesthetic side effects. Patient education in care of the tracheostomy is important postoperatively. Pharmacologic agents should be tried before tracheostomy unless a life-threatening cardiac arrhythmia or severe congestive heart failure exists and immediate reversal of complications is required.

In overweight patients, weight loss decreases the amount of apnea time. Dieting is very difficult for hypersomnolent, depressed patients and is often impossible until the apnea is under control. Some overweight individuals have hypoxemia during sleep when the ventilation pattern is normal. This is likely due to disturbed distribution of ventilation caused by the heavy thoracic cage's compression of the lungs or elevation of the diaphragm caused by excess abdominal adipose tissue. In this situation oxygen administration will help correct the nocturnal hypoxemia. Oxygen is thought to lengthen apneas but on balance does demonstrably reduce the degree and duration of nocturnal hypoxemia.

• • •

Regardless of the treatment plan chosen, the physician should objectively evaluate the therapy. Sleep evaluation should be repeated to document improvement or absence of therapeutic effect; changes in the patient's perception of symptoms are not very reliable. In the course of a given patient's illness, several sleep evaluations may therefore be required. Because of the mental depression accompanying sleep apnea, patients with this condition are easily discouraged. Family members and medical personnel must continue to be positive in their approach and make certain that patients keep follow-up appointments and pursue treatment over an extended period.

REFERENCES

1. Block, A.J., Boysen, P.G., Wynne, J.W., et al.: Sleep apnea, hypopnea and oxygen desaturation in normal subjects, N. Engl. J. Med. **300**:513, 1979.
2. Martin, R.J., Pennock, B.E., Orr, W.C., et al.: Respiratory mechanics and timing during sleep in occlusive sleep apnea, J. Appl. Physiol: Respir. Environ. Exercise Physiol. **48**:432, 1980.
3. Meyer, J.S., Sakai, F., Karacan, I., et al.: Sleep apnea, narcolepsy and dreaming: regional cerebral hemodynamics, Ann. Neurol. **7**:479, 1980.
4. Hill, M.W., Guilleminault, C., and Simmons, F.B.: Fiber-optic and EMG studies in hypersomnia—sleep apnea syndrome. In Guilleminault, C., and Dement, W.C., editors: In Sleep apnea syndromes, New York City, 1978, Alan R. Liss, p. 249.
5. Tilkian, A.G., Guilleminault, C., Schroeder, J.S., et al.: Hemodynamics in sleep-induced apnea: studies during wakefulness and sleep, Ann. Intern. Med. **85**:714, 1976.
6. Sackner, M.A., Landa, J., Forrest, T., et al.: Periodic sleep apnea: chronic sleep deprivation related to intermittent upper airway obstruction and central nervous system disturbance, Chest **67**:164, 1975.
7. Guilleminault, C., Eldridge, F.L., Tilkian, A., et al.: Sleep apnea syndrome due to upper airway obstruction. A review of 25 cases, Arch. Intern. Med. **137**:296, 1977.
8. Clark, R.W., Schmidt, H.S., Schaal, S.F., et al.: Sleep apnea; treatment with protriptyline, Neurology **29**:1287, 1979.
9. Sutton, F.D., Zwillich, C.W., Creagh, C.E., et al.: Progesterone for outpatient treatment of Pickwickian syndrome, Ann. Intern. Med. **83**:476, 1975.
10. Orr, W.C. Imes, N.K., and Martin, R.J.: Progesterone therapy in obese patients with sleep apnea, Arch. Intern. Med. **139**:109, 1979.
11. Motta, J., Guilleminault, C., Schroeder, J.S., et al.: Tracheostomy and hemodynamic changes in sleep induced apnea, Ann. Intern. Med. **89**:454, 1978.

Chapter 24

DISORDERS OF VENTILATORY CONTROL

David W. Hudgel

Disruption of the normal ventilatory control system may occur because of familial or environmental factors and as a complication of certain neurologic and respiratory diseases. The ventilatory control system consists of central and peripheral components. The purpose of this system is to (1) adjust ventilation to meet metabolic needs for oxygen and carbon dioxide elimination and (2) respond to mechanical loads placed on the respiratory system. Failure of the respiratory center or important peripheral receptors results in acute or chronic hypoventilation and its complications. Therapy is aimed at stimulating ventilation centrally, enhancing the input of peripheral receptors, or reducing the load placed on the respiratory system. Interestingly, intentional interruption of this system has been used to eliminate dyspnea in terminally ill patients with COPD.

The purpose of this chapter is to review the normal physiology of ventilation control, to describe the clinical expressions of abnormalities of this physiology, and to discuss the present status of therapy for these disorders.

Ventilation control physiology

The respiratory center is located near the dorsal surface of the medullopontine area of the brain stem, directly beneath the fourth ventricle. This center is really a group of nuclei, some with a stimulatory and some with an inhibitory influence on ventilation. The activity of these nuclei is specifically influenced by peripheral and other CNS inputs. The resulting efferent signal to respiratory muscles from the respiratory center is the culmination of (1) the inherent rhythmic activity of the central nuclei and (2) the input of peripheral receptors including CNS sources. Detailed discussion of the neurophysiology is beyond the scope of this chapter, but can be found in reviews of the subject.[1-3]

However, some discussion of the influence on ventilation of peripheral and CNS receptors is appropriate (Fig. 24-1). Ventilation is affected by cerebral activity. For instance, excitement or emotional distress leads to hyperventilation, for example, the hyperventilation syndrome characterized by acute respiratory alkalosis and its characteristic symptomatology.

Central and peripheral chemoreceptors have a major impact on ventilation, but they influence resting ventilation to only a minor degree. They enhance or suppress ventilation depending on pH or oxygenation status of blood and cerebro-spinal fluid. The central chemoreceptor, which senses carbon dioxide, is located in the medulla, near the respiratory center and fourth ventricle. The carotid bodies, located at the bifurcation of the carotid arteries, are responsible for about 50% of the ventilatory stimulation produced by carbon dioxide. The stimulus to ventilation is not carbon dioxide per se, but changes in pH. Thus the central chemoreceptor responds to pH changes in the cerebrospinal fluid and the carotid body responds to pH changes in the blood. In humans, the carotid body is the only oxygen receptor. The carotid body senses changes in oxygen tension in the blood, stimulating ventilation during hypoxemia and suppressing it during hyperoxemia. In most important physiologic systems more than one control mechanism or receptor is usually involved, as, for example, for carbon dioxide.

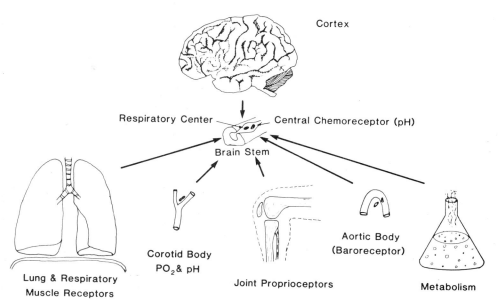

FIG. 24-1. Peripheral and CNS ventilatory receptors.

When damage or disease affects the carotid body, no back-up system exists for dealing with hypoxemia; carotid body dysfunction thus becomes manifested as a disorder of ventilatory control.

Lung and thoracic cage and/or respiratory muscle receptors also influence ventilation. The pulmonary stretch receptor is a classic example: lung distention leads to apnea due to vagal inhibition of respiratory center output. On the other hand, airway irritant receptor stimulation leads to rapid shallow breathing. It is not clear whether interstitial receptors, (i.e., J receptors) affect ventilation, but it is conceivable that increased minute ventilation would be beneficial during pulmonary edema or interstitial inflammation.

In animals, passive movement of hind limbs causes hyperventilation, a response likely mediated by joint proprioceptors. This mechanism could play a role in the hyperpnea of exercise. Ventilation follows metabolic rate quite closely. A decrease in body temperature, semistarvation, hypothyroidism, and sleep are known to decrease ventilation and the ventilatory response to other stimuli such as hypoxemia or hypercapnia, while ventilatory responses to chemical stimuli are potentiated during states where metabolic rate increases, such as hyperthermia, eating, hyperthyroidism, and exercise.

Genetic factors also appear to influence ventilatory control mechanisms. An adolescent asthmatic has been described who was not dyspneic even though cyanotic when wheezing.[4] Another child suffered recurrent episodes of respiratory failure during upper respiratory tract infections.[5] These children had very depressed responses to hypoxia, as did most of their healthy immediate family members. It was concluded that these patients could not respond appropriately to a respiratory insult producing hypoxemia because of a genetically depressed hypoxic drive. Endurance athletes and patients with COPD who routinely hypoventilate have low responses to chemical stimuli. Likewise, their healthy family members also have low responses to chemical stimuli.[6,7] One's ventilatory response to a stress on the respiratory system may be at least partially determined by genetic factors.

The aortic body is responsible for the cardiovascular response to changes in the chemical composition of the blood, especially to hypoxemia. This response is abnormal in familial and acquired dysautonomia states.

In addition to mechanisms of ventilatory drives mentioned alone, resistive and elastic loading of the respiratory pump, the lungs, and the thoracic cage influence ventilation. Resistive loading occurs with any condition that produces increased RAW, such as occurs in patients with COPD, asthma, or an isolated lesion in the upper airways. Elastic loads are encountered with any interstitial or alveolar process and with obesity. These conditions all cause an increase in the work of breathing. In healthy individuals a low or moderate level of loading will produce a compensatory increase in respiratory drive. For instance, the asthmatic changes respiratory drive in relation to fluctuating levels of airways obstruction. If the load becomes extreme, the subject will choose to hypoventilate and retain carbon dioxide. However, once hypoxemia occurs, the person will increase ventilation in an attempt to compensate.

Abnormalities of ventilation control

Abnormalities of ventilatory control result from (1) any interruption or depression of afferent receptor input to the respiratory center, (2) abnormalities within the respiratory center itself, (3) disorders in the efferent pathway, or (4) abnormalities of the lungs, thoracic cage, and respiratory muscles. Unfortunately, the medical profession does not know enough about many of the various syndromes to classify them accurately in this manner, but an attempt to do so in this chapter may lend some order to discussion of these pathophysiologic states.

Disorders of afferent limb. Carotid body function may be impaired by any disease state that alters carotid artery blood flow and blood flow within the carotid body itself and interrupts the neural activity in the carotid body or in the pathway from the carotid body to the brain stem. Carotid artery occlusion and endarterectomy near the carotid bifurcation, cervical injuries, poliomyelitis, Arnold-Chiari malformation, and familial and acquired dysautomonia all affect input to or from the carotid body. In addition, the carotid body adapts and thereby becomes unresponsive to chronic hypoxemia as in cyanotic congenital heart disease, living at high altitude, or chronic hypoxemic pulmonary disease. Similarly, decreases in carotid body function also partially affect the response to hypercapnia, since the carotid body is responsible for approximately half this response. Disorders that alter carotid body responses to chemical stimuli usually do not interfere with resting ventilation unless an additional load or stress is placed on the ventilatory system.

Some patients with COPD also have an abnormality in carotid body functioning. These patients—the so-called blue bloaters—hypoventilate, develop cor pulmonale and congestive right heart failure, and are usually overweight. Interestingly, they are less dyspneic than other COPD patients. It has been postulated that the decreased ventilatory responsiveness in these patients is inherited and predisposes them to abnormal ventilation when faced with the mechanical stress of their disease. On the other hand, the abnormal responsiveness at least may be partially acquired, secondary to chronic hypoxemia, since long-term oxygen administration will improve their responsiveness to hypoxemia.[8]

Although the hypoventilating COPD patient has diminished hypoxic and hypercapnic responsiveness, some still remains. Elimination of the hypoxic response will cause further hypoventilation, that is, too much oxygen will suppress ventilation. Since these patients have minimal hypercapnic drive, the acute carbon dioxide retention that occurs because of this hypoventilation does not stimulate ventilation. "CO_2 narcosis" and coma may follow.

Patients with chronic bronchial asthma tend to have a decreased response to hypoxia but a normal response to hypercapnia, implying that there may be specific carotid body dysfunction in these patients.[9,10]

Abnormalities of ventilatory control may be caused by interruption of pulmonary, diaphragm, or thoracic cage receptors. Patients with high spinal cord injuries or cordotomy may be affected by the mechanism. Poliomyelitis patients have damage to the reticular formation, which appears to affect afferent as well as motor pathways.

Respiratory center abnormalities. Brain stem injury or disease may affect the afferent and efferent pathways to and from the respiratory center as well as respiratory center function per se. Temporary abnormalities such as congestive heart failure and hypoxemia may also depress respiratory center function by unknown mechanisms.

The classic defect of the respiratory center is primary hypoventilation, also known as Ondine's curse.[11,12] This syndrome was first reported following surgical damage to the cervical spinal cord and medulla oblongata. It may also occur secondary to neurologic diseases or infectious damage of the brain stem. However, in most patients no pathologic defect is found. These patients have chronic hypoxemia and hypercapnia without an increased alveolar-arterial oxygen gradient. Pulmonary function tests are usually normal, and administration of 100% oxygen will normalize the arterial oxygen tension. These patients can also correct the arterial blood gas abnormality by voluntary hyperventilation. Response to exercise is suboptimal with very little increase in alveolar ventilation and a worsening of the Pao_2 and $Paco_2$ status. These patients have essentially no ventilatory response to hypoxia or hypercapnia; consequently, they develop cor pulmonale, right heart failure, and erythrocytosis due to the hypoxemia. They are often intellectually impaired and experience loss of memory. Approximately half these patients will develop obstructive apnea during sleep and thereby experience further hypoxemia.[13] Diagnostic and therapeutic activities should be directed toward ventilation during both wakefulness and sleep. These patients may be diagnosed in infancy, but some patients with the idiopathic variety of the disease develop severe right heart failure and erythrocytosis in adulthood. Responses to hypoxemia or hypercapnia are severely diminished or almost nonexistent.

Some research indicates that infants with sudden infant death syndrome

(SIDS) may have abnormalities of ventilatory control, possibly in the respiratory center. These infants have apneas during sleep and have been shown to have a decreased ventilatory response to inhaled carbon dioxide during sleep.[14]

Sedative hypnotic, tranquilizing, and analgesic medications also depress respiration and respiratory drive centrally. Patients with pulmonary, neuromuscular, or ventilatory control abnormalities must be given these medications with extreme caution since even "subtherapeutic" doses may lead to acute respiratory failure.

Likewise, general anesthetic agents such as halothane, nitrous oxide, and thiopental have been shown to depress ventilatory drive. When these agents are used in patients with abnormal ventilatory control, the operative and postoperative periods must be monitored very closely to guarantee that hypoventilation and respiratory failure do not occur.

Efferent pathway abnormalities. It is possible for the receptors to sense a ventilatory stimulus appropriately and for the respiratory center to increase activity, but the muscles of respiration must be activated for increased ventilation to occur. Phrenic nerve damage or its involvement in an inflammatory or cancerous process will impair function of the diaphragm, the major muscle of respiration. Generalized neuromuscular or primary skeletal muscle diseases also will interfere with diaphragm function. Some individuals may have inefficient transfer of phrenic neural activity to muscle activity or, in turn, into inspiratory force.

Disorders of ventilatory control thus occur because of afferent, central, or efferent defects. In the majority of patients the possible site of abnormality can be detected by careful evaluation. For instance, a patient with asthma may present with recurrent episodes of cyanosis during episodes of mild airflow obstruction. Evaluation of hypoxic and hypercapnic drives in such a patient might reveal a markedly depressed hypoxic response and a minimally decreased hypercapnic response. This would suggest a defect in carotid body function, which is normally responsible for all the hypoxic and a portion of the hypercapnic response. Another example is an adult with florid right heart failure and erythrocytosis. Evaluation might reveal arterial blood gas values consistent with hypoventilation. Hypoxic and hypercapnic drive analysis would show nearly complete absence of response. Such a patient demonstrates a central dysfunction consistent with primary hypoventilation.

Treatment

Therapy for disorders of ventilation control is in its infancy. Because of a lack of a full understanding of the biochemistry of the respiratory center and peripheral receptors, objective application of pharmacology has not been possible. Although several pharmacologic agents are known to be effective in these disorders, their use has not been based on a full understanding of the mechanism of action. And unfortunately, many anatomic defects, results of trauma, or neuromuscular diseases are irreversible and to date untreatable.

Medroxyprogesterone has been shown to stimulate daytime ventilation and improve the responses to hypoxia and hypercapnia in patients with obesity-hypoventilation or Pickwickian syndrome (see Chapter 23). It also diminishes some of the sleep hypoxemia in these patients and those with chronic mountain sickness. By producing a mild metabolic acidosis, aceta-zolamide also stimulates ventilatory drive. It might be useful in states with a baseline hyperventilation, subsequent respiratory alkalosis, and decreased respiratory drives, such as in acute asthma and high altitude acclimatization. Aspirin has similar properties. Aminophylline may stimulate ventilatory drives in some patients.[15]

Patients with central hypoventilation have not responded well to respiratory stimulants such as medroxyprogresterone, acetazolamide, or aspirin. In acute respiratory failure these patients do respond to parenterally administered respiratory stimulants such as doxapram, but obviously this treatment is only practical for the short term. Oxygen administration, at least during sleep, is important to prevent right heart failure and erythrocytosis in these patients. Some patients with severe hypoventilation have been successfully treated with diaphragm pacing.[13] If sleep evaluation demonstrates obstructive apnea, this must be specifically treated also.

In terminally ill, very dyspneic COPD patients, carotid body denervation has been used to relieve dyspnea. Since this procedure will decrease resting ventilation and eliminate the patient's ability to recognize worsening hypoxemia, it should only be considered for patients whose pulmonary status is deteriorating despite aggressive medical therapy of the underlying pulmonary disease. Carotid body denervation has also been used to treat asthma. Claims that this procedure improves bronchoconstriction are not founded. It is detrimental to eliminate an asthma patient's ability to recognize hypoxemia, since this may precipitate acute respiratory failure or other hypoxemic complications.

REFERENCES

1. Biscoe, T.J.: Carotid body: structure and function, Physiol. Rev. **51**:437, 1971.
2. Mitchell, R.A., and Berger, A.J.: Neural regulation of respiration, Am. Rev. Respir. Dis. **111**: 206, 1975.
3. Wasserman, K., chairman: Recent advances in carotid body physiology (Symposium), Fed. Proc. **39**:2626, 1980.
4. Hudgel, D.W., and Weil, J.V.: Asthma associated with decreased hypoxic ventilatory drive: a family study, Am. Intern. Med. **80**:622, 1974.

5. Moore, G.C., Zwillich, C.W., Battaglia, J.D., et al.: Respiratory failure associated with familial depression of ventilatory response to hypoxia and hypercapnia, N. Engl. J. Med. **295**:861, 1976.

6. Scoggin, C.H., Doekel, R.D., Kryger, M.H., et al.: Familial aspects of decreased hypoxic drive in endurance athletes, J. Appl. Physiol. **44**:464, 1978.

7. Mountain, R., Zwillich, C.W., and Weil, J.V.: Hypoventilation in obstructive lung disease: the role of familial factors, N. Engl. J. Med. **298**:521, 1978.

8. Bradley, C.A., Fleetham, J.A., and Anthonisen, N.R.: Ventilatory control in patients with hypoxemia due to obstructive lung disease, Am. Rev. Respir. Dis. **120**:21, 1979.

9. Hudgel, D.W., Capehart, M., and Hirsch, J.E.: Ventilation response and drive during hypoxia in adult patients with asthma, Chest **76**:294, 1979.

10. Richter, T., West, J.R., and Fishman, A.P.: The syndrome of alveolar hypoventilation and diminished sensitivity of the respiratory center, N. Engl. J. Med. **256**:1165, 1957.

11. Hunt, C.E., Matalong, S.V., Thompson, T.R., et al.: Central hypoventilation syndrome, Am. Rev. Respir. Dis. **118**:23, 1978.

12. Glenn, W.W.L., Gee, J.B.L., Cole, D.R., et al.: Combined central alveolar hypoventilation and upper airway obstruction. Treatment with tracheostomy and diaphragm pacing, Am. J. Med. **64**:50, 1978.

13. Shannon, D.C., Kelly, D.H., and O'Connell, K.: Abnormal regulation of ventilation in infants at risk for sudden-infant-death syndrome, N. Engl. J. Med. **297**:747, 1977.

14. Dowell, A.R., Heyman, A., Sieker, H.O., et al.: Effect of aminophylline on respiratory-center sensitivity in Cheyne-Stokes respiration and in pulmonary emphysema, N. Engl. J. Med. **273**:1447, 1965.

15. Smith, T.F., and Hudgel, D.W.: Ventilation and inspiratory muscle activity responses to hypoxia and hypercapnia in childhood asthmatics, J. Pediatr., in press.

Chapter 25

THE PNEUMOCONIOSES

Roger S. Mitchell

Definition and etiology

A pneumoconiosis is any change in the lung caused by inhaled dusts.

Various occupations in which pulmonary lesions have been reported include the following:

Aluminum pneumoconiosis
Ammunition maker
Fireworks maker

Asbestosis
Asbestos weaver
Brake manufacturer
Clutch manufacturer
Filter maker
Floor tile maker
Insulator
Lagger
Mill worker
Miner or miller
Roofer
Shipbuilder
Steam fitter

Baritosis (barium)
Barite miller and miner
Ceramics worker
Fluorescent lamp maker
Glassmaker
Metallurgist

Missile worker
Neon sign maker
Nuclear energy worker
Phosphor maker
Propellant manufacturer
Toxicologist
X-ray tube maker

Beryllium disease
Alloy maker
Bronze maker
Ceramics worker
Demolition person
Electronic tube maker
Extraction worker
Fettler
Flame cutter
Foundryman
Grinder
Metalworker
Metallizer
Polisher
Scarfer

Coal workers' pneumoconiosis
Coal miner
Motorman
Roof bolter
Tipple worker
Trimmer

Kaolinosis (clay)
Brick maker
Ceramics worker
China maker
Miner
Potter

Siderosis (iron)
Ship breaker
Welder

Silicosis
Abrasives worker
Bentonite mill worker
Brick maker
Ceramics worker
Coal miner

Diatomite worker
Enameler
Fettler
Filter maker
Foundryman
Miner or miller
Motorman
Paint maker
Polisher
Quarry man
Sandblaster
Shotblaster
Stonecutter
Stone driller
Well driller

Talcosis (certain talcs)
Ceramics worker
Cosmetics worker
Miner or miller
Papermaker
Plastics worker
Rubber worker

The simple fact that even prolonged exposure to a dust can be documented does not necessarily mean that a discernible pulmonary disorder or disability has occurred. Any harmful effect resulting from dust exposure is determined by a knowledge of the nature, duration, and intensity of the exposure, the particle size of the potentially hazardous dust, and whether the individual also smokes cigarettes. *Individual susceptibility to pulmonary injury,* for example, differences in pulmonary clearance efficiency, may play an important role.

Standards of safe working conditions in most nations today are based on maximum allowable concentrations, permissible concentrations, or target levels. Over the last 20 to 30 years these levels have been steadily lowered because of the following considerations: (1) experience with illnesses, (2) deaths of workers, and (3) feasibility. The goal of standards listed in Table 25-1 is the level to which workers may be exposed for 40 hours a week for a working *lifetime* without appreciable harm.

In determining whether an individual has a symptom- or disability-producing occupational disease, a complete and detailed work history is essential. General job terminology is much less desirable than the worker's per-

TABLE 25-1. Examples of currently acceptable threshold limits of dust

Substance	m.r.p.c.f.*
Silica	
Crystalline (quartz)	5
Amorphous, including natural diatomaceous earth	20
Silicates (<1% crystalline silica)	
Asbestos	5
Talc	20
Portland cement (inert)	50
Coal dust	2

*Millions of respirable particles per cubic foot of air.

sonal job description. It is not enough to know, for example, that the patient was a foundry worker; the physician must learn whether the individual operated a shake-out section or an iron torch in the casting-cleaning department of the foundry. Such a distinction is significant because the person who operates a shake-out section is often exposed to high concentrations of finely divided dusts containing fibrogenic free silica; the iron torch operator, on the other hand, is usually exposed only to high concentrations of benign iron oxide fumes. A patient may say he is a sandblaster, but what does he use as an abrasive? Sand that contains a high concentration of free crystalline silica? Steel shot? Silicon carbide? Aluminum oxide? Details about welding are also important for several reasons. Some metals are known to cause disease. Cadmium, for instance, may produce a chemical pneumonitis. Dangerous exposure to ozone or to silica may result from welding; for example, gas shielded arc welding can produce excessive concentrations of ozone, a chemical highly damaging to the lungs; some welding fumes contain silica, but iron oxide fumes are essentially harmless.

In many instances it is desirable for the physician to obtain specialized advice on the potential disease-producing hazards of a given occupation from the state department of industrial or occupational hygiene. At times a specific on-site investigation of the hazards of a specific task is desirable. An additional problem is the frequency with which people tend to change jobs.

The *particle size* is important because particles of more than 5 μm seldom penetrate to the alveoli. When they become submicronic (i.e., less than 0.5 μm) in size, on the other hand, some may enter the lungs and pass right out again like a gas. In short, particles larger than 5.0 μm are most likely to be deposited in the nasopharynx; those from 0.5 to 5 μm are most likely to be deposited in the nonciliated pulmonary surfaces—the alveolar walls—and are labeled "respirable."

The following is a partial list of occupational dust diseases:

1. Inert pneumoconioses
   - a. Iron: siderosis
   - b. Tin: stannosis
   - c. Barium: baritosis
   - d. Cement
   - e. Fiberglass
2. Active pneumoconioses caused by silica or silica content (i.e., fibrosis and other pathology producing)
   - a. Silica
   - b. Certain silicates, including kaolin
   - c. Diatomaceous earth
   - d. Asbestos
   - e. Bauxite
   - f. Talc
3. Active pneumoconioses caused by dusts other than silica:
   - a. Aluminum and aluminum oxide
   - b. Coal*
   - c. Graphite
   - d. Nickel carbonyl
   - e. Tungsten carbide
   - f. Beryllium
   - g. Cadmium
   - h. Cerium

SILICOSIS

Silicosis was first suspected by Hippocrates. Agricola described the fatal effects of silica dust in 1556, but the subject was given scant attention until the late nineteeth century. About 3000 new cases per year are diagnosed in the United States at present. The disease occurs particularly in persons engaged in underground mining, foundry work, and sandblasting. The duration of exposure needed to produce silicosis varies from as little as 18 months to as long as 30 years, depending on the intensity of the exposure. The disease process, once started, continues to worsen for at least 1 to 2 years after exposure ends.

The inhaled free crystalline silica or silicon dioxide particles are ingested by macrophages, which are then destroyed; some pass into the lymphatics, which drain into the hilar nodes. More macrophages are produced; they ingest the liberated silica particles and are in turn destroyed. Collagen formation and hyalinization ensue, producing silicotic nodules measuring 2 to 5 mm. These nodules microscopically show fibrous whorls, are avascular and laminated, and contain silica particles that can be seen with lateral illumination. As the process progresses, the nodules coalesce and, when large enough, may undergo aseptic necrosis (i.e., cavitate). They tend to be distributed in the peribronchial and perivascular spaces that have perilymphatic drainage. Bronchiolar smooth muscle atrophy is frequently seen.

---

*Coal, especially anthracite, sometimes contains an appreciable amount of silica.

Simple silicosis is essentially an x-ray change consisting of nodulation with no single nodule greater than 9 mm. Subjects with simple silicosis in the absence of other pulmonary diseases such as chronic bronchitis and emphysema do not have symptoms or functional impairment that can reliably be related to their silicosis.

Complicated silicosis is the advanced stage of the disease and is characterized by the presence of lumpy densities, usually associated with parenchymal fibrosis. In complicated silicosis, cough, expectoration, repeated chest infections, nonpleuritic chest pain, wheezing, dyspnea on exertion, ventilatory restriction, and airways obstruction *may* be present. In time the small nodules are replaced by large conglomerate masses 1 cm or larger and the condition is labeled progressive massive fibrosis (PMF)

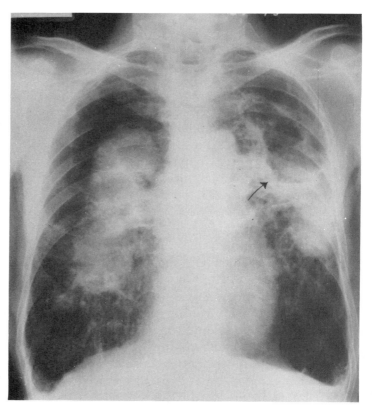

FIG. 25-1. Progressive massive fibrosis (PMF): advanced silicosis with superimposed tuberculosis. Note very large cavity with air fluid level, left lung. Also note central masses and peripheral emphysema. *(Courtesy Medical Illustration Service, Veterans Administration Hospital, Denver, Colorado.)*

(Fig. 25-1). In the late stages the lungs commonly become severely restricted and sometimes obstructed, diffusion is impaired, and hypoxemia supervenes—all of which results in respiratory insufficiency, pulmonary hypertension, cor pulmonale, congestive right heart failure, and death. The complication of superimposed tuberculosis and the nontuberculous mycobacterioses greatly accelerates the onset of disability and death in silicosis.

A characteristic radiographic feature of some cases of silicosis is the finding of so-called *eggshell nodes* at the hila: they are enlarged, numerous, and characterized by calcification only in their periphery—a virtually pathognomonic sign of silicosis, but seen in only approximately 5% of cases (Fig. 25-2).

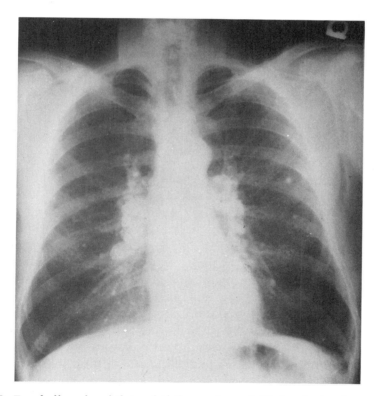

FIG. 25-2. Eggshell nodes, bilateral: hilar nodes calcified only in their periphery; characteristic of both advanced silicosis and coal workers' pneumoconiosis. *(Courtesy Medical Illustration Service, Veterans Administration Hospital, Denver, Colorado.)*

The *treatment* of advanced, disabling silicosis is not very effective; it consists mostly in relieving the hypoxemia with oxygen-enriched air and treating the congestive heart failure with digitalis, diuretics, and salt restriction. The inhalation of aluminum powder to neutralize the effects of inhaled silica was once recommended but is now recognized as having no demonstrable benefit.

By far the most important consideration is *prevention*, which includes the use of wet drilling methods to keep down inhalable dust concentrations, adequate ventilation, effective and tolerable masks, and regular monitoring of dust counts in the mines. Routine annual chest radiographic examinations and change of occupation when the presence of simple silicosis is well established are helpful in preventing the progression to PMF.

Silica and silicon dioxide react synergistically with mycobacteria; not only is their growth accelerated on culture media, but host immunity to them is reduced. Fully developed silicotuberculosis is difficult to treat even with the most effective antituberculosis chemotherapy. Patients with silicosis who react to tuberculin (i.e., 10 mm induration or more to intermediate-strength PPD-T) should be given INH as preventive therapy for 2 years after careful exclusion of the presence of active tuberculosis, especially by sputum microbiology.

ASBESTOSIS

Asbestos, a commercial term, is a mixture of hydrous silicates of magnesium, sodium, and iron in various proportions and in fibrous form. There are two major types: the *amphiboles* (crocidolite, amosite, anthophyllite) and *chrysotile*. Crocidolite fibers, long, thin, and straight in comparison with the others, which are larger and serpentine, are more prone to cause harm: the reason for this difference is not understood. Asbestos is used industrially in many ways, including the manufacture of clutch facings, brake linings, auto undercoating, roofing, insulation, and fire-resistant textiles. The heat generated by applying brakes converts a high percentage of asbestos brake lining into forsterite, an amorphous and essentially benign form of asbestos. The risk of mining asbestos is reduced, because the mining is mostly open pit and the crude ore comes out in large clumps. Certain procedures such as drilling and milling are quite hazardous unless wet drilling, proper ventilation, and proper masks are used. The adverse effects are dose related and may not become manifest for many years after exposure has occurred. The asbestos fiber causes a physical type of tissue irritation, morphologically seen as a diffuse, nonnodular, pulmonary fibrosis involving the terminal airways, alveoli, and pleurae (Fig. 25-3). Asbestos bodies may also be found in the sputum (rarely in pleural fluid), but they may

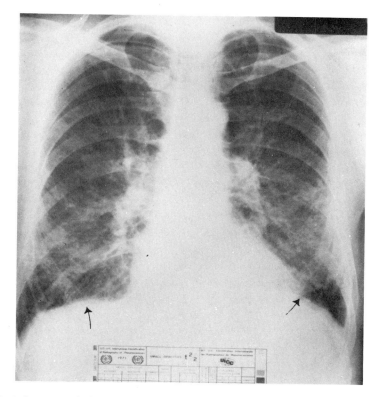

FIG. 25-3. Asbestosis: bilateral parenchymal fibrosis, especially in lower lungs, with diaphragmatic calcifications, bilateral. *(Courtesy Medical Illustration Service, Veterans Administration Hospital, Denver, Colorado.)*

also be found in the absence of asbestotic disease. Symptoms, especially dyspnea and dry cough, tend to occur before radiographic changes are clearly manifest. Changes are noted particularly in the parietal pleurae and in the lower lungs. Pleural effusions, including bilateral effusions, are common but often overlooked. The process may progress even long after exposure has ended. Physiologic changes include airway obstruction, restriction, and impaired diffusion caused by the widespread fibrosis. Other complications of asbestos exposure are bronchogenic carcinoma, confined almost exclusively to cigarette smokers, and pleural and peritoneal mesothelioma (Fig. 25-4).

TALCOSIS

Talc (or soapstone) is a hydrated magnesium silicate widely mined and milled for use as a dusting powder and as a constituent of paints, ceramics, asphalt, roofing materials, insecticides, and cosmetics. Whether talc per se

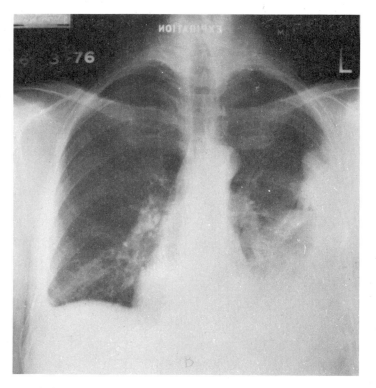

FIG. 25-4. Mesothelioma: left pleura, with hydropneumothorax and obliteration right costophrenic angle. *(Courtesy Medical Illustration Service, Veterans Administration Hospital, Denver, Colorado.)*

(free of fibers) can cause disease is not known. It is generally agreed that the disease of talc workers is attributable to *tremolite fibers* and possibly to chrysotile and anthophyllite (i.e., asbestiform) as well. Exposure may produce rather massive fluffy densities, especially in the midlungs, without significant symptoms or physiologic disturbance. There is a distinct risk, however, of disabling or fatal progressive fibrosis. Inhaled in high concentrations, talc may produce an acute bronchoconstriction that may be fatal in children. Pathologically, the process is initially a granulomatous reaction containing doubly refractile particles engulfed in macrophages; this is followed by interstitial fibrosis and endarteritis. Corticosteroids may cause symptomatic relief in severe cases.

COAL WORKERS' PNEUMOCONIOSIS

Coal workers' pneumoconiosis (CWP) is defined as the accumulation of coal dust in the lungs and the reaction of the tissues to its presence. It should not be confused with *black lung,* which is a legal or lay term meaning any chronic respiratory disease in a coal miner. The reason for making this distinction is that black lung compensation benefits are now given to surface coal miners as well as underground coal miners with respiratory disability after 25 or 30 years of exposure without the necessity of confirmation of CWP by chest radiograph. This is the result at least in part of disagreements over the interpretation of chest radiographs of miners.

Although some *silica* is present in some coal dusts, especially the anthracite and higher ranks (grades) of coal, and the radiographic appearances of silicosis and CWP are indistinguishable, the consensus of informed opinion is that contaminating silica does not play a major role in causing simple CWP. This opinion is based on two facts: (1) pure carbon exposure in humans can produce a disease radiographically and pathologically similar to CWP and (2) the pathology of CWP is quite different from that of silicosis.

The initial pulmonary reaction to coal dust is the *coal macule,* which ranges in size from 1 to 5 mm. Coal macules are located in the secondary lobule, especially in the upper lobes. They are found in black pigment deposited around respiratory bronchioles, often with a zone of air space (focal emphysema) surrounding them. Early CLE emphysema has the same location and appearance and may be difficult to distinguish from coal macules except for the presence of pigment. *Coal nodules* are almost always seen in a background of coal macules. They tend to start in the same location, are larger—up to 20 mm before they coalesce, are palpable on the cut surface of lung as opposed to coal macules, and contain variable amounts of reticulin and collagen.

When more than 13% (some say 18%) of the lung ash at autopsy proves to be silica, the case is diagnosed as silicosis. In addition, silica is believed to play a key role when simple CWP progresses to PMF.

CWP was first described in Great Britain in the 1830s, although the mining of coal goes back another 1400 years or so. CWP is now found in only a small percentage of current U.S. miners; a higher percentage is found in former miners. The frequency of CWP has been falling off because of improved dust control in the mines in recent years. In the past, it took 15 to 20 years of exposure to acquire the disease. Today, the risk from even 35 years exposure is minimal, except in small, poorly minitored and ventilated mines.

The diagnosis is based on a detailed and reliable history of exposure (including dust counts made in the involved mines and the nature of the miner's work, i.e., intensity of exposure in the mines) *and* experienced interpretation of a chest film of good quality showing at least some fine nodulation.

An elaborate system of reading the chest film for all pneumoconioses has been developed and is known as the ILO '80 Classification System. Each lung is divided into three zones. The fine nodulations are classified as predominantly rounded or irregular and rated as 1, 2, or 3 according to the profusion or numbers of the shadows. The process progresses from simple to complicated when any opacity measures at least 1 cm (Category A), when one or more opacities combined measure more than 5 cm but less than one third of one lung (Category B), and when one or more large opacities added together have a diameter exceeding one third of one lung (Category C).

The onset of symptoms and physiologic deficits (impairment of gas transfer, restriction, and airways obstruction) reliably attributable to the presence of coal dust is delayed in almost all cases until the appearance of complicated CWP. Coal workers with or without radiographic evidence of simple CWP often have the symptoms, signs, and physiologic findings of COPD, but careful studies of miners and controls indicate that the incidence of COPD is far more related to cigarette smoking than to coal mining.

Death caused by CWP is usually related to the development of restriction (i.e., fibrosis), usually with some degree of airways obstruction, hypoxemia, pulmonary hypertension, and cor pulmonale. Tuberculosis and mycobacteriosis are rare complications today.

Treatment of CWP is essentially nonexistent. *Prevention* depends on dust monitoring and control, adequate ventilation of the mines, wet drilling, effective and tolerable masks, annual chest radiographic examinations, and termination of employment of those with Category 2 or more CWP.

OTHER PNEUMOCONIOSES INVOLVING SILICA

Shaver's disease is caused by the inhalation of fumes containing aluminum oxide and silica produced by fusing bauxite powder in iron pots at over 2000° C. It occurred almost exclusively in a small region near Niagara Falls in Canada. The course of the disease was rapid with severe dyspnea, spontaneous pneumothoraces, severe respiratory insufficiency, and death.

Diatomite or diatomaceous earth contains amorphous silicon dioxide and is mined in several parts of the world, especially in coastal California. It is used to manufacture abrasive polish, insulation, and cleaning materials. In the calcined or flux calcined form it can produce a severely disabling pneumoconiosis because of contamination with free crystalline silica.

Caplan's syndrome was first described in Welsh coal miners with rheumatoid arthritis. It consists of large "cannonball" infiltrates in both upper lungs, generally with no or mild pulmonary symptoms. The nodules are morphologically similar to rheumatoid nodules. These lesions have more recently been found in hard rock miners and even in a few nonminers with the rheumatoid diathesis in many other parts of the world (see Chapter 31).

BERYLLIUM

Beryllium has become an important and useful metal because of its lightness and tensile strength. It has been used, for example, in the phosphors used in fluorescent lighting tubes, in the cement used to manufacture false teeth bridgework, in the solid fuels for space flight, and in ceramics and various alloys. Because of the hazards involved, it is currently used mostly in nuclear physics, since it reduces the speed of fission reactions, and for windows in x-ray tubes. The raw ore is not hazardous until it has been processed into the pure metal or one of its salts. Inhalation of purified beryllium may cause an acute rhinitis, tracheobronchitis, or pneumonitis, usually after a brief but heavy exposure. The interval between exposure and onset may vary up to several weeks. Although some 80% of people afflicted recover completely, the resulting pneumonia or edemalike processes produce severe hypoxemia; the patient will require supplementary oxygen and, at times, mechanical ventilation. Mortality is around 10%; some 10% of patients progress to the chronic form.

Beryllium granulomas may occur in the skin.

Chronic *beryllium granulomatosis* is a systemic disease that produces granulomas throughout the body, especially in the lungs. It has occurred as late as 15 years after initial exposure. The exposure may be slight and even indirect, as, for example, the wife of a beryllium worker exposed to beryllium oxide dust on his workclothes. There is considerable variation in individual susceptibility, with only a small fraction of the population being highly susceptible. The disease apparently occurs only after exposure to processed beryllium such as beryllium oxide and not after exposure to beryllium ores. The disease has an insidious onset characterized by persistent, severe, dry cough, severe weight loss, and severe dyspnea on exertion; other less common symptoms include a low-grade fever and anorexia. The chest radiographic findings resemble the miliary form of sarcoidosis, including hilar adenopathy. Severe, almost pure diffusion impairment with no ventilatory impairment or restriction is the striking physiologic picture. The morphology is almost indistinguishable from miliary sarcoidosis, except that the lesions and, in fact, many involved and uninvolved organs contain a significant amount of beryllium. Response to corticosteroids is often dramatically but only temporarily beneficial.

OTHER MISCELLANEOUS PNEUMOCONIOSES

Arc welder's siderosis probably should not be classified as a disease, since symptoms, abnormal signs, and disability do not occur and autopsy shows no tissue changes. The chest radiograph shows a fine miliary stippling caused by the deposition of iron pigment. When the welding process includes minerals other than iron (e.g., silicon dioxide, silicates, aluminum), it becomes hazardous. Acute welder's lung is apparently a pneumonitis occurring in response to high concentrations of ozone, usually caused by the presence of aluminum.

Tungsten carbide, or hard metal, workers are exposed to a very fine powder and may develop interstitial fibrosis or airways obstruction possibly because of cobalt content.

Nickel carbonyl, emitted during nickel processing and used as a catalyst in petroleum, plastic, rubber, and nickel plating industries, may cause acute pneumonitis and/or bronchiolitis; it is also associated with an increased incidence of lung cancer.

Uranium miners are unavoidably exposed to silica. In addition, especially when they also smoke cigarettes, they have a high risk of lung cancer, significantly higher than cigarette smoking alone would cause.

• • •

All physicians should watch for occupational or environmental causes of chest symptoms and radiographic changes. It is also possible that such exposures may precipitate pulmonary collagenoses such as lupus erythematosus and scleroderma.

SUGGESTED READINGS

AMA Council on Occupational Health: The pneumoconioses: diagnosis, evaluation, and management, Arch. Environ. Health **7**:131, 1963.

Bechlake, M.R.: Asbestos related diseases of the lung and other organs: their epidemiology and implications for clinical practice, Am. Rev. Resp. Dis. **114**:187, 1976.

Caldwell, D.M.: The coalescent lesion of diatomaceous earth pneumoconioses, Am. Rev. Tuberc. **77**:644, 1958.

Coates, E.O., and Watson, J.H.L.: Diffuse interstitial lung disease in tungsten carbide workers, Ann. Intern. Med. **75**:709, 1971.

Enterline, P.E.: Epidemiology of coal workers' pneumoconiosis, Ind. Med. Surg. **39**:115, 1970.

Gaensler, E.A., and Kaplan, A.I.: Asbestos pleural effusion, Ann. Intern. Med. **74**:178, 1971.

Hackett, R.L., and Sunderman, F.W., Jr.: Pulmonary alveolar reaction to nickel carbonyl: ultrastructural and histochemical studies, Arch. Environ. Health **16**:349, 1968.

Hardy, J.L., and Leahy, J.E.: Recognition of occupational lung disease, Clin. Notes Respir. Dis. **6**(4):3, 1967.

Heuck, F., and Hoscheck, R.: Cer-pneumoconiosis, Am. J. Roentgenol. Radium. Ther. Nucl. Med. **104**:777, 1968.

Higgins, I.T.T., and Oldham, P.D.: Ventilatory capacity in miners: a five-year follow-up study, Br. J. Ind. Med. **19**:65, 1962.

International Union Against Cancer: IUAC/Cincinnati classification of the radiographic appearances of pneumoconioses, Chest **58**:57, 1970.

Kleinfeld, M., Messite, J., Kooyman, O., et al.: Welders' siderosis: a clinical, roentgenographic, and physiological study, Arch. Environ. Health **19**:70, 1969.

Lane, E., and Anderson, W.H.: The dyspneic miner and the 1969 Federal Coal Mine Health and Safety Act (The "Black Lung Act"), Am. Rev. Respir. Dis. **103**:880, 1971.

Langer, A.M., Selikoff, I.J., and Sastre, A.: Chrystolite asbestos in the lungs of persons in New York City, Arch. Environ. Health **22**:348, 1971.

Lapp, H.L., Seaton, A., Kaplan, K.C., et al.: Pulmonary hemodynamics in symptomatic coal miners, Am. Rev. Respir. Dis. **104**:418, 1971.

Meyer, E.C., Kratzinger, S.F., and Miller, W.H.: Pulmonary fibrosis in an arc welder, Arch. Environ. Health **15**:462, 1967.

Michel, R.D., and Morris, J.F.: Acute silicosis, Arch. Intern. Med. **113**:850, 1964.

Miller, A.A., and Ramsden, F.: Carbon pneumoconiosis, Br. J. Ind. Med. **18**:103, 1961.

Milne, J., Christophers, A., and de Silva, P.: Acute mercurial pneumonitis, Br. J. Ind. Med. **27**:334, 1970.

Mitchell, R.S., ed.: Manual on Coal Workers' Pneumoconiosis, NIOSH, In press, 1981.

Morgan, W.K.C.: The prevalence of coal workers' pneumoconiosis, Am. Rev. Respir. Dis. **98**:306, 1968.

Morgan, W.K.C., Burgess, D.B., Jacobson, G., et al.: The prevalence of coal workers' pneumoconiosis in U.S. coal mines, Arch. Environ. Health **27**:221, 1973.

Morgan, W.K.C., and Seaton, A.: Occupational lung diseases, Philadelphia, 1975, W.B. Saunders Co.

Morrow, C.S.: The results of chemotherapy in silicotuberculosis, Am. Rev. Respir. Dis. **82**:831, 1960.

Nadel, J.A.: Physiology of coal workers' pneumoconiosis, Ind. Med. Surg. **39**:119, 1970.

Naeye, R.L., Mahon, J.K., and Delinger, W.S.: Effects of smoking on lung structure of Appalachian coal workers, Arch. Environ. Health **22**:190, 1971.

National Academy of Sciences: Mineral resources and the environment: supplementary report: coal workers' pneumoconiosis—medical considerations, some social implications, Washington, D.C., 1976, The Academy.

Phibbs, B.P., Sundin, R.E., and Mitchell, R.S.: Silicosis in Wyoming bentonite workers, Am. Rev. Respir. Dis. **103**:1, 1971.

Solomon, A.: Radiology of asbestosis, Environ. Res. **3**:320, 1970.

Trapp, E., Renzetti, A.D., Jr., Kobayashi, R., et al.: Cardiopulmonary function in uranium miners, Am. Rev. Respir. Dis. **101**:27, 1970.

Ziskind, M., Jones, R.N., and Weill, H.: Silicosis, Am. Rev. Respir. Dis. **113**:643, 1976.

Chapter 26

AIR POLLUTION AND THE LUNGS

Roger S. Mitchell

Air pollution resulting from the burning of coal has been recognized as an unpleasant nuisance for at least 400 years. Widespread realization that air pollution is a threat to life, health, and the economy and recognition that air pollution arises from many sources in addition to coal, however, is relatively new and presents a major problem of modern living. Actually, discharge of wastes of all kinds into air and water, that is, using the air and lakes and streams as a sewer, is as old as the human race. The chief reasons why it has only relatively recently become a recognized problem in the civilized world are the population explosion, the increasing tendency of people to concentrate in urban areas, and the introduction—and, until recently, the uninhibited expansion—of fossil fuel-powered means of transportation.

No one can doubt that air pollution can kill. At least 10 acute air pollution disasters have been recognized and well documented in various parts of the world, including the United States, in the last few years. The 1952 sulfur dioxide and particulate disaster in London, which was responsible for over 4000 deaths, was a major factor in focusing attention on the problem.

At times people may think that they can relax, since these disasters happen so seldom and, furthermore, tend to adversely affect mostly the elderly and the infirm, especially those with chronic heart and lung conditions. The trouble with this attitude is that the threat of immediate death from an acute air pollution disaster does not begin to tell how every individual may suffer from this problem.

The various ways in which urban, industrial, or community air pollutants may cause adverse effects are presented in the following list:

Metal, paint and rubber corrosion	Bad odors
Crop damage	Disease aggravation—heart and lungs
Weather alteration	Disease cause—eyes, lungs, and heart
Visibility impairment	"Greenhouse effect"

256

The "greenhouse effect" is the stimulation of plant growth from excess carbon dioxide and the resultant warming effect on the immediate environment.

Major sources of air pollution include:

Production, processing, and use of petroleum products
Chemicals, metal processing, ceramics from factories
Backyard, industrial, and community incineration
Combustion of coal
Chemical solvents
Certain agricultural practices

Many of the known constituents of urban air pollution are:

Primary emissions	Reaction products
Sulfur oxides	Oxidants: ozone and other
Nitrogen oxides	free radicals
Carbon monoxide	Peroxyacetyl nitrates (PAN)
Carbon dioxide	Fly ash
Hydrocarbons	Formaldehyde
Organic solvents	Benzo(a)pyrene and numerous
Fluorides	other polycyclic aromatic
Insecticides	hydrocarbons
Lead	**Materials of natural origin**
Radioactive dusts	Allergens
	Soil dust
	Radioactive isotopes
	Asbestos fibers
	Rubber particles from tires

Air pollutants are capable of the following adverse effects on human lungs:

Cause bronchial irritation, excess mucus secretion, cough
Increase resistance to airflow
Paralyze cilia temporarily
Lower resistance to respiratory infections
Aggravate chronic lung (and heart) disease by interference with oxygen transport (CO)
Induce carcinogenesis (?)

An urban factor increases the risk of lung cancer, holding smoking constant. This may or may not be something in polluted urban air, according to current opinion.

Other factors that influence the effect of air pollutants are:

Temperature of burning
Geography
Precipitation
Meteorology, including sunlight, wind, humidity, clouds, and fog
Cigarette smoke
Particle size (see Chapter 24)

Air pollution appears to play at least a partial causative role in *chronic bronchitis, emphysema,* and *COPD.* The causes of these diseases, almost certainly multiple, are not precisely known. It is known, however, that they are more common in men than in women and in cigarette smokers than in non-smokers. The cigarette relationship complicates the problem from the standpoint of consideration of the role of air pollution. Polluted air is inhaled through the nose and is thus partially filtered, but it is inhaled constantly. Cigarette smoke is inhaled directly through the mouth without being filtered by the nose—which, incidentally, is a highly effective filter—but the inhalation is intermittent.

These diseases are much more closely related epidemiologically to cigarette smoking than to air pollution. Strictly speaking, cigarette smoking may be regarded as a highly concentrated form of personal air pollution.

Evidence associating air pollution with the causation of chronic bronchitis is more convincing than that associating it with emphysema.

Children who grow up in cities have more chest infections and poorer lung function than do children from rural areas. This is of considerable interest, since many observers believe that respiratory infections and damage early in life play a significant role in the later development of chronic bronchitis and emphysema.

Persons with COPD suffering from acute exacerbations have shown significant improvement in airflow when removed from Los Angeles air to rooms ventilated with thoroughly filtered clean air. Ozone has been shown to impair oxygen diffusion into the lungs of humans.

So-called *Tokyo-Yokohama asthma* is a severe wheezing bronchitis clearly related to heavy industrial air pollution; it occurs almost exclusively in cigarette smokers. Permanent impairment can occur if the subject remains in the unfavorable environment.

So-called *New Orleans asthma* was originally believed to be another example of wheezing bronchitis caused by a special type of industrial air pollution; however, it is now thought to be most likely a form of true allergic asthma with a common but as yet unidentified cause.

PAN is a free radical formed by the interaction of sunlight, hydrocarbons, and nitrogen oxides from automobile exhausts. It is the substance known to inhibit enzyme activity in plants, causing the death of plants and trees along highways in southern California. In minute quantities undetectable by humans, it has been shown experimentally to impair exercise performance in healthy people.

Carbon monoxide has hemoglobin affinity 245 times that of oxygen; hence even small concentrations tend to block oxygen transport to the brain and heart. Driving through commuter traffic in downtown Los Angeles can produce a blood level high enough to cause symptoms even in a nonsmoker; commuters who smoke get even higher concentrations. It is strongly suggested that such elevated carbon monoxide levels increase the frequency of angina attacks as well as the risk of dying after an acute myocardial infarction. Carbon monoxide may also be involved in the pathogenesis of atherosclerosis.

The medical scientific community is in broad general agreement that the evidence—epidemiologic, physiologic, pathologic, and experimental pathologic—indicates that air pollution may be harmful to human health. The severity of air pollution is worsening; it takes months or years after the decision to do something about it has been made before any substantial improvement can be achieved. In support of this statement, in the Los Angeles area almost all sources of air pollution other than those emanating from automobiles and trucks have been fairly well controlled for the past several years, yet that area still has a severe air pollution problem. This was the final proof needed that the automobile is and has been the major source of the Los Angeles type of air pollution. Air pollution's persistence despite major efforts at control of automobile emissions and use reflects an almost insoluble problem. Progress has been and is being made toward controlling automobile pollution, aided greatly by the growing scarcity of petroleum.

• • •

In summary, urban air pollution—carbon monoxide and oxidants in particular—can aggravate preexisting chronic lung and heart diseases and, in combination with cigarette smoke, can play a causative role in chronic bronchitis and emphysema. Urban air pollution is also offensive to the eye, nose, and spirit. It will continue to increase unless something is done.

SUGGESTED READINGS

Aronow, W.S., Harris, C.N., Isbell, M.W., et al.: Effect of freeway travel on angina pectoris, Ann. Int. Med. **77:**669, 1972.

Bates, D.V.: Air pollutants and the human lung. The James Waring Memorial Lecture, Am. Rev. Respir. Dis. **105:**1, 1972.

Carnow, B.W., Senior, R.M., Karsh, R., et al.: The role of air pollution in chronic obstructive pulmonary disease, J.A.M.A. **214:**894, 1970.

Cohen, S.I., Perkins, N.M., Ury, H.K., et al.: Carbon monoxide uptake in cigarette smoking, Arch. Environ. Health **22:**55, 1971.

Goldsmith, J.R.: Health effects of air pollution, Basics Respir. Dis. **4:**1, 1975.

Goldsmith, J.R.: The new airborne disease community air pollution: community air pollution, Calif. Med. **113:**13, 1970.

Lambert, P.M.: Smoking, air pollution, and bronchitis in Britain, Lancet **1:**853, 1970.

Mitchell, R.S., Judson, F.N., Moulding, T.S., et al.: Health effects of urban air pollution, J.A.M.A. **242:**1163, 1979.

Uoshida, K., Takatsuka, Y., Kitabatake, M., et al.: Air pollution and its health effects in Yokkaichi area: review on Yokkaichi asthma, Mie Med. J. **18:**195, 1969.

Woolcock, A.J., Blackburn, C.R.B., Freeman, M.H., et al.: Studies of chronic (nontuberculosis) lung disease in New Guinea populations: the nature of the disease, Am. Rev. Respir. Dis. **102:**575, 1970.

Young, W.A., Shaw, D.B., and Bates, D.V.: Effect of low concentrations of ozone on pulmonary function in man, J. Appl. Physiol. **19:**765, 1964.

Chapter 27

SARCOIDOSIS

Marvin I. Schwarz

Sarcoidosis is a multisystem granulomatous disease with worldwide distribution and undetermined etiology. The southeastern United States has an especially high incidence, particularly among the black population. Siltzbach found the attack rate of sarcoidosis in black neighborhoods of New York City to be 64 per 100,000, as opposed to 7 per 100,000 in predominantly white neighborhoods of the city. However, in Sweden, where blacks are few in number, the attack rate is 64 per 100,000. The disease appears most commonly between 10 and 40 years of age, with the peak incidence between 20 and 30 years of age. Women are affected more than men.

Pathology

The typical histologic lesion of sarcoidosis is a noncaseating granuloma composed of epitheloid and occasional Langhans' type giant cells. Inclusion bodies of the Schaumann or crystalline type are often found. The fate of this granulomatous lesion is either complete resolution without structural change or hyaline fibrosis causing alteration in target organ function. The sarcoid granuloma is identical to that seen in berylliosis, farmer's lung, regional enteritis, and the noncaseating granulomas occasionally seen in tuberculosis and fungal diseases. In addition, nodes that are drainage sites for certain chronic infections or malignant disorders demonstrate histologic features indistinguishable from sarcoidosis.

Immunology

Humoral immunity. One of the clinical hallmarks of sarcoidosis is a quantitative increase in all three major immunoglobulins (IgM, IgG, IgA), particularly in patients with early active disease. In addition, total hemolytic complement activity is increased. And, as an expression of this nonspecific increase in serum immunoglobulins, 40% to 60% of patients with sarcoidosis have a positive serum rheumatoid factor. Positive rheumatoid factors are more commonly seen in women than in men and are not related to the presence of a sarcoidal arthritis. IgM is markedly elevated in patients with erythema nodosum, and a persistently elevated IgG indicates chronic disease in most patients. The enhanced antibody response in sarcoidosis is also reflected by the finding of increased titers to mycoplasmal pneumonia, herpeslike virus (Epstein-Barr), and the measles, herpes simplex, and rubella viruses. This capacity for overproduction of antibodies does not interfere with the expected antibody response to infectious agents.

Cellular immunity. Skin test reactivity in patients with sarcoidosis is absent or diminished when compared with a control population. Classically, tuberculin reactivity is depressed after the onset of sarcoidosis, but the incidence of sarcoidosis is not related to the individual's previous skin test reactivity. The majority of patients with active disease have decreased skin reactivity to tuberculin and other antigens including trichophytin, mumps, and candidiasis. The status of the reactivity of the skin tests has no prognostic value; if active tuberculosis develops in a patient with sarcoidosis, the tuberculin test usually becomes positive. Patients with sarcoidosis can temporarily revert to positive tuberculin reactivity when vaccinated with BCG or when tuberculin sensitivity is passively transferred. In addition, cortisone, when administered orally or when added to the tuberculin skin test, can produce a positive skin test in previously nonreactive subjects—the so-called *paradoxical response*. In Hodgkin's disease, by contrast, another pathologic state associated with anergy, skin test reactivity cannot be actively or passively transferred.

Another method to measure the ability to develop delayed type sensitivity is by sensitization of the skin to dinitrochlorobenzene (DNCB). Studies have shown that in active sarcoidosis, skin reactivity to DNCB is depressed, whereas patients with healed sarcoidosis react. Lymphocytes from patients with active sarcoidosis undergo a higher rate of spontaneous blastic transformation when compared with controls but demonstrate a decreased responsiveness to phytohemagglutinin. The cells' failure to respond to phytohemagglutinin corresponds well to failure of DNCB sensitization and to the presence of extrathoracic dissemination of the disease. Recently, peripheral T cell lymphopenia has been reported in acute sarcoidosis corroborating the above findings. In addition, increased amounts of activated T cells are found in the bronchoalveolar lavage of patients with sarcoidosis, suggesting that the lung is the focus of activity of the cellular immune system.

Clinical picture

General symptoms include fatigue, weakness, malaise, fever, and weight loss. Symptoms arising from specific organ involvement are mentioned under separate headings below. In some series, up to 40% of sarcoidosis patients are asymptomatic and are discovered only by routine chest radiography.

Thorax. The lungs and mediastinal lymph nodes are involved in over 90% of patients with proven sarcoidosis (Fig. 27-1). Dyspnea and cough are the most common complaints, and hemoptysis is occasionally seen, although 40% of patients with chest radiographic findings may be asymptomatic. The most common radiographic presentation of sarcoidosis is bilateral hilar and mediastinal node enlargement. This may be an isolated finding or may be associated with diffuse alveolar and/or interstitial infiltrates. The initial lesions may spontaneously resolve or progress to a predominantly interstitial infiltration with partial or complete resolution of the nodal enlargement. If a patient has interstitial infiltrates and no hilar lymph node enlargement or other systemic involvement, the diagnosis of sarcoidosis may be difficult to

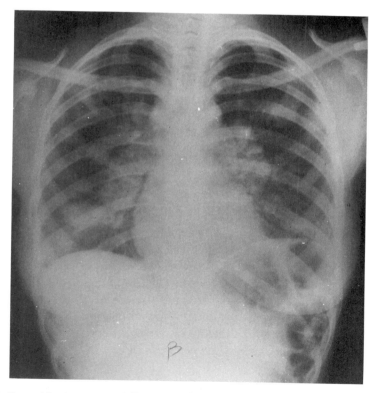

FIG. 27-1. Sarcoidosis: acute, diffuse, both lungs, with alveolar and interstitial infiltrates and gross hilar and mediastinal involvement. *(Courtesy Medical Illustration Service, Veterans Administration Hospital, Denver, Colorado.)*

make without lung biopsy. As the granulomatous process progresses, fibrosis occurs and the upper lobes retract, leaving dense bands of fibrous tissue and a tendency to form empty spaces. Within these cavitylike structures, saprophytic colonization with *Aspergillus* may occur, producing the characteristic radiographic picture of fungus ball. In addition, pleural disease, frank cavitation of nodules, scattered calcifications, endobronchial disease, and even eggshell calcification of mediastinal nodes are occasionally seen.

Skin. The most characteristic dermatologic lesion of sarcoidosis is a raised maculopapular eruption that can be found anywhere on the body and has a special predilection for previous trauma sites, for example, scars and tattoos. The presence of this form of cutaneous sarcoidosis implies a more chronic course for the systemic disease. Erythema nodosum, which frequently accompanies early disease (hilar nodes with or without pulmonary infiltrates), implies a more benign self-limiting course. Löfgren's syndrome, which consists of erythema nodosum, fever, arthralgia, and hilar and peripheral lymphadenopathy, is a common presenting symptom complex of acute sarcoidosis in Scandinavia and Europe.

Eyes. Ocular disease is seen in 20% of patients. The most common manifestations are conjunctival plaques, lacrimal gland enlargement, and uveitis. Uveitis may result in blindness, a complication reported in 3.5% of patients. Less common ocular complications include glaucoma and cataracts secondary to disease of the retina, sclera, and lens.

Reticuloendothelial system. Palpable adenopathy is found in 70% of patients with sarcoidosis; hepatosplenomegaly is found in 25%. Although these conditions rarely cause significant functional problems, prehepatic portal hypertension has been reported, and in the occasional case of massive sarcoid splenomegaly, splenectomy may be indicated.

Musculoskeletal system. A patient with acute sarcoidosis may see a physician because of arthralgia and, occasionally, polyarthritis. The occurrence of a chronic arthritis with periosteal bone resorption appearing as cysts may mimic rheumatoid disease and is usually associated with a chronic protracted course. Diffuse granulomatous myositis, an uncommon complication of sarcoidosis, also indicates progressive disease and a poor prognosis.

Exocrine glands. Uveoparotid fever, a combination of parotid gland enlargement, uveitis, fever, and occasional seventh nerve palsy, is a rare presentation of sarcoidosis. Sarcoid granulomas are also a rare cause of pancreatitis.

Kidneys. Hypercalcemia and hypercalciuria caused by increased absorption of dietary calcium as a result of increased sensitivity to vitamin D is seen in 15% to 30% of patients and may result in nephrocalcinosis, nephrolithiasis, and chronic renal disease. Occasionally, renal impairment results from extensive granulomatous infiltration of the renal parenchyma or an immune complex membranous glomerulonephritis.

Heart. Involvement of the ventricular septum and conduction system may lead to various arrhythmias and sudden death. With extensive granulomatous myocardial involvement, congestive failure may supervene. Pericardial effusions and ventricular aneurysms are also seen; in those patients who have clinically apparent cardiac disease, they often are the only manifestations of sarcoidosis and portend a poor prognosis.

CNS. CNS involvement may result in a basal granulomatosis that can lead to hypothalamic hypopituitarism, hypothalamic hypothyroidism, hydrocephalus, lymphocytic meningitis, and cranial nerve palsies. Thyroiditis has been reported during the active phase of sarcoidosis.

Laboratory findings

Hemoglobin values below 11 gm/100 ml are seen in 22% of patients. Hemolytic anemia may rarely be autoimmune in nature (Coombs positive) or result from hypersplenism. Usually the anemia is similar to that seen in chronic systemic disease. Leukopenia is seen in 30% of cases and eosinophilia in 24%. Thrombocytopenia is an uncommon finding but may accompany hypersplenism. The erythrocyte sedimentation rate is frequently elevated. The hypergammaglobulinemia, altered skin test reactivity, and positive rheumatoid factors have been discussed. Abnormalities of liver function, particularly a moderate elevation of alkaline phosphatase, implies diffuse granulomatous hepatic involvement although the liver may be involved without abnormality of hepatic function tests. Elevation of the angiotensin converting enzyme (ACE) in the serum of patients with active sarcoidosis has recently been described. This enzyme appears to reflect the clinical activity of the disease. Elevation of ACE is fairly specific for sarcoidosis, but increased levels have also been seen with Gaucher's disease and leprosy.

Characteristically, pulmonary function testing reveals a restrictive pattern with preservation of flow rates and a reduction in the diffusing capacity for carbon monoxide. Arterial blood gases may be normal or reveal hypoxemia and hypocapnia (hyperventilation); the stress of exercise may accentuate these abnormalities. It is not unusual for a patient's pulmonary function to be entirely normal or for the physician to find only an isolated reduction in diffusing capacity in an early case. Endobronchial sarcoidal involvement may lead to impairment of airflow in the exceptional case.

Diagnosis

Although histopathologic confirmation is often required, the clinical picture may be quite diagnostic. Biopsies should be performed on accessible lesions of the skin or enlarged peripheral lymph nodes. Mediastinoscopy with biopsy of anterior mediastinal nodes is a time-honored procedure if more external tissue is not available. Limited or conventional thoracotomy with biopsy of hilar nodes and/or lung tissue has been standard practice for many years. In subjects with parenchymal disease on chest radiograph, the yield is 96%; in those with negative x-ray films, 44%. Recently, transbronchial biopsy has been advocated as the biopsy procedure of choice. However, biopsy of any kind may be omitted when the clinical picture leaves little or no doubt of the diagnosis of sarcoidosis.

The Kveim test consists of an intradermal injection of suspended, pulverized, and sterilized sarcoidal spleen or lymph node material followed by biopsy of the area some 6 to 12 weeks later; it has limited use because of the lack of standardization of the test material and the recently raised question of false-positive responses.

Treatment

The nonspecific, self-limiting symptoms of acute sarcoidosis such as fever, arthralgia, erythema nodosum, mild dyspnea, and cough may not require any treatment. The more serious manifestations such as severe cough or dyspnea, hypercalcemia, uveitis, involvement of the cardiac conduction system, impaired or worsening pulmonary function, arthritis, myositis, and CNS involvement should be treated with corticosteroids. The usual dosage is 30 to 60 mg prednisone daily for 7 to 14 days followed by tapering to the lowest effective dose for a total duration of 3 to 6 months.

SUGGESTED READINGS

Berger, K.W., and Relman, A.S.: Renal impairment due to sarcoid infiltration of kidney: report of case proved by renal biopsies before and after treatment with cortisone, N. Engl. J. Med. **252**:44, 1955.

Buckley, C.E., Nagaya, H., and Sieker, H.O.: Altered immunologic activity in sarcoidosis, Ann. Intern. Med. **64**:508, 1966.

Chusid, E.L., Shah, R., and Siltzbach, L.E.: Tuberculin tests during the course of sarcoidosis in 350 patients, Am. Rev. Respir. Dis. **104**:13, 1971.

Dauber, J.H., Rossman, M.D., and Daniele, R.P.: Bronchoalveolar cell populations in acute sarcoidosis, J. Lab. Clin. Med. **94**:862, 1979.

DeRemee, R.A., and Andersen, H.A.: Sarcoidosis: a correlation of dyspnea with roentgenographic stage and pulmonary function changes, Mayo Clin. Proc. **49**:742, 1974.

Gozo, E.G., Jr., Cosnow, I., Cohen, H.C., et al.: The heart in sarcoidosis, Chest **60**:379, 1971.

Israel, H.L.: Prognosis of sarcoidosis, Ann. Intern. Med. **73**:1038, 1970.

Kataria, Y.P., Sagone, A.L., LoBuglio, A.F., et al.: In vitro observations on sarcoid lymphocytes and their correlation with cutaneous anergy and clinical severity of disease, Am. Rev. Respir. Dis. **108**:767, 1973.

Leiberman, J.: Elevation of serum angiotension-converting-enzyme (ACE) level in sarcoidosis, Am. J. Med. **59**:365, 1975.

Maddrey, W.C., Johns, C.J., Boitnott, J.K., et al.: Sarcoidosis and chronic hepatic disease: a clinical and pathologic study of 20 patients, Medicine **49**:375, 1970.

Mariani, A.F., Clifton, S., Davies, D.J., et al.: Membranous glomerulonephritis associated with sarcoidosis, Aust. NZ J. Med. **8**:420, 1978.

Marshall, R., and Karlish, A.J.: Lung function in sarcoidosis: an investigation of the disease as seen at a clinic in England and a comparison of the value of various lung function tests, Thorax **26**:402, 1971.

Marshall, R., Smellie, H., Baylis, J.M., et al.: Pulmonary function in sarcoidosis, Thorax **13**:48, 1958.

Mayock, R.L., Bertrand, P., Morrison, C.E., et al.: Manifestations of sarcoidosis: analysis of 145 patients, with a review of nine series selected from the literature, Am. J. Med. **35**:67, 1963.

Mitchell, D.N., and Scadding, J.G.: Sarcoidosis, Am. Rev. Respir. Dis. **110**:774, 1974.

Oreskes, I., and Siltzbach, L.E.: Changes in rheumatoid factor activity during the course of sarcoidosis, Am. J. Med. **44**:60, 1968.

Poe, R.H., Israel, R.H., Utell, M.J., et al.: Probability of a positive transbronchial lung biopsy result in sarcoidosis, Arch. Intern. Med. **139**:761, 1979.

Sharma, O.P., James, D.G., and Fox, R.A.: A correlation of in vivo delayed-type hypersensitivity with in vitro lymphocyte transformation in sarcoidosis, Chest **60**:35, 1971.

Siltzbach, L.E.: Sarcoidosis: clinical features and management, Med. Clin. North Am. **51**(2):483, 1967.

Siltzbach, L.E., James, D.G., Neville, E., et al.: Course and prognosis of sarcoidosis around the world, Am. J. Med. **57**:847, 1974.

Stone, D.J., and Schwartz, A.: A long-term study of sarcoid and its modification by steroid therapy, Am. J. Med. **41**:528, 1966.

Ueda, E., Kawabe, T., Tachibana, T., et al.: Serum angiotension-converting enzyme activity as an indicator of prognosis in sarcoidosis, Am. Rev. Respir. Dis. **121**:667, 1980.

Winnacker, J.L., Becker, K.L., and Katz, S.: Endocrine aspects of sarcoidosis, N. Engl. J. Med. **278**:427, 483, 1968.

Chapter 28

NONCARDIAC PULMONARY EDEMA

Charles Scoggin

Noncardiac pulmonary edema is a type of lung congestion that occurs in the absence of cardiac malfunction. In contrast to cardiac pulmonary edema, the findings of heart failure are absent (Table 28-1). No left ventricular gallop is present, neck veins are not distended, and the pulmonary artery wedge pressure is normal (i.e., less than 18 cm of water). In general, the pathophysiology of noncardiac pulmonary edema remains speculative. Current research techniques are limited, and it is difficult to say with assurance how much of the lung congestion is caused by disruption of the endothelial membrane of the pulmonary capillaries and how much is caused by increased intravascular pressure from such factors as microthrombi or pulmonary venular constriction. Regardless of the mechanism, the outcome is essentially the same: gas exchange is impaired and arterial hypoxemia is the result.

Etiology

In each form of noncardiac pulmonary edema a major precipitating factor is obvious from the clinical setting in which it occurs.

High altitude. High altitude pulmonary edema (HAPE) is a unique form of this syndrome associated with exposure to altitudes greater than 8000 feet. It usually occurs within 24 to 36 hours after ascent to high altitude and generally affects the young, the vigorous, and the healthy. Parenthetically, individuals native to high altitude may develop the syndrome upon reascent to altitude after a sojourn at low altitude. Extremely cold weather coupled with vigorous activity seems to predispose persons to HAPE but exceptions occur; this association remains uncertain. It has been speculated that overperfusion of certain areas of the lungs leads to localized increases in hydrostatic pressure, thus producing the patchy pulmonary edema seen radiographically in HAPE. HAPE's occurrence in the normal lung of individuals with unilateral pulmonary artery atresia of the other lung lends support to

TABLE 28-1. Differentiation of noncardiac and cardiac pulmonary edema

	Noncardiac	Cardiac
Cardiac enlargement	0	+
Left ventricular S_3 gallop	0	+
Engorgement of neck veins	0	+
Pulmonary arterial wedge pressure elevated (>18 cm H_2O)	0	+

this hypothesis. It is also possible that alterations in coagulability of the blood could lead to microvascular obstruction, pulmonary venous hypertension, and transudation of fluid into the extravascular space.

The symptoms of HAPE are shortness of breath, cough, and nonpleuritic chest pain. Fine rales may or may not be present. The chest film discloses a fluffy alveolar infiltrate that is readily confused with pneumonia. Examination of the sputum should help differentiate the two conditions. Death is rare but has been reported.

Drug overdose. Pulmonary edema is a well-recognized consequence of narcotic overdose. It can occur not only with heroin but with a variety of other narcotics, and it has been associated with oral as well as intravenous drug abuse. Salicylate overdose is an important and often overlooked cause. A neurogenic mechanism has been postulated. The typical person so afflicted is an elderly, confused individual with unexplained pulmonary congestion. Pulmonary edema due to drug overdose should be treated by measures directed at providing adequate oxygenation and reversing the effects of the causative agent, for example, with antagonists such as nalorphine for narcotics.

Neurogenic. Patients who have suffered severe head trauma or who have experienced seizures, an intracranial hemorrhage, or some profound infection may develop acute pulmonary edema. A possible mechanism for neurogenic pulmonary edema relates to increased sympathetic discharge; this may lead to either pulmonary venous hypertension or a shift of the systemic blood volume to the pulmonary circulation.

Smoke inhalation. Smoke inhalation may lead to noncardiac pulmonary edema by direct damage to the alveolar-capillary membrane. The clinical picture often is not evident immediately but may develop several hours after exposure. Observation for 12 to 24 hours after exposure is therefore indicated. Corticosteroid therapy may offer protective advantage.

Toxic gas inhalation. Inhalation of toxic gases such as chlorine, nitrogen oxides, sulfur oxides, ozone, phosgene, and paraquot may cause noncardiac pulmonary edema by direct injury to the alveolar-capillary membrane. As in

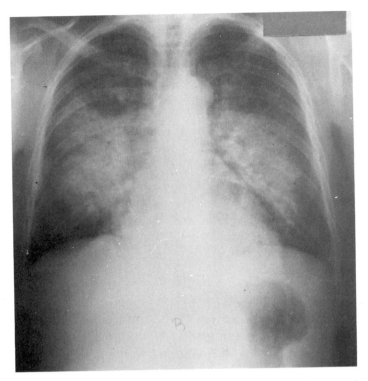

FIG. 28-1. Uremic pneumonitis, indistinguishable from other forms of pulmonary edema, except that the heart is only marginally enlarged and the apices and costophrenic angles are essentially clear. *(Courtesy Medical Illustration Service, Veterans Administration Hospital, Denver, Colorado.)*

smoke inhalation, the full-blown clinical picture may be delayed for several hours. Because of this frequent delay in onset, individuals who have been exposed should be observed for at least 12 to 24 hours following inhalation.

Uremia. In some patients with adequate left ventricular function and without fluid overload, pulmonary edema labeled *uremic pneumonitis* (Fig. 28-1) has occurred in the setting of renal failure. Increased capillary permeability caused by circulating toxic substances is the presumed mechanism. Dialysis to correct the uremia is the treatment of choice.

Aspiration. Inhalation of gastric contents, particularly when hydrochloric acid is present, may cause severe pulmonary edema. In this setting, physical damage to the alveolar-capillary membrane is again presumably the mechanism. The use of corticosteroids and antibiotics in this condition remains controversial. If evidence of infection—for example, purulent sputum—is present, then antibiotics are usually empirically begun. If aspiration has occurred while the patient is institutionalized, antibiotic therapy for anaerobic organisms and gram-negative infection should be included.

Near drowning. People who have inhaled large amounts of either fresh or sea water often develop the picture of pulmonary edema, immediate or delayed. An alteration in alveolar-capillary permeability is the presumed mechanism. As in smoke and toxic gas inhalation, the delayed appearance of pulmonary edema necessitates that victims of near drowning be watched for at least 24 hours to ensure that respiratory distress does not develop.

Diagnosis

Patients with noncardiac pulmonary edema who are conscious often complain of shortness of breath, cough, and nonpleuritic chest pain. Fine to coarse rales may be heard. Patients often appear cyanotic; however, signs of left ventricular failure and systemic volume overload are absent. Arterial blood gases reveal hypoxemia. If gas exchange is severely hindered or respiration impaired as in narcotic overdose, hypercapnia and respiratory acidosis will also be present. If the patient is hypotensive, arterial pH may be decreased because of lactic acidosis. The chest radiograph will disclose the characteristic fluffy alveolar pattern associated with all forms of pulmonary edema; however, the cardiac shadow is normal in size and contour and Kerley's B lines are absent. When doubt persists, the most reliable way of confirming the diagnosis of noncardiac pulmonary edema is by direct measurement of the pulmonary artery wedge pressure by flow-directed Swan-Ganz catheter. If the wedge pressure is normal, then pulmonary congestion is not due to cardiac failure. It may also be difficult to differentiate noncardiac pulmonary edema from infection (e.g., pneumonitis). The clinical setting in which pulmonary congestion occurs is very helpful in differentiating the two conditions. In addition, as in HAPE, examination of the sputum may also be helpful.

Treatment

Treatment of noncardiac pulmonary edema is directed toward alleviation of the inciting event and maintenance of adequate arterial oxygenation. Management of these patients is much like the management of patients with ARDS (see Chapter 6). Patients with pulmonary edema secondary to narcotic overdose should have a narcotic antagonist administered. When pulmonary edema occurs in association with increased intracranial pressure, pulmonary congestion may resolve as intracranial pressure is decreased. High altitude pulmonary edema usually responds to oxygen therapy alone or evacuation to a lower altitude. Corticosteroids, salt-poor albumin, and diuretics have all been recommended, but their use remains controversial. Rarely, it may be necessary to institute mechanical inhalation to provide adequate oxygenation. PEEP may be useful in improving arterial oxygenation while allowing reduction of the amount of inspired oxygen.

SUGGESTED READINGS

Hackett, P.H., Creagh, C.E., Grover, R.F., et al.: High-altitude pulmonary edema in persons without the right pulmonary artery, N. Engl. J. Med. **302:**1070, 1980.

Heffner, J., Starkey, T., and Anthony, P.: Salicylate-induced noncardiogenic pulmonary edema, West J. Med. **130:**263, 1979.

Scoggin, C.H., Hyers, T.M., Reeves, J.T., et al.: High-altitude pulmonary edema in the children and young adults of Leadville, Colorado, N. Engl. J. Med. **297:**1269, 1977.

Snashall, P.D.: Pulmonary oedema, Br. J. Dis. Chest **74:**1, 1980.

Staub, N.C.: Pulmonary edema—hypoxia and overperfusion, N. Engl. J. Med. **302:**1085, 1980.

Staub, N.C.: "State of the art" review. Pathogenesis of pulmonary edema, Am. Rev. Respir. Dis. **109:**358, 1974.

Chapter 29

THE DIAPHRAGM

Michael Shasby

Normal anatomy and physiology

The diaphragm is a dome-shaped musculotendinous sheet separating the thoracic and abdominal cavities (see Fig. 29-1). Its muscle fibers originate from the sternum, ribs 7 through 12, and the first two to three lumbar vertebrae and insert into a central tendon. The tendon itself is shaped like an Australian boomerang with its apex pointing toward the sternum. Posteriorly, two crura arise from the first three lumbar vertebrae on the right and the first two on the left and unite anterior to the aortic hiatus to form the medial arcuate ligament. Laterally, the fibers originate from ribs 7 through 12 and ascend to the central tendon, which is inferior to and contiguous with the pericardium. Anteriorly, the fibers originate from the xiphoid process.[1]

The diaphragm has three large apertures for the aorta, vena cava, and esophagus and several smaller ones for the epigastric vessels and splanchnic nerves.[2] A space may occur anteriorly between the muscle fibers originating from the xiphoid process and from the seventh rib; it is called a *foramen of Morgagni*. When a defect is the muscle fibers occurs posteriorly, it is called a *foramen of Bochdalek*.

The normal diaphragmatic contour is a smooth dome. When this is replaced by arcuate elevations in healthy subjects, it is termed *scalloping*. However, Felson found this in only 5.5% of a large series of subjects; absence of the usual smooth contour should not readily be accepted as a normal variant.[2]

On a posteroanterior chest radiograph the cupola of the right hemidiaphragm is at the level of the fifth rib anteriorly or the sixth anterior interspace. In 91% of persons the right hemidiaphragm is one-half interspace higher than the left. The lower hemidiaphragm is associated with the position of the systemic ventricle in children with cardiac anomalies, and the lower position of the left hemidiaphragm is attributed to the position of the left ventricle.[3]

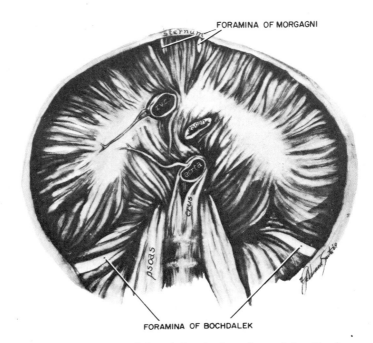

FIG. 29-1. Anatomy of the abdominal surface of the diaphragm.

Movement of the hemidiaphragms is not symmetric in most healthy persons, although the discrepancy in movement is usually less than 2 cm.[4,5] Mean inspiratory movement of the hemidiaphragms was 3.3 cm on the right and 3.5 cm on the left in a large series of healthy subjects. Movement of less than 3 cm did not imply pathology by itself.[3]

Motor innervation of the diaphragm originates in spinal motor neurons at the levels of the third through fifth cervical vertebrae and travels to the diaphragm by the phrenic nerves. The motor neurons receive excitatory and inhibitory stimuli from the medullary respiratory center as well as stimuli from higher brain areas for activities such as cough, defecation, and talking.[6] The phrenic nerves also convey afferent sensory information from proprioceptive fibers in the diaphragm and are important in mediating the sensation of dyspnea.[7]

Abnormal anatomy and physiology

When the normal muscle fibers of the diaphragm fail to develop, they are replaced by a thin membranous sheet called an *eventration*. The eventration can be complete and occupy an entire hemidiaphragm or exist as a partial segment of an otherwise normal hemidiaphragm. Complete eventration occurs primarily on the left side and may be radiographically indistinguishable from a paralyzed hemidiaphragm. The chest radiograph shows elevation of the hemidiaphragm with reduced or even paradoxic motion on fluoroscopy. In infants, a complete eventration can permit translocation of abdominal organs into the chest, compromising respiratory function and creating a surgical emergency.[8] Eventrations in adults are usually asymptomatic but may permit gastric and colonic volvulus with resultant gastrointestinal symptoms. Radiographically, the distended stomach and colon are apposed to the interior surface of the diaphragm and distinguish this condition from a hernia.[2]

Most eventrations in adults are partial and located in the anteromedial portion of the right hemidiaphragm.[9] Radiographically, they appear as a soft tissue mass in that area; anatomically, they are usually occupied by liver. This can be confirmed with a liver scan. These are rarely symptomatic and rarely need repair.

Herniation of abdominal viscera into the chest can occur through a normal hiatus, congenital defects, or traumatic rents in the diaphragm. The most common diaphragmatic hernia is an esophageal hiatus hernia. Although an acquired defect in the esophageal hiatus may play a role in the pathogenesis of these hernias, obesity and pregnancy appear to be at least as important. Sliding or direct esophageal hernias involve displacement of the gastroesophageal junction into the thorax. Clinical symptoms and morbidity are related to reflux of gastric acid onto the esophageal mucosa; this is related more to the competence of the gastroesophageal sphincter than to the hernia per se.[10] Radiographically, the sliding hernia appears as a soft tissue density in the posteroinferior mediastinum; not infrequently, an air-fluid level may be seen within the shadow. Therapy of these hernias is directed at reducing the reflux of gastric acid, but when complications occur, surgical intervention is indicated.

Rolling or paraesophageal hernias involve displacement of part of the gastric fundus into the chest; the gastroesophageal junction remains intra-abdominal. Although less common, these hernias are more likely to strangulate and become a surgical emergency. Radiographically, this may appear as two air-fluid levels, one in the posterior mediastinum and one below the diaphragm.[11]

Although the esophageal hernias are most frequent in adults, herniation of abdominal contents through a foramen of Bochdalek is more frequent in infants and not infrequently constitutes a surgical emergency. Clinically evident hernias occur on the left side in 80% to 90% of cases and vary in the extent of defect. After surgical correction of the hernia the compressed lung may develop normally or may remain hypoplastic, particularly in the lower lobe.[12]

In adults most of the posterior diaphragmatic defects are small and contain either retroperitoneal fat, omentum, or part of the spleen or kidney. Intraperitoneal or retroperitoneal injection of air may aid in the diagnosis and obviate the need for surgery.[13]

Hernias through a foramen of Morgagni are the least frequent and usually occur on the right side, since the left is protected by the pericardium. Radiographically, they appear as a well-defined opacity at the right cardiophrenic angle. Most contain hepatic tissue and are asymptomatic, but when bowel herniates into one the incidence of complications approaches 15%.[14]

Penetrating or *nonpenetrating trauma* to the diaphragm may also cause diaphragmatic hernia. Although these represent only 5% of diaphragmatic hernias, they account for 90% of strangulated hernias and should not be overlooked.[15]

Neoplasms of the diaphragm are rare; about 40% are benign. The benign neoplasms are usually asymptomatic and consist of a variety of mesenchymal tumors including lipomas, fibromas, angiofibromas, neurofibromas, and neurilemmomas. Radiographically, they appear as a small irregularity of the diaphragm.

Malignant diaphragmatic tumors can be primary or metastatic. The primary tumors are usually mesenchymal sarcomas that cause patients chest pain, cough, or gastrointestinal discomfort. The radiographic appearance is similar to that of a benign lesion. Tumors metastasize to the diaphragm primarily by contiguous spread; hematogenous metastases are rare.

Other anatomic anomalies of the diaphragm include diaphragmatic cysts and accessory diaphragms.[3]

Abnormal position and movement

Most conditions that cause abnormal position of the diaphragm are accompanied by abnormal movement. COPD is the most common cause of abnormal position and movement and is discussed in the section on **Abnormal function**. Bilateral paralysis is the epitome of abnormal diaphragmatic movement and presents radiographically as fixed elevation of both hemidiaphragms. The diaphragm accounts for most of the vital capacity during quiet breathing; hence, bilateral paralysis is usually accompanied by severe dyspnea and particularly orthopnea.[16] In contrast, unilateral paralysis is usually asymptomatic.

Bilateral paralysis can result from interruption of the nerve supply to the diaphragm anywhere from the phrenic nucleus in the cervical spinal cord to the motor end plate on the diaphragm itself. Guillain-Barré syndrome and myasthenia gravis are the most common neurologic diseases to cause paralysis of the diaphragm.[17] Cervical cord trauma in the phrenic nucleus will paralyze the diaphragm, as will a variety of other neurologic diseases including amyotrophic lateral sclerosis, multiple sclerosis, botulism, therapy with aminoglycoside and polymyxin antibiotics, and organophosphate poisoning.[16]

Although the diaphragm is not totally paralyzed in primary muscle disease, the paresis is functionally similar and has a radiographic appearance similar to bilateral paralysis. The weakened muscle does not contract well, and the same symptoms of dyspnea and especially orthopnea predominate. Both Duchenne's muscular dystrophy and myotonic dystrophy can involve the diaphragm, although not usually until late in the disease.[18,19] Metabolic and endocrine myopathies such as glycogen storage disease and thyrotoxicosis can produce a weakened diaphragm, as can inflammatory myopathies such as polymyositis, scleroderma, and systemic lupus erythematosis. Acute diaphragmatic paresis can also occur with hypokalemia or hypophosphatemia.

The diagnosis of bilateral diaphragmatic paresis is suggested by inward motion of the abdominal wall on inspiration and can be confirmed by fluoroscopy or measurement of transdiaphragmatic pressures.[16] Ventilatory support is usually indicated when the vital capacity is reduced to two times the predicted tidal volume or the maximal inspiratory pressure is less than 20 cm of water.[17]

As noted above, *unilateral diaphragmatic paralysis* is usually asymptomatic and almost always caused by interruption of the phrenic nerve. The most common cause is bronchogenic or metastatic carcinoma, and a thorough investigation for such a lesion should be made in anyone with unilateral paralysis. The second most common cause is idiopathic; this most often involves the right hemidiaphragm in males.[20] The diagnosis of unilateral paralysis is made fluoroscopically: upon sudden inspiratory sniffing, the paralyzed side rises and the normal side descends. Upon expiratory sniffing the reverse occurs. One or both of these maneuvers will almost invariably allow the physician to make the diagnosis. It is essential to realize that both elevation in repose and descent with quiet inspiration may be seen with hemidiaphragmatic paralysis.[21]

Hemidiaphragmatic motion may be abnormal with disease in contiguous tissues, for example, subphrenic abscess, pneumonitis, atelectasis, lobar collapse, and pulmonary infarction. Bronchial obstruction with air trapping and pneumothorax can produce paradoxic motion of the hemidiaphragm, but not with sniffing.

An uncommon form of disturbed diaphragmatic motion is diaphragmatic flutter or myoclonus. Involuntary contractions at a frequency of approximately 100/min occur and may be superimposed on a normal tidal volume.

The symptoms may resemble palpitations; at least one patient responded well to phenytoin.[22]

Abnormal function

The most common form of diaphragmatic dysfunction is seen in patients with COPD.[23] The tension the diaphragm can develop is greater at low than at high lung volumes. The hyperinflated lungs of COPD patients put the diaphragm at a marked disadvantage on its length-tension curve and cause it to work much less efficiently. In addition, the hyperinflation increases the radius of curvature of the diaphragm and by Laplace's law reduces the transdiaphragmatic pressure at any given diaphragmatic tension; this reduces the pressure needed to inflate the lung. In addition, as hyperinflation caused by emphysema increases, diaphragmatic contraction becomes less vertical and more horizontal, thereby pulling in the lower chest rather than displacing the diaphragm into the abdomen (see Chapter 10).

COPD also increases the resistive load on the inspiratory muscles, which decreases their metabolic efficiency.[24] The wasted ventilation of COPD also decreases the efficiency of diaphragmatic work. Both these render the diaphragm more easily fatigued. The force-velocity characteristics of the diaphragm are also changed in COPD, although the exact etiology is not known; this is manifest as a slower rate of change in pressure during contraction. Because flow rates are generally less in patients with COPD, this is probably of less significance than it would be in patients with normal airways.[22]

As with any skeletal muscle the diaphragm is subject to changes in nutrition, and, in fact, diaphragmatic mass shows a close correlation with total body mass. In the late stages of COPD, shortly before the onset of severe respiratory failure, most patients begin to lose weight, and nutrition becomes a significant problem. In this catabolic state, muscle tissue is sacrificed for energy needs and the disadvantaged inspiratory muscles are further weakened, hastening the onset of respiratory failure.

REFERENCES

1. Leak, L.V.: Gross and ultrastructural morphologic features of the diaphragm, Am. Rev. Respir. Dis. **119S**(Pt. 2):3, 1979.
2. Felson, B.: Chest roentgenology, Rev. ed., Philadelphia, 1973 W.B. Saunders Co.
3. Fraser, R.G., and Paré, J.A.P.: Diagnosis of diseases of the chest. Philadelphia, 1977, W.B. Saunders Co.
4. Simon, G., Bonnel, J., Kazantzis, G., et al.: Some radiological observations on the range of movement of the diaphragm, Clin. Radiol. **20**:231, 1969.
5. Alexander, C.: Diaphragm movements and the diagnosis of diaphragmatic paralysis, Clin. Radiol. **17**:79, 1966.
6. Von Euler, C.: On the neural organization of the motor control of the diaphragm, Am. Rev. Respir. Dis. **119S**(Pt. 2):45, 1979.
7. Rochester, D.F., and Braun, N.M.T.: The diaphragm and dyspnea, Am. Rev. Respir. Dis. **119S**(Pt. 2):77, 1979.

8. Paris, F., Blasco, E., Canto, A., et al.: Diaphragmatic eventration in infants, Thorax **28:**66, 1973.
9. Vogl, A., and Small, A.: Partial eventration of the right diaphragm (congenital diaphragmatic herniation of liver), Ann. Intern. Med. **43:**61, 1955.
10. Cohen, S., and Harris, L.D.: Does hiatus hernia affect competence of the gastroesophageal sphincter? N. Engl. J. Med. **284:**1053, 1971.
11. Menuck, L.: Plain film findings of gastric volvulus herniating into the chest, Am. J. Roentgenol. **126:**1169, 1976.
12. Morris, J.J., Black, F.O., and Stephenson, H.E., Jr.: The fate of the unexpanded lung in congenital diaphragmatic hernia, Dis. Chest **48:**649, 1965.
13. Le Roux, B.T.: Supraphrenic herniation of perinephric fat, Thorax **20:**376, 1965.
14. Betts, R.A.: Subcostosternal diaphragmatic hernia, Am. J. Roentgenol. **75:**269, 1956.
15. Keshishian, J.M., and Cox, P.A.: Diagnosis and management of strangulated diaphragmatic hernias, Surg. Gynecol. Obstet. **115:**626, 1962.
16. Derenne, J.P.H., Macklem, P.T., and Roussos, C.H.: The respiratory muscles: mechanics, control and pathophysiology, Am. Rev. Respir. Dis. **118:**119, 373, 581, 1978.
17. O'Donohue, W.J., Baker, J.P., Bell, G.M., et al.: Respiratory failure in neuromuscular disease, J.A.M.A. **235:**733, 1976.
18. Inkley, S.R., Oldenburg, F.C., and Vignos, P.J.: Pulmonary function in Duchenne muscular dystrophy related to stage of disease, Am. J. Med. **56:**297, 1974.
19. Harper, P.S.: Myotonic dystrophy, vol. 9, Philadelphia, 1979, W.B. Saunders Co.
20. Riley, E.A.: Idiopathic diaphragmatic paralysis, Am. J. Med. **32:**404, 1962.
21. Mitchell, R.S.: Phrenic nerve interruption in the treatment of pulmonary tuberculosis. II. Complications and sequelae of phreniclasis, Am. Rev. Tuberc. **60:**168, 1949.
22. Phillips, J.R., and Eldridge, F.L.: Respiratory myoclonus (Leeuwenhoek's Disease), N. Engl. J. Med. **289:**1390, 1973.
23. Rochester, D.F., Arora, N.S., Braun, N.M.T., et al.: The respiratory muscles in chronic obstructive pulmonary disease (COPD), Bull. Eur. Physiopathol. Respir. **15:**951, 1979.
24. Rochester, D.F., and Briscoe, A.M.: Metabolism of the working diaphragm, Am. Rev. Respir. Dis. **119S:**101, 1979.

Chapter 30

MEDIASTINAL DISEASES

Richard H. Simon

The tissues of the mediastinum can be affected by a wide range of disease processes. Discussed in this chapter are those diseases that primarily involve the mediastinum and that are not traditionally covered under other subject headings.

Anatomy

The mediastinum is an anatomically complex space within the chest that contains important elements of various organ systems. The mediastinum's lateral borders are formed by the parietal pleura of the pulmonary cavities. It is bounded anteriorly by the sternum and posteriorly by the thoracic vertebrae and the medial portion of the posterior rib cage. It extends superiorly to the thoracic inlet and inferiorly to the diaphragm. The mediastinum can be divided anatomically into anterior, middle, and posterior compartments to aid in the differential diagnosis of mediastinal masses based on location. The *anterior mediastinum* is the tissue located behind the sternum and in front of the anterior margin of the pericardium, ascending aorta, and brachiocephalic vessels. It includes the thymus, anterior lymph nodes, and connective tissue. The *middle compartment* consists of those structures behind the anterior compartment and anterior to the posterior surfaces of the pericardium and trachea; it contains the heart and great vessels, trachea and mainstem bronchi, phrenic and proximal vagus nerves, and lymph nodes. The *posterior mediastinum* is the space that extends behind the pericardium and trachea and contains the esophagus, descending aorta, sympathetic chain, distal vagus nerves, thoracic duct, and additional lymphatics.

MEDIASTINITIS

Bacterial infection of the mediastinum usually can be traced to a specific source. The most common cause is esophageal perforation, which can result from trauma during gastrointestinal endoscopy, erosion from a foreign body, necrosis of an esophageal carcinoma, or failure of a surgical anastomosis. Rarely, perforation is spontaneous or associated only with vomiting. The mediastinum also can be infected by direct extension of suppuration from adjacent spaces. Abscesses in oropharyngeal tissues can descend the fascial planes of the neck and involve the mediastinum. The initial site of infection may be the tonsils or a dental root or it may arise from perforation of a pyriform sinus during a difficult endotracheal intubation. Postoperative wound infection of a median sternotomy incision may penetrate to the mediastinal tissues. Rarely, infection may extend into the mediastinum from sites in the lung, pleural space, or pericardium.

Chest pain, fever, severe prostration, dysphagia, and shortness of breath are the principal symptoms of bacterial mediastinitis. Examination may reveal a mediastinal friction rub. A characteristic crunching sound, often synchronous with the heart, may be heard if pneumomediastinum has resulted from perforation of the esophagus. Also, in this situation, the examination may reveal signs of pneumothorax or empyema. The chest radiograph invariably shows widening of the mediastinum and possibly pneumomediastinum, pleural effusion, or pneumothorax. The suspicion of esophageal rupture may be confirmed radiologically by detecting extravasation of swallowed contrast material. Successful treatment of bacterial mediastinitis requires adequate drainage of all involved spaces including the original site of infection. The choice of antibiotics should be guided by the results of bacterial cultures. Anaerobic organisms are frequently involved when the mediastinitis is secondary to oropharyngeal or esophageal infection.

The mediastinum can be involved in other infectious processes. Histoplasmosis and primary tuberculosis (particularly in children) are the two most common infectious causes of mediastinal lymph node enlargement. Occasionally the nodes becme large enough to compress airways and cause obstruction. Late calcification of healed histoplasmosis or tuberculosis is the most frequent cause of the calcifications so commonly seen on chest radiographs. These calcified granulomas on rare occasion erode into an airway and cause hemoptysis. The resulting broncholiths can then be expectorated as "lung stones" or chalky sputum.

Fibrosing mediastinitis is a rare disease in which an intense fibrotic proliferation occurs within the connective tissue of the mediastinum. In a minority of patients, inactive histoplasmosis and, rarely, tuberculosis have been identified as the underlying cause. In a few patients the drug methysergide has been implicated. However, in most cases no etiologic agent is found. The dense fibrous tissue can obstruct the superior vena cava, pulmonary veins, and major airways or constrict the pericardium. Tissue biopsy is required to differentiate fibrosing mediastinitis from diffuse infiltration of the mediastinum by malignant tumor. Surgical lysis of the fibrous bands is technically difficult and usually of only temporary benefit. Glucocorticoid therapy is rarely effective.

MEDIASTINAL MASSES

The number of possible causes of masses in the mediastinum is large because of the many different types of tissue located there. In some patients the diagnosis is obvious because the patient is known to have a disease that includes a mediastinal mass as one possible manifestation. For example, the cause of mediastinal enlargement in a patient with bronchogenic carcinoma is most likely extension of a tumor to the mediastinal lymph nodes. However, in many cases the diagnosis is not obvious, and a specific evaluation must be undertaken.

A majority of adult patients with mediastinal masses are asymptomatic. The mass is detected fortuitously, usually by radiologic studies performed for unrelated reasons. The remaining patients seek medical attention because the mass has caused symptoms either by encroaching upon adjacent structures or by producing systemic effects such as weight loss, fatigue, or anorexia. In a few patients the symptoms are due to a variety of paraneoplastic syndromes associated with some mediastinal tumors. The presence of symptoms provides both diagnostic and prognostic information; 95% of asymptomatic masses in adults are benign, while only 47% of masses in the symptomatic cases are benign.

The physical examination of the patient with a mediastinal mass may reveal evidence of compression or distortion by the mass. Impingement on an airway lumen may cause a localized wheeze or signs of distal atelectasis or infection. Superior vena caval obstruction will be manifested by distension of the venous system in the head, neck, and arms. Involvement of the recurrent laryngeal nerve causes hoarseness from paralysis of a vocal cord; involvement of the superior sympathetic ganglia causes Horner's syndrome. A complete examination may detect evidence of the same disease process outside the mediastinum and thus facilitate diagnosis. For example, the detection and biopsy of an enlarged peripheral lymph node may yield the diagnosis of lymphoma and explain the mediastinal widening.

The single most valuable test to evaluate a mediastinal mass is the posteroanterior and lateral chest radiograph. Most important, it can localize the mass to the anterior, middle, or posterior mediastinal compartment. This assignment to a specific area narrows the diagnostic possibilities. The order of frequency of the various types of mediastinal masses differs considerably for each of the mediastinal spaces. In evaluating the chest radiograph, it is extremely helpful if an older film can be obtained for comparison. A mass unchanged for several years is most likely not a malignant tumor.

In some patients the precise location of a mass relative to normal structures cannot be determined by conventional radiography. Occasionally it may be difficult to determine if the mass is in the mediastinum or in the adjacent lung parenchyma. Oblique views may provide the answer. When doubt remains, conventional tomograms usually clarify the anatomy. CAT scans often allow very precise localization and, in addition, can provide information on the tissue composition of the mass; the technique often reveals if the mass is cystic, vascular, composed of adipose tissue, or contains calcium. At present, as in other body areas, additional critical studies comparing CAT scans with less expensive techniques are needed.

Other diagnostic procedures that are useful in selected cases include barium contrast esophageal and gastrointestinal studies, fluoroscopy, angiography, bronchoscopy, esophagoscopy, and radionuclide scans. However, despite recent advances in these and other diagnostic techniques, most primary mediastinal neoplasms still require biopsy for definitive diagnosis. When tissue is required, the superior and right midde mediastinum can be approached by mediastinoscopy through a suprasternal notch incision. The left middle mediastinum is better evaluated through a left parasternal approach. If neither of these techniques allows adequate access to the mass, a thoracotomy is indicated. Because the risks from biopsy are low and the chance of malignancy significant, the evaluation of any mediastinal mass should be pursued until a specific diagnosis is obtained.

In the following sections the most common causes of mass lesions in each of the anatomic compartments of the mediastinum will be discussed. The need for surgery in either diagnosis or treatment of each condition will not be stressed. Except where stated, this discussion assumes that the same disease process that causes the mediastinal lesion is not readily detectable in tissues outside the mediastinum.

Anterior mediastinum

The most common causes of anterior mediastinal masses, in decreasing order of frequency, are thymomas, germ cell neoplasms, lymphoma, and intrathoracic thyroid tissue. Of these masses, only small asymptomatic thyroids do not require surgical excision. Hence, all patients with masses fitting this description should have a radioactive iodine scan to rule out intrathoracic thyroid. All the other tumors require biopsy for diagnosis; further noninvasive evaluation of the tumor mass is rarely necessary. Thymomas and teratomas can cause paraneoplastic syndromes (see below), and evidence of them should be sought during routine evaluation of a patient with an anterior mediastinal mass.

Thymomas appear with equal frequency in both sexes and at any age, with the peak incidence between 40 and 60 years. The patient may have pain and cough from compression of adjacent structures or symptoms of various syndromes associated with thymomas; the two most frequent are myasthenia gravis and red blood cell aplasia. Diseases less frequently associated with thymoma are Cushing's disease, hypogammaglobulinemia, Whipple's disease, and a variety of collagen vascular disorders. Thymomas have smooth or lobulated borders and may contain calcium. They should be treated by total surgical excision. Postoperative radiation should be given to the 20% to 50% of patients with invasive tumors.

Germ cell neoplasms are the next most common tumors of the anterior mediastinum. They are separated into teratomas, seminomas, embryonal cell carcinomas, and choriocarcinomas. Of the teratomas, 70% are benign; the other germ cell tumors are always considered malignant. Teratomas, with their variable components of ectoderm, endoderm, and mesoderm, may appear cystic or show calcifications on x-ray film or CAT scan. The other germ cell tumors appear as homogeneous loculated masses. If the mediastinum is the only site involved, total surgical excision should be attempted. The germ cell tumors respond variably to radiation and chemotherapy.

Mediastinal lymph node involvement with lymphoma is usually part of a more widespread disease. However, in a distinct group of patients the tumor is confined to the mediastinum. The anterior compartment is the most frequent site but the disease can involve any of the nodal groups in the mediastinum. Nodular sclerosing Hodgkin's disease is the most frequent cell type. Of the non-Hodgkin's lymphomas, the diffuse, poorly differentiated cell type predominates.

Intrathoracic thyroid tissue is most often located in the anterior compartment but also occurs in the posterior mediastinum. Unlike the more frequent substernal extension of a cervical goiter, it is either totally independent of the cervical thyroid or connected only by a thin fibrous band. It frequently causes deviation of the trachea visible on chest radiograph. Almost all patients are euthyroid although occasional patients have Grave's disease. The diagnosis can be confirmed by demonstrating uptake of radioactive iodine on scan. If the patient is asymptomatic, the tissue does not need to be surgically excised.

Middle mediastinum

The most common causes of middle mediastinal masses are enlarged lymph nodes from either tumors or benign conditions, pericardial or bronchogenic cysts, and foramen of Morgagni hernias. The evaluation depends heavily on the location of the mass. Effort should be made to diagnose noninvasively the benign conditions that do not require surgical treatment.

Enlarged paratracheal or parabronchial lymph nodes occur in histoplasmosis, tuberculosis, and, rarely, in other granulomatosis infections. Calcification often occurs with healing and indicates the mass's benign nature. Rim or eggshell calcifications are virtually diagnostic of a pneumoconiosis due to silica or coal dust. Mediastinal node enlargement in sarcoidosis is usually accompanied by large, bilateral hilar and paratracheal nodes; this pattern often virtually confirms the diagnosis. Tissue biopsy is required when there is any suspicion of lymphoma or carcinoma.

Herniation through the foramen of Morgagni usually appears as a mass located just behind the sternal xiphoid in the right cardiophrenic angle. It may contain large or small bowel or omentum. In patients with masses in this location, barium contrast studies should be obtained to demonstrate hollow viscus herniation, if present. A CAT scan demonstrating a low absorption number compatible with adipose tissue is diagnostic of omental herniation. The other common nonmalignant causes of middle mediastinal masses are congenital pericardial and bronchogenic cysts. Most patients with mediastinal cysts require surgery to differentiate them from malignant conditions. Further experience with new techniques such as the CAT scan and two-dimensional ultrasonography may enable physicians to differentiate between benign and malignant lesions in asymptomatic patients. At present, however, most patients continue to require surgery for diagnosis.

Pericardial cysts are found most often in the right cardiophrenic angle and occasionally communicate with the pericardium. They appear as homogeneous masses with a distinct, smooth margin. They can assume a teardrop appearance when they extend between the right middle and lower lobes of the lung. They are rarely symptomatic although they may reach considerable size.

Bronchogenic cysts can arise from trachea, carina, or mainstem bronchi. They most freqently appear as masses with smooth margins displacing the esophagus posteriorly at the level of the tracheal bifurcation. Air-fluid levels may be seen on the chest radiograph if the cyst communicates with the airway lumen. Symptoms arise from compression of adjacent structures or from infection.

In obese patients or those with exogenous glucocorticoid excess, mediastinal fat can hypertrophy and appear as a mass lesion. The radiograph may show diffuse mediastinal widening or a mass in the area of the pericardial fat pads. The diagnosis can be established by a CAT scan that demonstrates the fat content of the mass; no further evaluation is necessary.

The remaining and all too frequent cause of a middle mediastinal mass is malignancy. When the mediastinal widening is due to lymph node metastases, detection and study of evidence of the primary disease outside the mediastinum is indicated initially. Malignant lymphoma and carcinoma of the lung, breast, gastrointestinal tract, and kidneys are the most frequent tumors that metastasize to the mediastinal nodes. If no primary lesion is detected by history, physical examination, or routine laboratory tests, surgical biopsy of the mediastinal mass is indicated. An exhaustive, expensive search for a primary lesion by radiography including radionuclide scans should not be carried out before biopsy unless the initial screening blood tests or urinalysis detects an abnormality at a specific site.

Additional causes of masses in the middle mediastinum are carcinoma of the trachea and aneurysms of the ascending aorta and other great vessels in the mediastinum.

Posterior mediastinum

The most common causes of masses in the posterior compartment are neurogenic tumors, diaphragmatic hernias, diseases involving the esophagus, and aneurysms of the descending aorta. Many of these conditions can be diagnosed and treated noninvasively, and the evaluation should be directed first at detecting these diseases.

A barium swallow should be obtained in all patients who have a mass in the area of the esophagus. This will permit better localization of the mass and will enable diagnosis in many cases. A large sliding hiatal hernia can present as a smooth-margined mass in the retrocardiac area just above the diaphragm. The diagnosis will be suggested if the mass contains an air-fluid level and can be confirmed by barium swallow. Foramen of Bochdalek hernias are rarely seen in adults.

A smooth fusiform mass in the location of the esophagus may be due to gross dilatation of that organ. The enlargement may be secondary to congenital achalasia or to stricture of the distal esophagus with proximal dilatation from esophagitis, scleroderma, or carcinoma of the gastroesophageal junction. Alternatively, the mass may be caused by the neoplastic tissue of an esophageal carcinoma. Congenital enteric cysts also may appear as a mass anywhere along the esophagus. In all these conditions the barium swallow is the most cost-effective initial study with which to evaluate the abnormality.

When a posterior mediastinal mass with smooth margins is contiguous with the descending aorta, further diagnostic procedures are indicated to differentiate between aneurysm, neoplasm, and cyst. If the physician suspects that the mass is an aneurysm, an angiogram should be obtained to confirm this diagnosis and allow proper planning of surgery. In doubtful cases the less invasive CAT scan performed with the injection of contrast material can accurately differentiate between aneurysms and nonvascular masses. If an aneurysm is found, an angiogram is necessary before surgery.

Masses lying along the vertebral column are most commonly due to neurogenic tumors and require tissue biopsy for diagnosis. They usually appear as rounded homogeneous masses with smooth margins. The tumors can arise from any component of neural tissue. Peripheral nerves give rise to neurolemmomas (Schwannomas) and neurofibromas. In 25% of patients with mediastinal neurofibromas, the mediastinal mass is only one manifestation of more generalized neurofibromatosis. Both these tumors can extend through the intervertebral foramina and compress the spinal cord, causing neurologic symptoms. Malignant degeneration to a neurosarcoma occurs in about 25% of these tumors.

Ganglioneuromas arise from the sympathetic chain and are seen in children and young adults. Although benign, the tumors may reach considerable size before the patient appears with symptoms due to compression of spinal cord, esophagus, or trachea. These tumors occasionally release catecholamines into the circulation in amounts sufficient to produce symptoms. Malignant neuroblastomas also arise from the ganglion cell but are seen usually in children. A few of these tumors spontaneously revert to benign ganglioneuromas. Chemodectomas and pheochromocytomas are neurogenic tumors that arise from paraganglion cells and can appear as mediastinal masses. Both these tumors can produce hormones.

All benign neurogenic tumors require complete surgical excision even if the patient is asymptomatic. This allows firm diagnosis, eliminates the chance of future problems from encroachment upon vital structures, and is prophylactic against malignant degeneration. Preoperative myelography may be required to assess the degree of extension into the spinal column. Malignant tumors are often responsive to radiation therapy.

Other causes of masses in the posterior mediastinum are thoracic duct cysts, diseases of the thoracic spine, and extramedullary hematopoesis.

SUGGESTED READINGS

Andrews, C.E., and Morgan, W.K.C.: Tumors of the mediastinum, pleura, chest wall, and diaphragm. In Baum, G.L., editor: Textbook of pulmonary diseases, ed. 2, Boston, 1974, Little, Brown and Co., pp. 803-812.

Berry, B.E., and Ochsner, J.L.: Perforation of the esophagus. A 30 year review, J. Thorac. Cardiovasc. Surg. **65**:1, 1973.

Goodwin, R.A., Jr.: Disorders of the mediastinum. In Fishman, A.P., editor: Pulmonary diseases and disorders, New York City, 1980, McGraw-Hill Book Co., pp. 1479-1489.

Jones, K.W., Pietra, G.G., and Sabiston, D.C., Jr.: Primary neoplasms and cysts of the mediastinum. In Fishman, A.P., editor: Pulmonary diseases and disorders, New York City, 1980, McGraw-Hill Book Co., pp. 1490-1521.

Leigh, T.F., and Weens, H.S.: Roentgen aspects of mediastinal lesions, Semin. Roentgenol. **4**:59, 1969.

Marston, E.L., and Valk, H.L.: Spontaneous perforation of the esophagus: review of the literature and report of a case, Ann. Intern. Med. **51**;590, 1959.

McLoud, T.C., Wittenberg, J., and Ferrucci, J.T., Jr.: Computed tomography of the thorax and standard radiographic evaluation of the chest: a comparative study, J. Comp. Assist. Tomogr. **3**:170, 1979.

Sanders, J.H., Jr., Malone, S., Neiman, H., et al.: Thoracic aortic imaging without angiography, Arch. Surg. **114**:1326, 1979.

Chapter 31

INTERSTITIAL LUNG DISEASE

Marvin I. Schwarz

The interstitial lung diseases (ILD) are a heterogeneous group of lung disorders that are characterized clinically by the insidious onset of exertional dyspnea, radiographically by interstitial infiltrates on the chest film, physiologically by a restrictive ventilatory defect, and pathologically by alveolar wall inflammation resulting in fibrosis.

Etiologically, ILD can be separated into five major groups: (1) the pneumoconioses, (2) drug induced (see opposite page), (3) the collagen vascular diseases (see Chapter 32), (4) primary diseases (see opposite page), and (5) an idiopathic group that represents well over 50% of ILD. This chapter will examine the idiopathic group.

ILD was originally described by Hamman and Rich in 1935.[1] They reported patients who rapidly developed cor pulmonale and died within 6 months of onset of dyspnea. Postmortem examination revealed alveolar wall fibrosis and the secondary vascular changes of pulmonary hypertension. Case reports of acute interstitial fibrosis of the lung, the "Hamman Rich syndrome," immediately followed, but it soon became apparent that the acute course was an exception and that an indolent clinical picture was more characteristic. The mean survival is 4 years, although the range is wide and many patients are alive 10 years after the onset of ILD. ILD is labeled in the literature by several different terms (see opposite page).

Liebow and colleagues have classified ILD according to its predominant histologic appearance[2] (see the chart on page 290).

Desquamative interstitial pneumonia (DIP) consists of hyperplasia of the type II alveolar lining cells. The alveolar lumens become packed with large mononuclear cells; some are desquamated type II cells, but most are alveolar macrophages. During this stage of ILD minimal amounts of collagen and both acute (neutrophils and eosinophils) and chronic (plasma cells and lymphocytes) inflammatory cells are also seen within alveolar walls and lumens.

In *usual interstitial pneumonia* (UIP) the alveolar walls are thickened by chronic inflammatory cells and variable amounts of fibrous tissue; in addi-

288

COMMONLY USED DRUGS THAT CAN CAUSE ILD

1. Nitrofurantoin
2. Gold
3. Gleomycin
4. Cyclophosphamide
5. Methotrexate
6. Busulfan
7. Carmustine (bischloronitrourea [BCNU])

OTHER PRIMARY PULMONARY DISORDERS ASSOCIATED WITH DIFFUSE INTERSTITIAL INFILTRATES

1. Sarcoidosis (third stage)
2. Pulmonary histiocytosis X
3. Chronic farmers' lung
4. Pulmonary hemosiderosis
5. Lymphangitic carcinomatosis
6. Neurofibromatosis
7. Tuberous sclerosis
8. Familial pulmonary dysplasia
9. ARDS

SYNONYMS FOR IDIOPATHIC ILD

1. Hamman Rich syndrome
2. Acute interstitial fibrosis of the lung
3. Interstitial fibrosis
4. Cryptogenic fibrosing alveolitis
5. Idiopathic pulmonary fibrosis
6. Honeycomb lung
7. Interstitial pneumonitis

tion, alveolar lining cell hyperplasia and alveolar wall necrosis with hyaline membrane formation may be present. In UIP, as the fibrous connective tissue replaces alveolar walls, marked distortion of the alveolar architecture and eventual honeycombing (mural fibrosis) occur. At this stage the inflammatory infiltrate is markedly reduced. In the lung parenchyma, collections of lymphocytes are commonly seen in both DIP and UIP. It has now become apparent that in many cases of ILD, features of DIP, UIP, and mural fibrosis can appear in different or adjacent sections of lung tissue. For these reasons several investigators believe that DIP, UIP, and mural fibrosis are different stages of the same disease process.[3]

The main feature of *lymphocytic interstitial pneumonia* (LIP) is a monotonous mass of lymphocytes that infiltrates and thickens alveolar walls. This entity must be differentiated from lymphomatous involvement of the lung; it can be established by the absence of pathologically involved mediastinal lymph nodes. LIP has been associated with hypergammaglobulinemic states such as Sjögren's syndrome and may lead to mural fibrosis.[4] Bronchiolitis obliterans and diffuse alveolar damage are usually seen in association with DIP and UIP and represent an organizing exudate within the terminal bronchioles.

The attack rate of ILD is unknown. Sexual, racial, seasonal, and geographic predisposition are lacking. In most series the mean age of patients at onset of symptoms is between 40 and 50 years, although ILD has been re-

HISTOPATHOLOGIC CLASSIFICATION OF ILD

1. Desquamative interstitial pneumonia (DIP)
2. Usual interstitial pneumonia (UIP)
3. Lymphocytic interstitial pneumonia (LIP)
4. Bronchiolitis obliterans and diffuse alveolar damage (BIP) (seen in DIP, UIP, and LIP)
5. Giant cell interstitial pneumonia (GIP) (rare)

ported in children as well as in persons aged 70 and over. Dyspnea of varying degrees is reported by all patients with ILD and, in fact, may predate the chest radiographic changes. Cough is less commonly seen but, when present, is nonproductive. Some patients have fever, arthralgias, and symptoms of upper respiratory infection. Examination may be entirely normal; chest examination frequently demonstrates bibasilar dry "Velcro" rales, which correlates best with the presence of fibrosis. Digital clubbing is more commonly seen in far advanced cases but may precede the onset of dyspnea or radiographic abnormalities. Other uncommon clinical features include digital vasculitis, Raynaud's phenomena, and discoid lupus.

The chest radiograph may be normal initially in a small percentage of patients but typically demonstrates lower zone bibasilar reticular or reticular-nodular interstitial infiltrates. As the disease advances, lung volume is reduced and radiographic evidence of pulmonary hypertension appears. In far advanced cases, radiographic honeycombing (small cystic spaces especially at the lung bases) may become apparent. These areas may rupture and produce bronchopleural fistula and pneumothorax. In the DIP phase of ILD, a fine lower zone alveolar pattern with radiation from the hilum has been described, although infrequently seen. Another complication of far advanced ILD with mural fibrosis is scar carcinoma. This may be a localized adenocarcinoma or a diffuse bronchoalveolar carcinoma.

The erythrocyte sedimentation rate may be elevated in early cases. A Coombs positive hemolytic anemia and idiopathic thrombocytopenia purpura have been reported in a few patients with ILD.[5,6] A significant number of patients with ILD (20% to 60%) will have either rheumatoid or antinuclear antibodies of low to moderate titer in their serum.[7,8] In addition, in those patients with active inflammatory histopathologic findings as opposed to mural fibrosis, circulating immune complexes will be present.[9]

Pulmonary physiologic studies demonstrate that these patients' lungs have become stiff, resulting in a reduction in both vital capacity and total pulmonary compliance. As the process continues, total lung capacity is reduced, the hallmark of a restrictive ventilatory defect. Unless complicated by airway disease, flow rates are well maintained. The diffusing capacity for carbon monoxide will be reduced, and $\dot{V}/Q$ mismatching will supervene. Resting arterial blood gases in the typical case demonstrate a compensated respiratory alkalosis, hyperventilation due to increased dead space ventilation, and hypoxemia due to $\dot{V}/Q$ mismatching and a widened alveolar-arterial oxygen tension difference. These abnormalities are accentuated by exercise. In early cases of ILD with minimal symptoms and questionable or negative chest radiographs, patients' routine pulmonary function testing including lung volumes, diffusing capacity, and resting arterial blood gases may be within normal limits. Vital capacity may be slightly reduced. It is only after the stress of exercise that hypoxemia, a widened alveolar-arterial oxygen tension difference, and increased dead space ventilation become apparent. Physiologic testing is not only important in establishing the presence and severity of disease initially, but it is also useful in following the disease's course and the results of therapy.[10-13]

Since inflammation precedes the fibrotic state in ILD, gallium 67 radionucleotide scanning has been used to differentiate fibrotic from inflammatory disease.[14] The increased uptake correlates best with inflammation and, therefore, may be useful in the staging of ILD. Bronchoalveolar lavage fluid from ILD subjects demonstrates increased numbers of neutrophils in addition to elevation of IgG.[15] However, to establish a definitive diagnosis in most patients, lung tissue is acquired. The open lung biopsy is preferred because of the larger sample size and the opportunity for the surgeon to obtain a biopsy of areas of obvious involvement and avoid areas that may appear grossly normal. This ability decreases the sampling error that may occur with either a transthoracic or transbronchial biopsy. Since ILD is a persistent inflammatory process, grossly involved areas of the lung may demonstrate mural fibrosis, while others may show DIP or early UIP. This information is important in both prognosis and in deciding on a therapeutic regimen.

Although much is known about ILD's clinical course and pathophysiology, its pathogenesis remains obscure. Evidence suggests that immunopathogenetic mechanisms may be operative. Patients with ILD may have rheumatic complaints including arthralgias, Raynaud's phenomena, digital vasculitis, and skin rashes consistent with discoid lupus.[16-19] The finding of rheumatoid factor in 20% to 60% and antinuclear factor in 35% of patients further supports the immune pathogenesis of ILD.[7,8] Turner-Warwick reported the results of immunofluorescent staining of lung tissue from 33 patients with ILD; antibody formation was demonstrated in plasma cells and germinal follicles. More important was the observation that in 6 cases, all with high titers of circulating antinuclear factors, immunoglobulin and complement (immune complex) were deposited in alveolar walls and capil-

DISEASES WITH AUTOIMMUNE FEATURES ASSOCIATED WITH ILD

1. Rheumatoid arthritis
2. Systemic lupus erythematosis
3. Polymyositis and dermatomyositis
4. Scleroderma
5. Renal tubular acidosis with hypergammaglobulinemia
6. Hashimoto's thyroiditis
7. Pernicious anemia
8. Coombs positive hemolytic anemia
9. Idiopathic thrombocytopenic purpura
10. Sjögren's syndrome
11. Chronic active hepatitis

laries.[20] In a study of 35 patients with ILD (7 with DIP, 13 with UIP, and 15 with mural fibrosis), all the DIP and UIP patients demonstrated alveolar immune complex deposition (direct immunofluorescent technique), while only 2 of the 15 patients with mural fibrosis had a similar deposition.[21] Interestingly, the incidence of serum autoantibodies (rheumatoid and antinuclear factors) was similar in all three groups. This study demonstrated a strikingly high prevalence of alveolar wall immune complexes in patients with active inflammatory disease. In Turner-Warwick's cases, on the other hand, 21 of 33 patients had predominant fibrosis and therefore a low prevalence of immune complexes. Nagaya described a patient with ILD who demonstrated alveolar wall immune complexes by immunofluorescent technique in areas of the biopsy where inflammation was seen but not in areas where fibrosis predominated.[22]

As mentioned before, an identical clinical and histopathologic presentation may be seen in the collagen vascular diseases. In addition, ILD has been reported to occur in association with other diseases in which autoimmune phenomena have been implicated (see above).[23,24]

Circulating immune complexes (Raji cell technique) are present in patients with ILD who have an active inflammatory histologic picture as opposed to those with mural fibrosis.[9,25-27] The presence of circulating immune complexes correlated well with the pulmonary parenchymal deposition of immunoglobulin and complement. Gadek and associates have demonstrated that patients with ILD will have immune complexes in the supernatants of their bronchoalveolar lavage.[28]

The literature is replete with reports describing the response of patients with ILD to corticosteroid drugs. These studies are retrospective, limited in numbers of patients, not controlled, and use varying drug doses and lengths of therapy. Despite the above limitations, Stack and associates feel that the main factor influencing prognosis in ILD is the patient's response to corticosteroid drugs.[29] They found that only 16% of 69 patients responded well; their 5-year survival rate was 67%, as compared with 20% for the nonresponders. The initial doses utilized in this study were 20 to 40 mg prednisone for 2 to 8 weeks, after which the drug was withdrawn or reduced to a daily maintenance dose of 5 to 10 mg. The authors graded response by a substantial relief of dyspnea, a vital capacity that increased by more than 10%, and considerable or complete clearing of the chest radiograph. The one pretreatment factor that correlated best with responsiveness was the histologic appearance of the biopsy specimen. Subjects with minimal fibrosis, alveolar cell hyperplasia and desquamation, and alveolar wall infiltration with plasma cells and lymphocytes were more apt to benefit from corticosteroids than those who demonstrated dense fibrosis and honeycombing. These findings have been confirmed by others.[3,9,30,31] Scadding and Hinson reported 8 patients with ILD and active cellular disease diagnosed by lung biopsy; 1 had spontaneous remission, 3 had definite improvement with corticosteroid therapy, and 4 had treatment failures.[31] In 7 patients with primarily alveolar wall fibrosis, 5 demonstrated no improvement when receiving corticosteroid treatment, 1 had a spontaneous remission after an initial treatment failure, and the remaining patient had only slight improvement. Doses were between 20 and 40 mg prednisone for varying times. Liebow et al. and others describe an excellent response to corticosteroids in patients with ILD who primarily had a desquamative picture.[31-34] Long-term follow-up of these patients is not available, and since progression of desquamation to dense alveolar wall fibrosis has been documented, it would be important to know whether this natural course is influenced by corticosteroids.

In one series of 11 patients treated with corticosteroids who had primarily a desquamative appearance on lung biopsy, 6 demonstrated symptomatic improvement, 3 progressed to a fibrotic picture despite therapy, and 2 died of intercurrent disease after improvement with corticosteroid treatment.[35] Although it has become apparent that corticosteroid responsiveness at least in part depends on the underlying pathologic picture, a substantial number of cases with an identical histopathologic picture have dissimilar responses to therapy. Other factors to be considered are age, sex, race, duration of symptoms, and the presence of serum autoantibodies and circulating immune complexes. Nagaya and associates reported two patients with immune complex deposition in the lung who demonstrated dramatic responses to corticosteroids.[36] Dreisin and associates similarly have shown that subjects with ILD and circulating immune complexes (by the Raji cell technique) may be responsive to treatment.[9]

The suspected immunopathogenesis of ILD has led several investigators to add immunosuppressive agents to the treatment program of ILD. To date only a few promising cases have been reported.[37] Weese and colleagues report three cases with progressive ILD refractory to corticosteroid therapy, two of which were treated with azathioprine and one with cyclophosphamide.[37] The two subjects treated with azathioprine had stabilization of their disease despite the fact that they both demonstrated alveolar wall fibrosis. Winterbauer and associates demonstrated that 12 of 20 patients with ILD responded to a combination of prednisone and azathioprine.[38] Patients ill for less than 1 year and those with minimal amounts of fibrosis were more likely to respond; 8 of the 12 appeared to have a selective response to azathioprine.

• • •

Idiopathic ILD remains an enigma from the etiologic, pathogenetic, and therapeutic standpoints. Management is empiric, and the prognosis is variable; it is most favorable in the absence of extensive interstitial fibrosis. This disease spectrum is being recognized more frequently, however, and new research is being directed toward its solution.

REFERENCES

1. Hamman, L., and Rich, A.R.: Fulminating diffuse interstitial fibrosis of the lung, Trans. Am. Clin. Climatol. Assoc. **51**:154, 1935.
2. Liebow, A.A., and Carrington, C.B.: Alveolar diseases. The interstitial pneumonias. In Simon, M., editor: Frontiers of pulmonary radiology, New York City, 1969, Grune & Stratton, Inc., pp. 102.
3. Crystal, R.G., Fulmer, J.D., Roberts, W.C., et al.: Idiopathic pulmonary fibrosis: clinical, histologic, radiographic, physiologic, scintigraphic, cytologic, and biochemical aspects, Ann. Intern. Med. **85**:769, 1976.
4. Turner-Warwick, M.: Philip Ellman lecture. Immunologic aspects of systemic diseases of the lungs, Proc. R. Soc. Med. **67**:541, 1974.
5. Scadding, J.W.: Fibrosing alveolitis with autoimmune haemolytic anaemia: two case reports, Thorax **32**:134, 1977.
6. May, J.J., Schwarz, M.I., and Dreisin, R.B.: Idiopathic thrombocytopenic purpura occurring with interstitial pneumonitis, Ann. Intern. Med. **90**:199, 1979.
7. Gottlieb, A.J., Spiera, H., Teirstein, A.S., et al.: Serologic factors in idiopathic diffuse interstitial pulmonary fibrosis, Am. J. Med. **39**:405, 1965.
8. Turner-Warwick, M., and Haslam, P.: Antibodies in some chronic fibrosing lung diseases. I. Non organ-specific autoantibodies, Clin. Allergy **1**:83, 1971.
9. Dreisin, R.B., Schwarz, M.I., Theofilopoulos, A.N., et al.: Circulating immune complexes in the idiopathic interstitial pneumonias, N. Engl. J. Med. **298**:353, 1978.
10. Eisenberg, H., Bubois, E.L., Sherwin, R.P., et al.: Diffuse interstitial lung disease in systemic lupus erythematosis, Ann. Intern. Med. **79**:37, 1973.
11. Schwarz, M.I., Matthay, R.A., Sahn, S.A., et al.: Interstitial lung disease in polymyositis and dermatomyositis: analysis of six cases and review of the literature, Medicine **55**:89, 1976.
12. Colp, C.R., Riker, J., and Williams, M.H., Jr.: Serial changes in scleroderma and idiopathic interstitial lung disease, Arch. Intern. Med. **132**:506, 1973.
13. Walker, W.C., and Wright, V.: Pulmonary lesions and rheumatoid arthritis, Medicine **47**:501, 1968.
14. Line, B.R., Fulmer, J.D., Reynolds, H.Y., et al.: Gallium-67 citrate scanning in the staging of

idiopathic pulmonary fibrosis: correlation with physiologic and morphologic features and bronchoalveolar lavage, Am. Rev. Respir. Dis. **118**:355, 1978.

15. Hunninghake, G.W., Gadek, J.E., Kawanami, O., et al.: Inflammatory and immune processes in the human lung in health and disease: evaluation by bronchoalveolar lavage, Am. J. Pathol. **97**:149, 1979.

16. Patchefsky, A.S., Banner, M., and Freundlich, I.M.: Desquamative interstitial pneumonia: significance of intranuclear viral-like inclusion bodies, Ann. Intern. Med. **74**:322, 1971.

17. Fraire, A.E., Greenberg, S.D., O'Neal, R.M., et al.: Diffuse interstitial fibrosis of the lung, Am. J. Clin. Pathol. **59**:636, 1973.

18. Turner-Warwick, M.: Interstitial lung disease and digital vasculitis, Am. Rev. Respir. Dis. (Abstract) **115**:173, 1977.

19. Nagaya, H., and Sieker, H.O.: Pathogenetic mechanisms of interstitial pulmonary fibrosis in patients with serum antinuclear factor. Am. J. Med. **52**:51, 1972.

20. Turner-Warwick, M., and Haslam, P.: Antibodies in some chronic fibrosing lung diseases. II. Immunofluorescent studies, Clin. Allergy **1**:209, 1971.

21. Schwarz, M.I., Dreisen, R.B., Pratt, D.S., et al.: Immunofluorescent patterns in the idiopathic interstitial pneumonias, J. Lab. Clin. Med. **91**:929, 1978.

22. Nagaya, H., Elmore, M., and Ford, C.D.: Idiopathic interstitial pulmonary fibrosis: an immune complex disease? Am. Rev. Respir. Dis. **107**:826, 1973.

23. Mason, A.M.S., McIllmurray, M.B., Golding, P.L., et al.: Fibrosing alveolitis associated with renal tubular acidosis, Br. Med. J. **4**:596, 1970.

24. Turner-Warwick, M.: Fibrosing alveolitis and chronic liver disease, Q. J. Med. **37**:133, 1968.

25. Brentjens, J.R., O'Connell, D.W., Pawlowski, I.B., et al.: Experimental immune complex disease of the lung. The pathogenesis of a laboratory model resembling certain human interstitial lung disease, J. Exp. Med. **140**:105, 1974.

26. Johnson, K.J., and Ward, P.A.: Acute immunologic pulmonary alveolitis, J. Clin. Invest. **54**:349, 1974.

27. Reynolds, H.Y., Fulmer, J.D., Kazmierowski, J.A., et al.: Analysis of cellular and protein content of broncho-alveolar lavage fluid from patients with idiopathic pulmonary fibrosis and chronic hypersensitivity pneumonitis, J. Clin. Invest. **59**:165, 1977.

28. Gadek, J., Hunninghake, G., Zimmerman, R., et al.: Pathogenetic studies in idiopathic pulmonary fibrosis, Chest **75**:264, 1979.

29. Stack, B.H.R., Choo-Kang, Y.F.J., and Heard, B.E.: The prognosis of cryptogenic fibrosing alveolitis, Thorax **27**:535, 1972.

30. Liebow, A.A., Steer, A., and Billingsley, J.G.: Desquamative interstitial pneumonia, Am. J. Med. **39**:369, 1965.

31. Scadding, J.G., and Hinson, K.F.W.: Diffuse fibrosing alveolitis (diffuse interstitial fibrosis of the lungs). Correlation of history at biopsy with prognosis, Thorax **22**:291, 1967.

32. Klocke, R.A., Augerson, W.S., Berman, H.H., et al.: Desquamative interstitial pneumonia: a disease with a wide clinical spectrum, Ann. Intern. Med. **66**:498, 1967.

33. Ansari, A., Buechner, H.A., and Brown, M.: Desquamative interstitial pneumonia: report of a case and review of the literature, Dis. Chest **53**:511, 1968.

34. Tubbs, R.R., Benjamin, S.P., Reich, N.E., et al.: Desquamative interstitial pneumonitis: cellular phase of fibrosing alveolitis, Chest **72**:159, 1977.

35. Patchefsky, A.S., Israel, H.L., Hock, W.S., et al.: Desquamative interstitial pneumonia: relationship to interstitial fibrosis, Thorax **28**:680, 1973.

36. Nagaya, H., Buckley, C.E., and Sieker, H.O.: Positive antinuclear factor in patients with unexplained pulmonary fibrosis, Ann. Intern. Med. **70**:1135, 1969.

37. Weese, W.C., Levine, B.W., and Kazemi, H.: Interstitial lung disease resistant to corticosteroid therapy: report of three cases treated with azathioprine or cyclophosphamide, Chest **67**:57, 1975.

38. Winterbauer, R.H., Hammar, S.P., Hallman, K.O., et al.: Diffuse interstitial pneumonitis: clinicopathologic correlations in 20 patients treated with prednisone/azathioprine, Am. J. Med. **65**:661, 1978.

Chapter 32

LUNG INVOLVEMENT IN THE COLLAGEN VASCULAR DISEASES

Marvin I. Schwarz *and* **Talmadge E. King, Jr.**

All the defined collagen vascular diseases have been associated with serious pleural and/or pulmonary pathology.[1] The most common form of pulmonary involvement is a chronic interstitial pattern indistinguishable from idiopathic pulmonary fibrosis. The pleuropulmonary disease may be the initiating episode in patients with previously undiagnosed collagen vascular disease. Moreover, the pleuropulmonary manifestations may be the major cause of morbidity and mortality in these disorders.

RHEUMATOID ARTHRITIS

The pleuropulmonary complications associated with rheumatoid arthritis (RA) are (1) pleurisy with or without effusion, (2) UIP, (3) necrobiotic nodules (nonpneumoconiotic intrapulmonary rheumatoid nodules) with or without cavities, (4) Caplan's syndrome (rheumatoid pneumoconiosis), and (5) pulmonary hypertension secondary to rheumatoid pulmonary vasculitis.[1-3] In addition, cricoarytenoid arthritis may cause severe laryngeal stridor and upper airways obstruction. Most patients with pleuropulmonary involvement have clinical evidence of RA and high titer rheumatoid factor. However, the lung disease may precede the usual clinical manifestations of RA.[2]

Pleurisy with or without effusion is the most frequent thoracic complication of RA. Pleural disease may occur before, during, or after the onset of joint manifestations. Despite the higher incidence of RA in females, rheumatoid pleural disease has a striking predilection for males. The effusion is usually unilateral (right-sided predominance) and likely to be recurrent. As many as a third of patients are asymptomatic. However, pleural disease occasionally results in dense pleural thickening, necessitating decortication. Empyemas or pyopneumothorax, sometimes with large accumulations of pus, may be found with no apparent predisposing condition other than RA.[4]

296

Although it is difficult to predict which patients with RA will develop pleural disease, a higher incidence in those who have subcutaneous nodules and high titers of rheumatoid factor appears evident. The pleural fluid characteristically has a yellow-green color and is an exudate. A low pleural fluid glucose (less than 30 mg/100 ml) is characteristic of RA. High concentrations of total lipids and cholesterol giving the fluid a milky or opalescent appearance have been described, especially in long-standing effusions. Complement levels may be markedly reduced; however, this finding is not specific, since it can be found in other collagen vascular diseases.[5] The finding of a higher than serum concentration of rheumatoid factor is nonspecific, since this also occurs in malignant effusions, bacterial pneumonias, and tuberculosis. Cytologic examination usually reveals a predominance of mononuclear cells. The RA cell or ragocyte is not commonly found in the pleural fluid although it is commonly found in synovial fluid. The pleural biopsy most often reveals nonspecific inflammation, but occasionally rheumatoid granulomas may be seen. Although pleural disease is a frequent manifestation of RA, appropriate studies should be undertaken in all patients with RA who have pleural effusion to rule out other causes of empyema, tuberculosis, and malignancy. Repeated needle aspirations, corticosteroid therapy, and decortication may be necessary depending on the extent and natural course of the pleural process.

Interstitial pneumonitis occurs with increased frequency in patients with RA, especially in men, although the exact incidence is unknown. If radiographic screening of patients with RA is used to detect the presence of interstitial lung disease, the incidence is only 1.6%.[2] However, when pulmonary function tests are used, 41% of an unselected series of RA patients had abnormal pulmonary function, that is, restrictive ventilatory impairment, reduced diffusing capacity, and varying degrees of resting hypoxemia that worsened with exercise.[2,6] The majority of these patients had no pulmonary symptoms; 40% had a normal chest film.

No specific pattern of arthritis is associated with interstitial lung disease, although 50% of patients have subcutaneous nodules. UIP may precede the onset of arthritis by months or several years. Cough and dyspnea are often present, but other symptoms such as fever, pleuritic chest pain, and hemoptysis are less common. Finger clubbing is quite common. The chest radiograph shows diffuse interstitial infiltrates most marked in the lung bases. Histologic examination of tissue may be helpful diagnostically if rheumatoid nodules are present in the lung in addition to the interstitial pneumonitis.

The interstitial pneumonitis is characterized by alveolar wall fibrosis, interstitial and intra-alveolar mononuclear cell infiltration, and lymphoid nodules, eventually leading to extensive fibrosing alveolitis and honeycombing. Direct immunofluorescent staining of the lung tissue has demonstrated rheumatoid factor within alveolar walls and pulmonary capillaries, suggesting a possible immune mechanism in the pathogenesis of rheumatoid lung disease.[7] An association appears to exist between obliterative bronchiolitis and RA although the exact relationship is as yet undefined; this fact may explain the pathologic involvement of the small airways often seen in patients with rheumatoid interstitial lung disease.[8] Corticosteroid therapy is the treatment of choice for severe disease.

Necrobiotic nodules, which are morphologically identical to the subcutaneous nodule, are more common in men and may be single or multiple. Since the nodular form of rheumatoid lung disease may also precede the arthritic manifestations, it must be differentiated from other granulomatous diseases; any single nodule raises questions about the etiologic identification of a solitary pulmonary nodule (see Chapter 22). Radiographically, the nodules appear as well-circumscribed masses commonly located in the periphery of the lung. Cavitation is common, and changes in nodule size correlate with the activity of the joint disease. The lesions are usually asymptomatic unless cavitation occurs. Cough and/or hemoptysis and pleural effusion and/or bronchopleural fistula frequently accompany cavitary disease.[9] Spontaneous pneumothorax may occur in association with peripheral lung nodules. Histologically, the lung nodules are identical to the subcutaneous rheumatoid nodules.

Caplan's syndrome was originally described as multiple pulmonary nodules in coal miners with RA. A similar syndrome has been reported in sandblasters, asbestos workers, potters, boiler scalers, aluminum powder workers, and brass and iron workers—that is, persons exposed to silica, not coal mine dust, who also have RA. Rheumatoid pneumoconiosis is characterized by rounded densities, usually located in the lung periphery, that may evolve rapidly and can undergo cavitation and occasionally calcify. The rheumatoid pneumoconiotic nodule consists of layers of partially necrotic collagen and dust and occasionally contains foci of tuberculosis. The pulmonary disease may precede or coincide with the onset of arthritis. It must be differentiated from the PMF of advanced silicosis (see Chapter 25).

Pulmonary hypertension in patients with RA is most commonly caused by advancing fibrosing alveolitis but rarely is the result of primary pulmonary vasculitis. In a few reported cases of RA a predominant pulmonary arteritis with fibrotic intimal proliferation and medial hypertrophy within small muscular pulmonary arteries and minimal interstitial pneumonitis was noted.[10] It remains unclear whether such cases are a distinct variant of rheumatoid lung disease.

Cricoarytenoid arthritis is estimated to be present in 26% of adults with RA. Although most patients have only mild symptoms, they may occasionally have a respiratory emergency with severe laryngeal stridor and breathlessness.[11] The condition usually worsens when the arthritis worsens but can occur when the disease is inactive. Ear pain, dysphagia, foreign body sensation in the throat, dyspnea on exertion, and inspiratory stridor are suggestive symptoms. Response to anti-inflammatory drugs has been seen, but tracheostomy and unilateral arytenoidectomy may be required in severe cases.

Finally, because of the widespread use of gold in the treatment of RA, one must recognize that gold has been recently suggested as a cause of pulmonary fibrosis.[12]

SYSTEMIC LUPUS ERYTHEMATOSUS

In systemic lupus erythematosus (SLE) the lungs and pleurae are involved more frequently than in other collagen vascular diseases; the incidence varies from 50% to 70%. The pleuropulmonary manifestations of SLE are (1) pleurisy with or without effusion, (2) atelectasis, (3) acute lupus pneumonitis, (4) diffuse interstitial disease, (5) uremic pulmonary edema, (6) diaphragmatic dysfunction with loss of lung volume, and (7) infections.[1] Predominance in females is striking.

Pleuritis, with or without effusion, is the most common thoracic complication of SLE. Frequently bilateral, and usually small but occasionally massive, pleural effusion may be the first manifestation of SLE in one third of patients. The effusions are exudates with high protein concentrations, low complement, and normal glucose. They tend to be recurrent and may be associated with pericarditis.

Basilar linear or platelike *atelectasis* is also frequent and may be transient. Atelectactic changes are frequently associated with pleuritis, effusion, and/or diaphragmatic elevation. The basilar atelectasis is felt to result from prolonged pleuritis and splinting. Dyspnea, with numerous pulmonary function abnormalities, may occur with these seemingly minor radiographic changes.

Noninfectious pulmonary infiltrates are common in SLE. Patients with lupus infiltrates can be divided into those with an acute onset and those with chronic complaints. *Acute diffuse lupus pneumonitis* and an *acute diffuse hemorrhagic alveolitis* have been described in SLE.[13] These patients are often extremely ill with severe dyspnea, cough productive of scant sputum, fever, hypoxemia, pleuritis, and frank respiratory failure. A bilateral alveolar filling process is usually present on chest film. Cardiomegaly and pleural disease may also be present. Infectious processes are seldom found in these patients, and they consequently do not respond to antibiotic therapy. Symptomatic and radiographic response to corticosteroids is frequently rapid. Azathioprine has been administered successfully to a small group of patients not responding to corticosteroids alone.

In those patients surviving the acute illness, the chest radiograph clears completely in 50% of patients; the remaining patients progress to *chronic interstitial pneumonitis* with hypocapnia, hypoxemia, restrictive pulmonary defect, and impaired diffusing capacity.[14] The principal symptoms are dyspnea, nonproductive cough, and pleuritic chest pain; digital clubbing is uncommon. Physical findings include poor diaphragmatic movement and basilar rales.

The specific pathology of acute lupus pneumonitis is unclear. Although most autopsies have shown pathologic findings in lungs, the histopathologic features are not considered pathognomonic; UIP, advanced fibrosis, and chronic fibrinous pleuritis are the most common findings. Acute inflammation of small pulmonary arteries and arterioles is seen in lupus pneumonitis; other nonspecific changes include alveolar hyaline membranes, hemorrhage, and capillary thrombi.

Recently, Gibson and co-workers[15] reported the association of *diaphragmatic dysfunction with loss of lung volume* in SLE. The etiology of this disorder is believed to be diffuse myopathy affecting the diaphragmatic muscles. Dyspnea while patients were supine was a common manifestation of this process.

Significant renal disease is a frequent manifestation of SLE; consequently, *uremic pulmonary edema* may occur in this disease. Perihilar and lower lobe alveolar infiltrates with or without pleural effusions are the common radiographic findings.

Approximately half the patients with SLE have a complicating pleuropulmonary *infectious process*. Because infections are a frequent cause of morbidity and mortality in SLE, it is important that all patients who have renal disease or are receiving high-dose corticosteroid therapy and have an acute febrile illness with lung involvement be evaluated for a life-threatening pulmonary infection.

PROGRESSIVE SYSTEMIC SCLEROSIS (SCLERODERMA)

Progressive systemic sclerosis (PSS) is a multisystem disease characterized by atrophy and sclerosis. The disease occurs most often in women between 30 and 50 years of age. Although skin manifestations are prominent, it is the visceral involvement—renal, cardiovascular, or pulmonary—that determines survival. The esophagus is the organ most frequently involved.

The exact incidence of pulmonary disease is difficult to determine. Morphologic studies have demonstrated pleural and pulmonary involvement in 82% to 90% of patients with PSS. Radiographic changes are often not present when pulmonary function tests are abnormal. In a large series of cases, radiographic changes in the lungs were found in 25% and pulmonary symptoms in only 16% of patients.[16] However, pulmonary function was almost invariably abnormal. The pleuropulmonary complications associated with PSS are (1) diffuse interstitial fibrosis, (2) pulmonary vascular disease, (3) pleural disease, (4) aspiration pneumonitis, and (5) bronchiolar carcinoma.

Diffuse interstitial fibrosis is found in nearly all these cases postmortem. The most prominent symptoms are dyspnea on exertion and cough. Physical findings include characteristic "Velcro" rales and some limited expansion of the chest. The most common abnormality on chest film is an interstitial reticular pattern particularly involving the bases. Cystic lesions (honeycombing) occur as the disease progresses and at times result in spontaneous pneumothorax. Pulmonary function tests in patients with PSS usually reveal a restrictive pattern with reduced lung compliance and impaired diffusing capacity, often before any clinical or radiographic evidence of lung disease appears.

Pulmonary vascular resistance has been found to be increased in all patients with PSS undergoing cardiac catheterization.[17] In half the patients the *pulmonary hypertension* was associated with clinical signs of right ventricular hypertrophy and clinical evidence of cor pulmonale. Pulmonary hypertension may occur without pneumonitis or fibrosis. The CREST syndrome (calcinosis, Raynaud's phenomenon, sclerodactylia, telangiectasis) appears to be a subset of PSS with predominantly vascular manifestations. Intimal proliferation with progression to virtual luminal obliteration may occur in any size vessel; it usually occurs in small and medium pulmonary arteries.

Recurrent *aspiration pneumonia* may result from disturbances of esophageal motility and subsequent food retention. *Pleural disease* is not as common in PSS as in other collagen vascular diseases, although minor degrees of pleuritis are histologically present in up to 30% of patients. Pleural and pulmonary calcification is rare. The common belief that PSS skin involvement limits chest expansion has been disproved. PSS has been clearly shown to be associated with an increased risk of *bronchiolar carcinoma*.[1]

To date, therapy has been ineffective for sclerodermatous pleuropulmonary disease.

POLYMYOSITIS AND DERMATOMYOSITIS

Polymyositis is a diffuse inflammatory and degenerative disorder of striated muscle that causes symmetric weakness and atrophy, principally of the limb girdles, neck, and pharynx. When an erythematous skin rash accompanies the weakness and pain, the disorder is termed *dermatomyositis*. The disease is twice as common in females as in males and occurs at two age levels: before 10 years of age and between 40 and 50 years of age. Polyarthritis or polyarthralgia occurs in 35% of patients. Cardiac involvement is also common, with histologically verified myocarditis in 30% of patients. Hypergammaglobulinemia is frequently present; 20% of these patients have been shown to have rheumatoid factor and antinuclear antibodies. In addition, 50% to 60% have antibodies to a defined extractable nuclear antigen (PM-1 antibody).

The mechanisms for the development of pulmonary disease in polymyositis and dermatomyositis are (1) UIP, (2) aspiration pneumonia caused by esophageal pathology, (3) hypostatic pneumonia secondary to chest wall involvement and hypoventilation,[18] and (4) drug-induced hypersensitivity pneumonitis (e.g., methotrexate).

Interstitial pneumonitis has been well documented in patients with polymyositis; however, it occurs less frequently in these disorders than in other collagen vascular diseases. The exact incidence is unknown but appears to be approximately 5% of patients with polymyositis. The clinical presentation of this form of lung disease is quite variable. It may appear as an acute pneumonitis with a mixed alveolar-interstitial infiltrate in association with skin and muscle manifestations, or it may be a symptomatic finding on the chest radiograph. Schumacher and co-workers have identified a subset of these patients in which interstitial disease occurred in patients with articular manifestations of polymyositis and dermatomyositis.[19] The most common symptoms are gradual onset of dyspnea and cough with development of diffuse pulmonary infiltrates most prominent at the lung bases. Pathologically, the lesions are similar to those of idiopathic interstitial pneumonitis. In addition, pulmonary vascular inflammation, desquamation of alveolar lining cells, and bronchiolitis obliterans may be present. In approximately 40% of patients the pulmonary disease precedes the skin and muscle manifestations by 1 to 24 months. Also, the severity of muscle disease and the development of lung disease are not correlated. Clubbing is usually absent. Pleural disease is distinctly uncommon. Corticosteroids have caused remissions with stabilization or improvement in the symptomatic, radiographic, and physiologic abnormalities in 40% of patients. Other immunosuppressive agents, especially methotrexate, are frequently used to treat this disorder; consequently, *transient bilateral pulmonary infiltrates have been reported.*

SYSTEMIC NECROTIZING VASCULITIS: POLYARTERITIS NODOSA GROUP

Three subgroups comprise this disorder.[22]

Classic polyarteritis nodosa is a necrotizing vasculitis of small and medium muscular arteries. Renal disease, hypertension, polyarthralgia, and hepatic disease (with hepatitis B antigenemia) are quite common. However, allergic histories with eosinophilia and eosinophilic tissue involvement and granulomas are not characteristically found. More important, lung involvement is extremely uncommon.

Allergic granulomatosis closely resembles classic polyarteritis nodosa but with certain clearly distinguishing features: (1) lung involvement (the sine qua non of this syndrome), (2) allergic background and/or asthma with high levels of peripheral eosinophilia (usually greater than 1500/mm^3), (3) eosinophilic tissue infiltration, (4) granulomatous reactivity, and (5) involvement of capillaries and venules in addition to muscular arteries as in classic polyarteritis nodosa. Pulmonary radiographic findings include diffuse alveolar infiltrates that may be transient, nodular pulmonary densities that may cavitate, pleural effusions, and diffuse interstitial lung disease. Pathologically, the lung shows eosinophilic granulomas—necrotizing lesions with frequent involvement of the pulmonary arteries.

The *overlap syndrome* combines the features of the above diseases. Small vessels—capillaries and venules—as well as large and small arteries may be involved. Lung involvement may occur in this group and may range from small vessel leukocytoclastic vasculitis to granulomatous vasculitis of medium-sized pulmonary vessels.

Treatment of the polyarteritis nodosa group of systemic necrotizing vasculitis with corticosteroids has improved survival. In addition, the use of cyclophosphamide, either alone or in combination with preexisting corticosteroid therapy, is associated with a favorable response in some patients.[1]

SJÖGREN'S SYNDROME

Sjögren's syndrome occurs as an idiopathic symptom complex (keratoconjunctivitis sicca, xerostomia [oral dryness], and recurrent swelling of the parotid gland) or in association with rheumatoid arthritis (50% of patients), SLE, systemic vasculitis, dermatomyositis and scleroderma. Sjögren's syndrome shows a remarkable predominance in females (90%). The disease appears to result from an aggressive T- and B-lymphocyte infiltration of exocrine glands. Patients manifest hypergammaglobulinemia and non-organ-specific autoantibodies such as rheumatoid factor (75% to 100% of patients), antinuclear antibodies (66% of patients), antithyroid antibodies, and antibodies to other tissue cells. Diagnosis depends primarily on recognition of the symptom/sign complex. In addition, lip biopsy demonstrating destructive lymphoid infiltrates of the minor labial salivary glands and parotid scintigraphy is useful.

Pulmonary manifestations occur frequently in Sjögren's syndrome.[1] However, because of the high incidence of rheumatoid diseases associated with this disease, it is difficult to determine which are specific for this disorder. The pleuropulmonary manifestations of Sjögren's syndrome are as follows:

1. Pleurisy with or without effusion.
2. Interstitial fibrosis indistinguishable from that found in other collagen vascular diseases, which occurs in approximately 15% of patients with Sjögren's syndrome.
3. Dessication of the tracheobronchial tree secondary to lymphocytic infiltration of the mucous glands, resulting in mucous gland atrophy and plugging of the respiratory tract by inspissated secretions followed by atelectasis and secondary infections.[20]
4. Lymphoid interstitial lung disease is relatively uncommon; chest films usually reveal a diffuse reticulonodular or coarse nodular infiltrate. Pseudolymphoma, histiocytic or lymphocytic lymphoma, or Waldenström's macroglobulinemia may be seen in a small number of patients. A highly differentiated reticulum cell sarcoma or unclassifiable lymphoma is the most common malignant infiltrate.[21]

The treatment of this disorder is not clearly defined. Corticosteroid and/or cytotoxic therapy has had limited success.

OTHER COLLAGEN VASCULAR DISEASES

Ankylosing spondylitis is a chronic inflammatory disease with prominent involvement of the sacroiliac joints, spinal articulations, and paravertebral soft tissues. It is a common cause of back pain in young men, with an 8:1 male-to-female ratio, 80% to 90% histocompatibility antigen (HL-A B27) in white patients. Major pulmonary manifestations of ankylosing spondylitis are (1) chest wall restriction that results from fusion of the costovertebral joints (lung function is only minimally impaired, with the major findings being a slight to moderate reduction in total lung capacity and vital capacity with normal flow rates) and (2) fibrobullous, usually bilateral, upper lobe parenchymal involvement; this is a well-known although uncommon extraskeletal manifestation of the disorder.[23] Atypical pleural thickening and/or an interstitial infiltrate are the earliest manifestations, followed by cavity formation and extensive fibrosis with upper lobe retraction and bronchiectasis. Secondary infection with *Aspergillus fumigatus* or tuberculosis is a not uncommon complication; it is usually heralded by productive cough and intermittent, occasionally massive hemoptysis.

Behçet's disease is a multisystem disorder characterized by ulcers of the mouth and genitalia, relapsing iritis, joint manifestations, thrombophlebitis migrans, erythema nodosum, and CNS abnormalities. Pulmonary involvement is rare and is usually manifested by fleeting bilateral infiltrates with or without pleurisy. Severe hemoptysis may occur.[24]

Relapsing polychondritis is a disease of unknown etiology characterized by inflammation and destruction of cartilage. Most patients have vasculitis of large and small arteries. Aortic and respiratory tract involvement are the most common causes of death. Pulmonary disease occurs in patients who have recurrent involvement of the laryngotracheal structures, causing upper airways obstruction and secondary pneumonia. Hoarseness, cough, dyspnea, laryngeal tenderness, wheezing, and stridor should alert the physician to the possibility of this life-threatening complication.[5] Corticosteroids may be beneficial for treatment of the acute laryngeal inflammation.

Immunoblastic lymphadenopathy and *lymphomatoid granulomatosis* are two multisystem diseases of unclear classification with many features common to other collagen vascular diseases. Immunoblastic lymphadenopathy has generalized lymphadenopathy, hepatosplenomegaly, anemia, and polyclonal hypergammaglobulinemia as its major manifestations. Bilateral lower lobe interstitial pneumonia and bilateral, usually exudative pleural effusions are the main pulmonary complications; 50% of patients have hilar and mediastinal adenopathy.[25] Lymphomatoid granulomatosis is a necrotizing vasculitis with prominent lung involvement similar radiographically to Wegener's granulomatosis, with frequent cavitation. Hemoptysis is not uncommon, and pleural effusions may or may not be present.[26]

REFERENCES

1. Hunninghake, G.W., and Fauci, A.S.: Pulmonary involvement in the collagen vascular diseases, Am. Rev. Respir. Dis. **119**:471, 1979.
2. Walker, W.C., and Wright, V.: Pulmonary lesions and rheumatoid arthritis, Medicine **47**:501, 1968.
3. Petty, T.L., and Wilkins, M.: The five manifestations of rheumatoid lung, Dis. Chest **49**:75, 1966.
4. Dieppe, P.A.: Empyema in rheumatoid arthritis, Ann. Rheum. Dis. **34**:181, 1975.
5. Hunder, G.G., McDuffie, F.C., Huston, K.A., et al.: Pleural fluid complement, complement conversion, and immune complexes in immunologic and nonimmunologic diseases, J. Lab. Clin. Med. **90**:971, 1977.
6. Frank, S.T., Weg, J.G., Harkleroad, L.E., et al.: Pulmonary dysfunction in rheumatoid disease, Chest **63**:27, 1973.
7. Horatius, R.J., Abruzzo, J.L., and Williams, R.C.: Immunofluorescent and immunologic studies of rheumatoid lung, Arch. Intern. Med. **129**:441, 1972.
8. Geddes, D.M., Corrin, B., Brewerton, D.A., et al.: Progressive airway obliteration in adults and its association with rheumatoid disease, Q. J. Med **46**:427, 1977.

9. Jones, J.S.: An account of pleural effusions, pulmonary nodules and cavities attributable to rheumatoid disease, Br. J. Dis. Chest **72:**39, 1978.

10. Baydur, A., Mongan, E.S., and Slager, U.T.: Acute respiratory failure and pulmonary arteritis without parenchymal involvement: demonstration in a patient with rheumatoid arthritis, Chest **75:**518, 1979.

11. Löfgren, R.H., and Montgomery, W.W.: Incidence of laryngeal involvement in rheumatoid arthritis, N. Engl. J. Med. **267:**193, 1962.

12. Smith, W., and Ball, G.V.: Lung injury due to gold treatment, Arthritis Rheum. **23:**351, 1980.

13. Matthay, R.A., Schwarz, M.I., Petty, T.L., et al.: Pulmonary manifestations of systemic lupus erythematosis: review of twelve cases of acute lupus pneumonitis, Medicine **54:**397, 1974.

14. Eisenberg, H., Dubois, E.L., Sherwin, R.P., et al.: Diffuse interstitial lung disease in systemic lupus erythematosis, Ann. Intern. Med. **79:**37, 1973.

15. Gibson, G.J., Edmonds, J.P., and Hughes, G.R.V.: Diaphragm function and lung involvement in systemic lupus erythematosis, Am. J. Med. **63:**926, 1977.

16. Bianchi, F.A., Bistue, A.R., Wendt, V.E., et al.: Analysis of twenty-seven cases of progressive systemic sclerosis (including two with combined systemic lupus erythematosis) and a review of the literature, J. Chron. Dis. **19:**953, 1966.

17. Sackner, M.A., Akgun, N., Kimbel, P., et al.: The pathophysiology of scleroderm involving the heart and respiratory system, Ann. Intern. Med. **60:**611, 1964.

18. Schwarz, M.E., Matthay, R.A., Sahn, S.A., et al.: Interstitial lung disease in polymyositis and dermatomyositis: analysis of six cases and a review of the literature, Medicine **55:**89, 1976.

19. Schumacher, H.R., Schimmer, B., Gordon, G.V., et al.: Articular manifestations of polymyositis and dermatomyositis, Am. J. Med. **67:**287, 1979.

20. Strimlan, C.V., Rosenow, E.C., Divertie, M.B., et al.: Pulmonary manifestations of Sjögren's syndrome, Chest **70:**354, 1976.

21. Anderson, L.G., and Talal, N.: The spectrum of benign to malignant lymphoproliferation in Sjögren's syndrome, Clin. Exp. Immunol. **10:**199, 1972.

22. Fauci, A.S., Haynes, B.F., and Katz, P.: The spectrum of vasculitis: clinical, pathologic, immunologic, and therapeutic considerations, Ann. Intern. Med. **89:**660, 1978.

23. Rosenow, E.C., Strimlan, C.V., Muhm, J.R., et al.: Pleuropulmonary manifestations of ankylosing spondylitis, Mayo Clin. Proc. **52:**641, 1977.

24. Cadman, E.C., Lundberg, W.B., and Mitchell, M.S.: Pulmonary manifestations in Behcet syndrome: case report and review of the literature, Arch. Intern. Med. **136:**944, 1976.

25. Iseman, M.D., Schwarz, M.I., and Stanford, R.E.: Interstitial pneumonia in angio-immunoblastic lymphadenopathy with dysproteinemia. A case report with special histopathologic studies, Ann. Intern. Med. **85:**752, 1976.

26. Liebow, A.A., Carrington, C.R.B., and Friedman, P.J.: Lymphomatoid granulomatosis, Hum, Pathol. **3:**457, 1972.

Chapter 33

DEVELOPMENTAL ANOMALIES OF THE LUNGS AND THORAX

Michael D. Iseman

A wide variety of developmental anomalies can influence both the morphology and function of the respiratory system. Although these abnormalities may be part of a symptom complex, they more often come to the attention of the physician through a radiologic study. Therefore, strong emphasis will be given to the radiographic manifestations of these anomalies. When pertinent, abnormalities of physiology and other pathogenetic implications will be briefly reviewed. In view of the limited scope of this text, only the entities most commonly encountered in adults will be discussed.[1]

Anomalies of the lung parenchyma

BRONCHOPULMONARY SEQUESTRATION

This is a group of congenital malformations in which a portion of lung tissue develops that is anatomically separated from the normal lung. Significant airway connections with the tracheobronchial tree are usually missing, and the blood supply to this tissue is generally derived from systemic arteries. The two categories of sequestration are intralobar and extralobar.

The pathogenesis of these anomalies is uncertain. One of the more attractive theories suggests that sequestrations arise because of the appearance of an extra lung bud from the primitive foregut.[2] It has been postulated that although both varieties arise distal to the normal lung bud, the intralobar variety arises relatively close to the normal bud and the extralobar anomalies arise more distally. This theory would concur with the observation that the extralobar sequestrations more typically are supplied by infradiaphragmatic arteries, which arise from the aorta.

Intralobar

This form is distinguished by its inclusion *within* the pleural limits of a normal lobe. It is more commonly detected clinically because of its tendency to become recurrently infected. Typically it becomes manifest in association with a pneumonitis, although it may appear as an asymptomatic mass detected on routine radiography. Intralobar sequestrations are not discovered until age 20 or more in 50% of patients because of their invisibility until infected.[3] They are typically located in the medial aspect of a lower lobe in juxtaposition to the diaphragm.[4] Rarely, they may be found elsewhere. During an acute pneumonia the surrounding tissue may be involved as well, and the process may be indistinguishable from a routine pneumonia. However, if the pneumonia persists or recurs, or if on clearing an apparent uniloculated or multiloculated cystic defect appears in the area, the possibility of sequestration should be considered. *Infected* intralobar sequestrations typically have a connection with the tracheobronchial tree and may therefore show impressive air-fluid levels, mimicking bronchopleural fistulae. Whether these tracheobronchial anastomoses develop as a result of infection or the infections occur as a result of existing airway anastomoses is not clear. Bronchography may be useful in establishing the diagnosis. Management consists of antibiotic treatment of the acute inflammatory process and subsequent surgical extirpation.

Extralobar

In contrast to the intralobar variety, this anomalous portion of lung is invested in its own visceral pleura. Ninety percent of these lesions are located in the left hemithorax between the lower lobe and the diaphragm.[5] They rarely become infected (presumably because of the pleural barrier) and therefore usually appear as an asymptomatic mass on radiography.

Typically, extralobar sequestration is diagnosed in infancy. This is due, in part, to the fact that this lesion commonly appears as a radiopaque cyst. Further, a variety of congenital anomalies associated with extralobar sequestration may bring the patient to medical attention; these anomalies include diaphragmatic defects, a variety of bronchial and vascular disturbances, and a number of esophageal, colonic, and vertebral anomalies.[3]

BRONCHIAL CYSTS

During the embryologic development of the tracheobronchial tree from the primitive foregut, cystic structures lined with bronchial epithelium, but not in communication with the airways, may evolve. These bronchial cysts may become manifest in the neonatal period as rapidly expanding masses that produce cardiorespiratory embarrassment, or they may appear later in life as a consequence of infection or hemorrhage within the cyst. They may be located within the lung parenchyma or in the mediastinum. The cysts within the lung typically are located in the medial aspect of the lower lobes but may be found elsewhere.[6] They may appear as solitary or multiple, smooth, ovoid shadows several centimeters in diameter. Although the walls may contain mucous glands, cartilage, and connective tissue, calcification is rarely seen on plain film or tomography. Since they are usually filled with mucus, cysts are of uniform water density. They typically are stable in size over long periods unless infection occurs. With infection the lesion may enlarge or develop connections with the bronchial tree, in which case the secretions may partially evacuate, resulting in the appearance of an air-fluid level. Infected cysts are managed optimally with antibiotics and subsequent surgical excision.

OTHER ANOMALIES

A number of other congenital abnormalities may become manifest as radiographic, functional, or other disorders of the lungs. These include:

1. *Azygous lobe.* As the embryologic right lung bud grows cephalad, it usually courses lateral to the azygous vein in its posteroanterior path to empty into the superior vena cava. Occasionally, a portion of the bud passes mesial to the azygous vein, resulting in an invagination of the visceral pleura as the lung bud advances cephalad. In the posteroanterior radiography of the developed lung, this appears as a pleural line extending in a smooth arc concave to the mediastinum from the lung apex to the takeoff of the upper lobe bronchus. At the caudal end of this pleural line the vein appears as an ovoid density, thus giving the appearance of an inverted comma with a long tail. The azygous lobe occurs in roughly 1 of 200 adults and is of no physiologic or pathologic consequence. Its recognition is important primarily in avoiding confusion with bullous emphysema.

2. *Congenital lobar emphysema* (invariably one of the upper or the right middle lobe) usually becomes manifest in the infant as it rapidly expands and produces respiratory embarrassment by compressing all normal lobes. It is caused by a flabby noncartilaginous lobar bronchus or by an anomalous vessel partially occluding such a bronchus. Management consists of prompt removal.

3. *Congenital bronchiectasis* (see Chapter 16).

Anomalies of the pulmonary vasculature

UNILATERAL HYPERLUCENT LUNG

Also known as the Swyer-James or Macleod syndrome, this anomaly suffers from considerable controversy regarding its pathogenesis. Various authors have proposed that it may arise from developmental abnormalities of the pulmonary arteries,[7,8] the bronchial tree,[9] or both; others suggest that it may be an acquired condition associated with childhood infection.[10,11] It is probably a condition with several different causes. Obviously, the name refers to the radiographic appearance, yet this entity consistently entails significant functional and pathologic findings. Morphologic abnormalities of the airways including bronchiectasis, bronchitis, bronchiolitis, and obliteration of small airways are universally present. Extensive destructive emphysema is also usually found. The process may involve either an entire lung or just one lobe. Physiologically, impaired ventilation, perfusion, and compliance and increased Raw are found in the involved lung. The contralateral lung is usually quite normal. Patients may contact a physician because of recurrent pneumonia, hemoptysis, symptoms of chronic bronchitis or bronchiectasis, or simply an abnormal routine chest film. Demonstration by fluoroscopy or inspiratory-expiratory films of mediastinal shift away from the involved lung (caused by air trapping) is useful in making the diagnosis. Management generally consists in control of infection. Extirpation does not improve overall lung function and is thus rarely indicated.

THE SCIMITAR SYNDROME

This unusual condition has a wide variety of other names that refer to an assortment of associated anomalies. Because of the variable appearance of these other findings, the memorable quality of the name, and the fact that it is usually the presence of the "scimitarlike" anomalous pulmonary venous drainage that calls attention to this complex, it seems appropriate to continue use of this title. The scimitar shadow is formed by a confluence of the pulmonary veins of the right lung as they pass down toward the diaphragm. This may represent either total or partial venous return from the right lung. The vein usually passes through the diaphragm and empties into the inferior vena cava.[12] Associated abnormalities that *may* be present include hypoplasia of the right lung and pulmonary artery, dextrocardia, and systemic arterial blood supply to portions of the right lung. Patients are usually asymptomatic; in view of the minor physiologic derangement, removal is usually not indicated. Diagnosis generally can be made with the routine chest film, which shows the venous scimitar and, variably, reduced volume of the right lung, hypoplasia of the right pulmonary artery, and obscuration of the right heart border.

PULMONARY ARTERIOVENOUS FISTULAE

This term gives rise to confusion because of inexactitude regarding the vessels involved in the shunt, that is, pulmonary arteries and veins, bronchial arteries and veins, or systemic arteries and veins. Discussion here is limited to the congenital form associated with familial telangiectasia (Osler-Weber-Rendu disease), wherein multiple pulmonary artery to pulmonary vein fistulae (A-V F) are present.[13] It has been estimated that 60% of patients with A-V F suffer from familial telangiectasia.[14] Radiographically, these anomalies appear as single or multiple round or oval densities up to several centimeters in diameter, especially in the lower and medial lung fields (Fig. 33-1). Although the diagnosis may be inferred by identification of the feeding artery and existing vein, by changes in the size of a mass on fluoroscopy during Valsalva or Müller maneuvers, or by increasing intrapulmonary shunt with higher lung volumes,[15] definite diagnosis entails arteriography. Obviously, the presence of telangiectasia elsewhere in the body aids in diagnosis. Significant but relatively uncommon manifestations include cyanosis, erythremia, hemoptysis, and brain abscess. Other findings include dyspnea on exertion, clubbing, and local bruits that increase with inspiration. Symptoms, when present, usually appear in the second or third decade.[1] Surgical

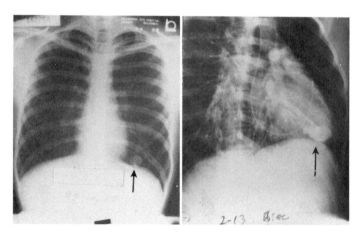

FIG. 33-1. Pulmonary arteriovenous fistula, left lower lobe. **A,** Two cm nodule at left base. **B,** Oblique film after injection of pulmonary artery with contrast medium. *(Courtesy Medical Illustration Service, Colorado General Hospital, Denver, Colorado.)*

intervention may be required for hemoptysis or high-output congestive heart failure (see Fig. 33-1).

Anomalies of the thorax

PECTUS EXCAVATUM

This anomaly of the thoracic cage is marked by depression of the lower sternum and the adjacent costal cartilages. The lowest point typically is at the junction of the xiphoid process and the body of the sternum. Because of its appearance the anomaly has also been termed *funnel chest*.

The pathogenesis is unclear, although it is felt that developmental anomalies of the diaphragm play a major role in this deformity. This disorder tends to be familial. Many such patients are asymptomatic, although complaints of limited exercise capacity and difficulty in coughing are common. The cosmetic defect creates significant psychological complications in some subjects. Other findings include functional heart murmurs, cardiac arrhythmias, and right axis deviation on the ECG. The chest radiograph may show displacement of the heart to the left, occasionally producing the erroneous impression of cardiomegaly. If the patient is significantly symptomatic or psychologically burdened by this disorder, surgical correction may be considered but is seldom functionally beneficial.

PECTUS CARINATUM

This disorder is marked by a midline or lateral protrusion of the anterior chest wall. An accompanying disproportionate growth of ribs produces an arcuate protrusion. Because of the prominent anterior profile of the chest the disorder has also been called *pigeon breast*. Symptoms include limited exercise tolerance and impaired cough, but these are usually less severe than with pectus excavatum. If symptoms or psychological ramifications are severe, surgical correction may again be considered, but with only occasional physiologic or cosmetic benefit.

REFERENCES
1. Landing, B.H., and Dixon, L.G.: Congenital malformations and genetic disorders of the respiratory tract (larynx, trachea, bronchi, and lungs), Am. Rev. Respir. Dis. **120**:151, 1979.
2. Flye, M.W., and Izant, R.J.: Extralobar pulmonary sequestration with esophageal communication and complete duplication of the colon, Surgery **71**:744, 1972.
3. DeParedes, C.G., Pierce, W.S., Johnson, D.G., et al.: Pulmonary sequestration in infants and children: a 20-year experience and review of the literature, J. Pediatr. Surg. **5**:136, 1970.
4. Ranninger, K., and Valvassori, G.E.: Angiographic diagnosis of intralobar pulmonary sequestration, Am. J. Roentgenol. **92**:540, 1964.

5. Wier, J.A.: Congenital anomalies of the lung, Ann. Intern. Med. **52:**330, 1960.
6. Rogers, L.F., and Osmer, J.C.: Bronchogenic cyst: a review of 46 cases, Am. J. Roentgenol. **91:**273, 1964.
7. Kent, D.C.: Physiologic aspects of idiopathic unilateral hyperlucent lung, with a review of the literature, Am. Rev. Respir. Dis. **90:**202, 1964.
8. Weg, J.G., Krumholz, R.A., and Hackleroad, L.F.: Unilateral hyperlucent lung: a physiologic syndrome, Ann. Intern. Med. **62:**675, 1965.
9. Prowse, O.M., Fuchs, J.E., Kaufman, S.A., et al.: Chronic obstructive pseudoemphysema: a rare cause of unilateral hyperlucent lung, N. Engl. J. Med. **271:**127, 1964.
10. Reid, L., Simon, G., Zorab, P.A., et al.: The development of unilateral hypertransradiancy of the lung, Br. J. Dis. Chest **61:**190, 1967.
11. Stokes, D., Sigler, A., Khouri, N.F., et al.: Unilateral hyperlucent lung (Swyer-James Syndrome) after severe mycoplasma pneumoniae infection, Am. Rev. Respir. Dis. **117:**145, 1978.
12. Frye, R.L., Marshall, H.W., Kincaid, O.W., et al.: Anomalous pulmonary venous drainage of the right lung into the inferior vena cava, Br. Heart J. **24:**696, 1962.
13. Hodgson, C.H., Burchell, H.B., Good, C.A., et al.: Hereditary hemorrhagic telangiectasia and pulmonary arteriovenous fistula: survey of a large family, N. Engl. J. Med. **261:**625, 1959.
14. Gomes, M.R., Bernatz, P.E., and Dines, D.E.: Pulmonary arteriovenous fistulas, Ann. Thorac. Surg. **7:**582, 1969.
15. Huseby, J.S., Culver, B.H., and Butler, J.: Pulmonary arteriovenous fistulas: increase in shunt at high lung volume, Am. Rev. Respir. Dis. **115:**229, 1977.

Chapter 34

PULMONARY DISEASES OF UNKNOWN ETIOLOGY

Michael D. Iseman

ALVEOLAR PROTEINOSIS

Pulmonary alveolar proteinosis (PAP) was first described in 1958.[1] This disease is characterized by extensive accumulation of an amorphous proteinaceous material within the distal air spaces of the lungs. Little, if any, disruption of the normal airway, air space, or vascular architecture occurs. The alveolar filling, when extensive, produces shunting and an increased risk of pulmonary infections, including those due to such opportunistic organisms as *Nocardia*. The disease typically afflicts adults between 20 and 50 years of age, although patients at both extremes of age are also seen. Patients may contact the physician if PAP is detected on routine chest radiograph or because of cough, breathlessness, diminished exercise tolerance, or the symptoms of a complicating infection. The chest radiograph typically reveals bilateral symmetric infiltrates that are widespread but most prominent in the perihilar regions (Fig. 34-1). The shadows are usually alveolar in quality with a variable reticular or interstitial component. The air bronchogram effect may be quite prominent. The classic picture is often quite suggestive of pulmonary edema; however, the absence of vascular redistribution, cardiomegaly, pleural effusions, and typical signs and symptoms are useful in excluding the latter. Mediastinal lymphadenopathy does not occur. Abnormal physical findings include diffuse rales; cyanosis and/or clubbing may also be present. Spirometry may often be normal in the beginning but may show a restrictive pattern later in the course. Arterial blood gases usually reveal impaired oxygen transport with resultant hypoxemia.

An increased shunt fraction (Qs/Qt > 14%) coupled with an elevated serum LDH level in a patient with diffuse lung disease is suggestive of

314

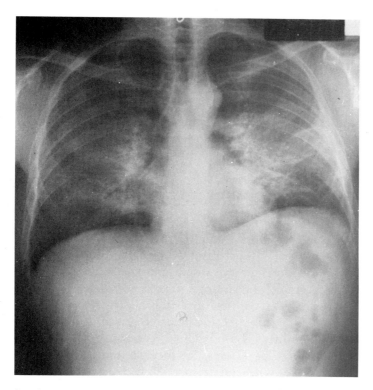

FIG. 34-1. Alveolar proteinosis: note "soft" fluffy shadows with air bronchogram and normal-sized heart. The process is diffuse here, but may be quite localized. *(Courtesy Medical Illustration Service, Veterans Administration Hospital, Denver, Colorado.)*

PAP, but both false-positive and false-negative findings occur.[2] Diagnosis of PAP may be supported further by characteristic findings in material recovered from the lung by segmental lavage.[3] These findings include (1) few alveolar macrophages, (2) large acellular eosinophilic bodies on a background of eosinophilic granules, and (3) proteinaceous material positive on stain by periodic acid–Schiff and negative to alcian blue. Confirmation of the diagnosis may be obtained by transbronchial or open lung biopsy.

Analysis of the material that fills the air spaces indicates that it is a lipoprotein similar to surfactant. It is speculated that proteinosis may reflect overproduction of a surfactantlike substance by the type II alveolar epithelial cells.[4,5] Recently, however, a striking increase in the concentration of immunoglobulin protein was also found in lavage effluents in six patients with PAP; it is possible that altered immunity plays a primary role in the pathogenesis of this disorder.[6]

Treatment consists of lung lavage with normal saline solution and chest percussion to facilitate the removal of the abnormal material from the air spaces and thus improve ventilation.[7,8] Aggressive diagnosis and management of superinfection are critical to the survival of the patient with PAP. Corticosteroids are of no benefit and are probably contraindicated because of increased risk of infection and the theoretic possibility that they may increase production of the sufactantlike material. Prognosis is quite variable but prolonged improvement and survival have been reported.[9]

PULMONARY ALVEOLAR MICROLITHIASIS

This is an extremely rare disorder characterized by deposition within the alveolar spaces of very small calcific spherules. The strong familial pattern emphasizes distribution among siblings, not between parent and child. Pathogenetic mechanisms remain unclear.[9] Early in the course of the disease the normal lung architecture is not disturbed, but progressive interstitial fibrosis with obliteration of the airways and vascular bed is likely to occur as the disease advances. Signs and symptoms are infrequent early in the illness, but dyspnea, cyanosis, clubbing, and cor pulmonale develop later. The disease has been noted in all age groups. Diagnosis may be made with great precision from the chest radiograph alone—it shows a diffuse, finely granular, extremely discrete dense micronodulation. In the beginning this may produce a diffuse hazy quality to the film, while later it may appear almost milky white. No effective treatment is known.

GOODPASTURE'S SYNDROME

Goodpasture's syndrome was first described in 1919. It is characterized by pulmonary hemorrhage and glomerulonephritis. It usually afflicts young adults, predominantly males. It typically is heralded by hemoptysis, associated with dyspnea on exertion, fatigue, malaise, fever, chills, and cough progressing over several weeks. The chest manifestations are followed by the onset of glomerulonephritis that, when untreated, usually progresses to uremia and death within 4 to 5 months.[10,11]

The chest radiograph typically reveals patchy, evanescent densities in the perihilar and lower lung zones, presumably the result of episodes of pulmonary hemorrhage. Reticular densities may evolve as well; these are believed to be caused by the incorporation of blood pigment within the interstitium. Other laboratory abnormalities include progressive anemia, proteinuria, hematuria, urinary casts, and the presence of hemosiderin-laden macrophages in the sputum.

The etiology and pathogenesis of this disorder are not clearly understood. Epidemiologic and anecdotal data suggest that some cases may be related to influenzal infection.[12] Immunohistologic studies have indicated that the majority of cases of Goodpasture's syndrome involve complement-fixing, cell-bound antibodies directed against basement membrane located within the lung and glomerulus of the kidney (the type II or cytotoxic immune reaction).

Diagnosis may be strongly inferred from the clinical presentation. Lung biopsy demonstrating linear deposition of IgG along the alveolar basement membrane or renal biopsy showing the typical picture of glomerular basement membrane immunoglobulin deposition confirms the diagnosis. The possibility of Goodpasture's syndrome without overt renal disease has been raised[13] and questioned.[14,15]

The differential diagnosis of pulmonary disease with hemorrhage and nephritis includes (1) Wegener's granulomatosis and related disorders, (2) polyarteritis nodosa, (3) systemic lupus erythematosis, (4) acute bacterial pneumonia with associated nephritis, (5) uremia with uremic pneumonitis or congestive heart failure, and (6) variant Goodpasture's syndrome—an entity similar to the classic syndrome in which a granular or lumpy pattern is seen, rather than a linear deposition of immunoglobulin along the glomerular or alveolar basement membrane, suggesting circulating immune complex disease. Studies in a few patients have, in fact, demonstrated circulating antibodies to glomerular basement membrane.[16]

The outcome in patients with Goodpasture's syndrome has been unfavorable, with death from renal failure or pulmonary hemorrhage usually occurring within a few months of onset. However, favorable outcome has recently been reported following bilateral nephrectomy,[17] treatment with massive doses of corticosteroids,[18] plasma exchange and immunosuppressive therapy,[19] and therapy with prednisone and cyclophosphamide.[20]

IDIOPATHIC PULMONARY HEMOSIDEROSIS

This disorder is characterized by recurrent pulmonary hemorrhages that may be manifest as hemoptysis and/or recurrent transient shadows on the chest radiograph. The disease characteristically afflicts the young but may also involve older adults. With continued hemorrhage, an iron-deficiency anemia develops because of a loss of iron in the sputum and deposition of iron in the interstitium of the lung where it is unavailable for hemoglobin synthesis. The disease typically follows an indolent course, with waxing and waning of the pulmonary hemorrhagic activity. Gradually, pulmonary fibrosis and hemosiderosis may result in restrictive lung dysfunction and the development of chronic cor pulmonale. In the beginning the chest film shows only the patchy air space densities associated with acute hemorrhage; however, as the disease continues, diffuse reticular markings appear. Clinically, patients complain of cough, hemoptysis, and fatigue. The physical findings are nonspecific; cyanosis, clubbing, and hepatosplenomegaly usually are late manifestations. Lymphadenopathy may be present in younger patients. Laboratory findings include variable iron-deficiency anemia and hemosiderin-laden macrophages in the sputum (a nonspecific finding associated with bleeding within the lung, most useful when the patient has radiographic infiltrates without a clear history of hemoptysis). Diagnosis usually requires lung biopsy. Histologic findings are *nonspecific*, that is, indistinguishable from any pulmonary hemorrhage by conventional studies. It is this absence of diagnostic features (e.g., vasculitis, inflammation, necrosis, granulomas, or immunologic abnormalities) combined with the clinical picture that constitute the diagnostic criteria for this disorder.[21] No therapy is presently available.

PULMONARY HISTIOCYTOSIS X

This complex includes Letterer-Siwe disease, Hand-Schüller-Christian (HSC) disease, and eosinophilic granuloma (EG). Because of overlapping clinicopathologic features and transitions from one form to another, these three diseases are generally regarded as part of a spectrum called histiocytosis X (HX). It should be noted that the features of EG are most common in patients with this disorder complex and that some physicians choose to refer to all these diseases as EG. The basic underlying mechanism is an inflammatory-type proliferation of the histiocytes (as opposed to the lipid storage–or metabolic-type histiocytoses).

Morphologically, the lung lesions appear initially as granulomatous infiltration of the interstitium and bronchial walls; the predominant cells are histiocytes, although eosinophils, lymphocytes, plasmacytes, and giant cells are usually present. Later, as the disorder progresses, coarse fibrotic changes may ensue, resulting in the nonspecific pattern of honeycomb lung.

Clinically, patients with HX may show a wide variety of manifestations including dyspnea, nonproductive cough, weight loss, fever, spontaneous pneumothorax, diabetes insipidus, and even asymptomatic detection on routine radiography. The disease typically appears in young adults, with a strong male preponderance. Physical findings are rarely helpful but may include painful bony lesions or exophthalmos. Results of pulmonary function tests show progressive restriction and impairment of diffusion.[22,23]

Radiographically, the early manifestations include a diffuse nodular infiltrate that, *unlike* many other interstitial processes, tends to be greater in the upper lung zones (see Fig. 34-2). As the disease advances the infiltrate changes to reticulonodular and then to coarse, destructive honeycombing. Notable is the tendency of the lungs in HX to retain their normal volume longer than in other interstitial, restrictive disorders. The diagnosis is suggested by the finding of a diffuse interstitial process in associa-

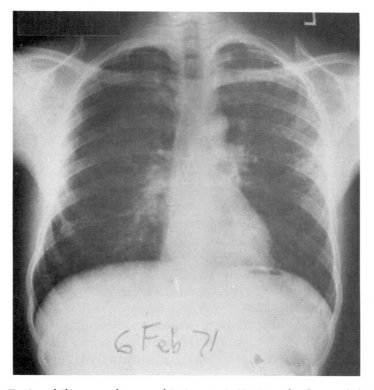

FIG. 34-2. Eosinophilic granuloma or histiocytosis X. Note the fine nodulation, some linear stranding, and the right-sided pneumothorax. *(Courtesy Medical Illustration Service, Veterans Administration Hospital, Denver, Colorado.)*

tion with spontaneous pneumothorax, bony lesions, diabetes insipidus, or exophthalmos. The similarities between this disorder and lymphangioleiomyomatosis (interstitial infiltrates, restrictive physiologic derangements, unusual preservation of lung volume on chest film, and increased risk of pneumothorax) should be noted. Some form of lung biopsy is necessary for confirmation.

The natural history of HX is variable. Agreement is lacking regarding the most appropriate treatment. However, a trial of glucocorticoid therapy seems justified, particularly in the early stages of the disease. Death typically results from progressive hypoxemia and consequent cor pulmonale.

LYMPHANGIOLEIOMYOMATOSIS

Lymphangioleiomyomatosis (LAM) is a rare disease affecting women in their childbearing years. It is manifested by an accumulation of atypical smooth muscle along the lymphatics of the lung, thorax, and abdomen.[24] The common clinical features include dyspnea, recurrent pneumothorax, hemoptysis, and chylous pleural effusions. The chest radiographic findings are variable. Initially, the film may be normal or show only a pleural effusion. Subsequently, diffuse reticulonodular shadows appear; as the process advances this reticulation becomes coarser, resulting in a striking honeycomb appearance. Pneumothorax may occur at any stage but is most common late in the course of the disease. An unusual, if not diagnostic, feature of the chest film of patients with LAM is the appearance of normal or increased lung volume in the presence of extensive, reticular, honeycomb shadows (see Histiocytosis X). This seeming radiographic paradox has its physiologic counterpart in the finding of severe, mixed obstructive and restrictive derangements. Typical findings include (1) reduced vital capacity by spirometry yet normal or increased volume by plethysmography (2) markedly reduced flow rates, and (3) grossly depressed diffusing capacity. The obstructive changes probably result from compromise of the conducting airways by exuberant growth of the atypical smooth muscle; this may also produce severe air trapping, focal emphysema, and a resultant risk of pneumothorax. Restriction results from both parenchymal destruction and pleural reaction. Hemoptysis is thought to result from occlusion of pulmonary veins. The striking reduction in diffusion is probably due to loss of alveolar membranes and V/Q imbalance.

The prognosis in LAM is unfavorable; patients typically have a slow progression over 2 to 10 years with death secondary to respiratory failure. Palliative therapy in the form of pleural decortication, surgical or chemical pleural symphysis, and thoracic duct ligation (to control chylothorax) may be considered. Corticosteroids are ineffective. Hormonal manipulation would appear an attractive avenue of investigation in LAM.

PULMONARY ANGIITIS AND GRANULOMATOSIS[25]

A number of rare idiopathic lung diseases are similar in their clinical and radiographic features, sharing to a variable degree vascular involvement and granulomatous changes on histologic examination. These include Wegener's granulomatosis, lymphomatoid granulomatosis, benign lymphocytic angiitis and granulomatosis, necrotizing sarcoid granulomatosis and bronchocentric granulomatosis.

Wegener's granulomatosis

First noted in 1936, Wegener's granulomatosis (WG) is an uncommon disorder that generally involves the upper respiratory tract, lungs, and kidneys. It occurs in all ages and both sexes, with a modest male preponderance. The pathologic features of WG consist of necrotizing giant cell granulomas with accompanying vasculitis and a focal segmental glomerulonephritis (not all glomeruli are involved and only portions of involved glomeruli are abnormal). Although classic WG usually includes the triad above, it may appear in a limited form in which only the lungs are involved[26]; on the other hand, organs in addition to the triad may be involved, including the CNS, the orbital structures, the middle ear, the peripheral joints, the skin, and the heart. Controversy exists as to whether WG is ever limited to the *upper* respiratory tract or whether this disorder, so-called *midline granuloma* (MG), is a distinct clinicopathologic entity. The pattern of involvement of the upper respiratory tract, as well as the sparing of the organs commonly involved by WG, suggests that MG should be regarded as a unique disorder. In addition, the accepted contemporary therapy for MG (local high-dose irradiation) differs considerably from that for WG (systemic chemotherapy).[27,28]

The clinical manifestations of WG are variable, although the typical course commences with sinusitis (nasal discharge, sometimes purulent from bacterial superinfection, pain, mucosal ulceration, and fever). Pulmonary symptoms and signs (cough, hemoptysis, or pleurisy) typically follow, although they may be simultaneous with or precede the upper respiratory changes. Constitutional symptoms such as fever, weakness, and weight loss are common. Renal disease usually becomes apparent after the respiratory tract illness; rarely, it may antedate respiratory manifestations.

The radiographic features of WG of the lung are not diagnostic but, taken in the context of other clinical findings, may be valuable in suggesting the diagnosis. Notable are the following features of the pulmonary infiltrates: bilateral, multiple, nodular or diffusely infiltrative, small or large, tendency to cavitate, transient but not usually fleeting, and infrequent and small pleural effusions. Hilar lymphadenopathy and reticular infiltrates are uncommon (see Fig. 34-3).

Originally believed to be universally lethal, contemporary management of WG with cytotoxic agents has resulted in high rates of remission. It is not clear which agents are best, although cyclophosphamide and chlor-

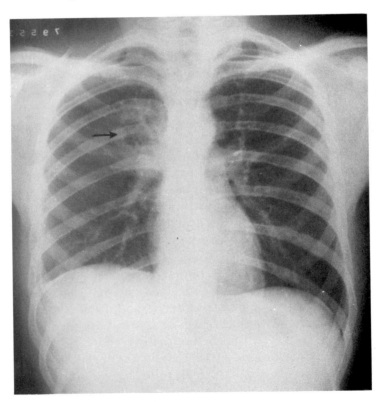

FIG. 34-3. Wegener's granulomatosis: 3 × 4 cm cavity in right upper lobe infiltrate, plus right pleural reaction. *(Courtesy Medical Illustration Service, Veterans Administration Hospital, Denver, Colorado.)*

ambucil are both effective.[28-31] Steroid therapy is apparently not only ineffective but possibly hazardous.

The inciting causes of WG are unknown; however, the histopathologic features of the kidneys suggest that the renal component is caused by immune complex deposition.[29]

Lymphomatoid granulomatosis

Lymphomatoid granulomatosis (LG) is clinically similar to WG. However, due to distinct differences in therapy and prognosis, it is important to distinguish between the two.[25,30,31] LG is a systemic angiocentric granulomatous vasculitis with a highly atypical lymphoreticular infiltrate ("lymphomatoid"). The lungs are almost universally involved with the variable abnormalities seen in the kidneys, skin, CNS, and peripheral nerves. Patients with LG typically are middle-aged (men or women) with cough, phlegm, fever, and dyspnea. The chest radiographic abnormalities most commonly seen are bilateral lower zone, softly marginated, floccular shadows that initially resemble bronchopneumonia sparing the hilar areas. These subsequently evolve toward more discrete nodose shadows that resemble metastatic soft tissue tumors. These shadows fluctuate in size and cavitate in about half the cases. Renal abnormalities are also found in nearly half the cases; the lesions generally are a focal granulomatous vasculitis without frank glomerulonephritis, as is seen in WG; also, renal failure is not a common finding in LG.

Response to therapy in LG is considerably less predictable than in WG. Although Israel contends that LG does not respond to chemotherapy,[31] Fauci suggests that, early in the course of the illness when only the lungs and skin are involved, patients respond well to cyclophosphamide.[30] Fauci further suggests that, in view of the fact that up to 25% of patients with LG eventually manifest a frank lymphoproliferative malignancy, consideration should be given to aggressive combined chemotherapeutic regimens similar to those used successfully in various lymphomas.[25] An interesting case of LG associated with retroperitoneal fibrosis and impaired cell-mediated immunity was reported in 1977.[32]

Benign lymphocytic angiitis and granulomatosis

Benign lymphocytic angiitis and granulomatosis (BLAG) is a putative entity similar to both WG and LG.[31] In a series of 11 patients the disease was largely restricted to the lungs (1 patient also had skin manifestations). The radiographic pattern is similar to WG and LG, typically consisting of multiple nodular shadows of variable size, often with cavitation. Histologically, BLAG is marked by richly cellular lesions composed of mature lymphocytes, plasma cells, and histiocytes. Israel contends that BLAG responds particularly well to chlorambucil. However, Fauci suggests that BLAG may indeed be an early or partial form of LG and that cyclophosphamide may be more efficacious and may prevent evolution of BLAG to the more ominous disorder, LG.[30]

Necrotizing sarcoid granulomatosis

In his 1972 review of pulmonary angiitis and granulomatosis, Liebow included the entity of necrotizing sarcoid granulomatosis (NSG).[25] He questioned at the time whether it was a necrotizing angiitis with sarcoid reaction or sarcoidosis with necrosis of the granulomas and vessels. The chest radiographic findings included multiple nodules ranging from miliary to large masses, ill-defined infiltrates, and—in 1 of 11 patients—hilar adenopathy. Typically, the patients complained of fever, sweats, malaise, cough, and pleuritic pain. Liebow considered the designation NSG a provisional one, speculating that it might only prove to be a variant of sarcoidosis. In 1975 Churg and colleagues reviewed 12 cases of NSG and concluded that the disorder did not behave like the other angiocentric granulomatoses, that it was a counterpart of nodular sarcoidosis, and that patients with NSG could be left untreated or treated with steroids alone; the one death in their series occurred in a patient treated with cyclophosphamide.[33]

Bronchocentric granulomatosis

In contrast to the other granulomatoses described above, which center on the pulmonary vessels, bronchocentric granulomatosis (BG) as described by Liebow primarily involves the airways, with vascular injury seemingly incidental to this process.[25] Further in contrast, extrapulmonary manifestations have not been reported. Pulmonary and constitutional symptoms seem less prominent with BG than with the other granulomatoses; instead, patients have an unpredictable collection of complaints including asthma, cough, purulent nasal discharge, migratory chest pain, and recurrent pneumonia. Some patients are asymptomatic. Noteworthy is the absence of fever. The radiographic findings also are quite variable, with both unilateral and bilateral shadows, migratory infiltrates over months and years, patterns in some suggestive of pneumonia or atelectasis, nodular or acinar shadows in others, and the appearance of hilar adenopathy in a few patients. In some patients the radiographic abnormalities appear to respond well to limited courses of steroids, although recurrence seems to be common. Diagnosis is usually made by biopsy.

REFERENCES

1. Rosen, S.H., Castleman, B., and Liebow, A.A.: Pulmonary alveolar proteinosis, N. Engl. J. Med. **258**:1123, 1958.
2. Martin, R.J., Rogers, R.M., and Myers, N.M.: Pulmonary alveolar proteinosis. Shunt fraction and lactic acid dehydrogenase concentration as aids to diagnosis, Am. Rev. Respir. Dis. **117**:1059, 1978.
3. Martin, R.J., Coalson, J.J., Rogers, R.M., et al.: Pulmonary alveolar proteinosis: the diagnosis by segmental lavage, Am. Rev. Respir. Dis. **121**:819, 1980.
4. Ramirez, J., and Harlan, W.R., Jr.: Pulmonary alveolar proteinosis: nature and origin of alveolar lipid, Am. J. Med. **45**:502, 1968.
5. Larson, R.K., and Gordinier, R.: Pulmonary alveolar proteinosis: report of six cases, review of the literature, and formulation of a new therapy, Ann. Intern. Med. **62**:292, 1965.
6. Bell, D.Y., and Hook, G.E.R.: Pulmonary alveolar proteinosis: analysis of airway and alveolar proteins, Am. Rev. Respir. Dis. **119**:979, 1979.
7. Kao, D., Wasserman, K., Costley, D., et al.: Advances in the treatment of pulmonary alveolar proteinosis, Am. Rev. Respir. Dis. **111**:361, 1975.
8. Rogers, R.M., Levin, D.C., Gray, B.A., et al.: Physiologic effects of bronchopulmonary lavage in alveolar proteinosis, Am. Rev. Respir. Dis. **118**:255, 1978.
9. Sosman, M.C., Dodd, G.D., Jones, W.D., et al.: The familial occurrence of pulmonary alveolar microlithiasis, Am. J. Roentgenol. **77**:947, 1957.
10. Benoit, F.L., Rulon, D.B., Theil, G.B., et al: Goodpasture's syndrome: a clinicopathologic entity, Am. J. Med. **37**:424, 1964.
11. Proskey, A.J., Weatherbee, L., Easterling, R.E., et al.: Goodpasture's syndrome: a report of five cases and review of the literature, Am. J. Med. **48**:162, 1970.
12. Wilson, C.B., and Smith, R.C.: Goodpasture's syndrome associated with influenza A2 virus infection, Ann. Intern. Med. **76**:91, 1972.
13. Mathew, T.H., Hobbs, J.B., Kalowski, S., et al.: Goodpasture's syndrome: normal renal diagnostic findings, Ann. Intern. Med. **82**:215, 1975.
14. Poskitt, T.R.: Goodpasture's syndrome (letter to editor), Ann. Intern. Med. **83**:283, 1975.
15. Bolton, W.K.: Goodpasture's syndrome (letter to editor), Ann. Intern. Med. **83**:284, 1975.
16. Martinez, J.S., and Kohler, P.F.: Variant "Goodpasture's syndrome"? The need for immunologic criteria in rapidly progressive glomerulonephritis and hemorrhagic pneumonitis, Ann. Intern. Med. **75**:67, 1971.
17. Nowakowski, A., Grove, R.B., King, L.H., et al.: Goodpasture's syndrome: recovery from severe pulmonary hemorrhage after bilateral nephrectomy, Ann. Intern. Med. **75**:243, 1971.
18. deTorrente, A., Popovtzer, M.M., Guggenheim, S.J., et al.: Serious pulmonary hemorrhage glomerulonephritis, and massive steroid therapy, Ann. Intern. Med. **83**:218, 1975.
19. Lockwood, C.M., Rees, A.J., Pearson, T.A., et al.: Immunosuppression and plasma-exchange in the treatment of Goodpasture's syndrome, Lancet **1**:711, 1976.
20. Teichman, S., Briggs, W.A., Knieser, M.A., et al.: Goodpasture's syndrome: two cases with contrasting early course and management, Am. Rev. Respir. Dis. **113**:223, 1976.
21. Thomas, H.M., and Irwin, R.S.: Classification of diffuse intrapulmonary hemorrhage (Editorial), Chest **68**:483, 1975.
22. Nadeau, P.J., Ellis, F.H., Jr., Harrison, E.G., Jr., et al.: Primary pulmonary histiocytosis X, Dis. Chest **37**:325, 1960.
23. Smith, M., McCormack, L.J., Van Ordstrand, H.S., et al.: "Primary" pulmonary histiocytosis X, Chest **65**:176, 1974.
24. Carrington, C.B., Cugell, D.W., Gaensler, E.A., et al.: Lymphangioleiomyomatosis. Physiologic-pathologic-radiologic correlations, Am. Rev. Respir. Dis. **116**:977, 1977.
25. Leibow, A.A.: The J. Burns Amberson lecture—Pulmonary Angiitis and Granulomatosis, Am. Rev. Respir. Dis. **108**:1, 1973.
26. Carrington, C.B., and Liebow, A.A.: Limited forms of angiitis and granulomatosis of Wegener's type, Am. J. Med. **41**:497, 1966.

27. Fauci, A.S., Johnson, R.E., and Wolff, S.M.: Radiation therapy of midline granuloma, Ann. Intern. Med. **84:**140, 1976.

28. Israel, H.L., and Patchefsky, A.S.: Treatment of Wegener's granulomatosis of lung, Am. J. Med. **58:**671, 1975.

29. Wolff, S.M., Fauci, A.S., Horn, R.G., et al.: Wegener's granulomatosis, Ann. Intern. Med. **81:**513, 1974.

30. Fauci, A.S.: Granulomatous vasculitides: distinct but related (letter to editor), Ann. Intern. Med. **87:**782, 1977.

31. Israel, H.L., Patchefsky, A.S., and Saldana, M.J.: Wegener's granulomatosis, lymphomatoid granulomatosis, and benign lymphocytic angiitis and granulomatosis of lung. Recognition and treatment, Ann. Intern. Med. **87:**691, 1977.

32. Hammar, S.P., Gortner, D., Sumida, S., et al.: Lymphomatoid granulomatosis: association with retroperitoneal fibrosis and evidence of impaired cell-mediated immunity, Am. Rev. Respir. Dis. **115:**1045, 1977.

33. Churg, A., Carrington, C.B., and Gupta, R.: Necrotizing sarcoid granulomatosis, Chest **76:**406, 1979.

Chapter 35

RESPIRATORY IMPAIRMENT/ DISABILITY EVALUATION

Lawrence H. Repsher

Definitions and criteria

Permanent pulmonary *impairment* refers to the decrement noted on various pulmonary function tests performed on a patient who is receiving optimal therapy for any chronic lung disease that is not anticipated to improve either spontaneously or after therapy. Pulmonary *disability* refers to this impairment's effect on an individual's ability to function at work and at home, taking into account sex, age, environment, job work requirements, education, availability of other work, and state of physical fitness.[1] The physician should be cognizant of many of these factors and may have an opinion regarding disability, but the ultimate decision on disability should be made by an independent administrative or judicial authority.

In assessing a person's impairment of work capacity due to chronic pulmonary disease, one should use the same general criteria for all patients rather than specific criteria for individual diseases, for example, coal worker's pneumoconiosis or byssinosis.[2] Specific diagnoses often have administrative importance concerning disability, for example, public health concerns with certain infectious diseases such as tuberculosis, rapidly progressive diseases such as lung cancer, and inherently unstable diseases such as labile bronchial asthma. However, these administrative concerns should not influence the assessment of an individual's current impairment or work capacity. The emphasis should be on estimating the individual's residual capacity for work rather than how much of the patient's original capacity has been lost.[3] The latter implies a precise knowledge of the patient's prior level of pulmonary function and work capacity, which, in most cases, is not available.

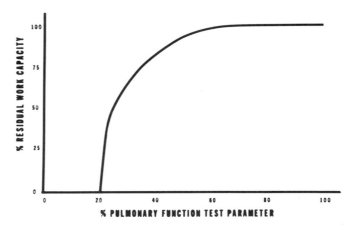

FIG. 35-1. Relationship between pulmonary impairment and residual work capacity.

Relationship between pulmonary impairment and residual work capacity

The relationship between the results of various pulmonary function tests and an individual's work capacity varies considerably from test to test and is often complex. However, this relationship is generally described by some variation of the curve demonstrated in Fig. 35-1. At maximum exercise capacity, the average healthy person is using only 60% to 70% of his or her MVV. Therefore, a substantial loss of ventilatory capacity must occur before overall work capacity is significantly reduced. After this substantial pulmonary reserve has been lost, overall work capacity progressively deteriorates. Death often occurs when residual pulmonary function drops to 10% or less of the predicted normal value.

Relative predictive value of residual work capacity of various pulmonary function tests

Some pulmonary function tests are of more value than others in predicting residual work capacity.[4,5] Many tests are too sensitive; these include frequency dependency of compliance, the closing volume, and measurements of Raw. Although effective in detecting mild or early pulmonary disease, these tests have little use in determining the severity of pulmonary impairment. The chest radiograph,[6] arterial blood gases at rest,[4] and the ECG[5] have also been found to have poor correlation with residual work capacity.

On the other hand, some tests have been found to have substantial predictive value for residual work capacity. Probably the best of these are the FEV_1 and the single breath D_{LCO}.[4,7] It is not surprising that these tests have significant predictive value. The primary function of the lungs in enabling the body to perform muscular work is to take up oxygen from the atmosphere and diffuse it to the hemoglobin of the pulmonary capillary blood. An essential reciprocal function is the removal of carbon dioxide from the pulmonary capillary blood and its excretion into the atmosphere. In this process chronic pulmonary disease can cause rate-limiting interference with lung function at two points[8,9]: disease that primarily affects the conducting airways of the lungs, reducing overall ventilatory capacity (reflected in the FEV_1), and disease that interferes with the diffusion of gases between the alveoli and the hemoglobin of the pulmonary capillary blood (reflected in the single breath D_{LCO}). Chronic pulmonary disease frequently impairs both these measures of pulmonary function. However, in individual cases, relatively pure impairment of the gas transfer function (interstitial lung disease [ILG]) or relatively pure impairment of the ventilatory function of the lungs (bronchial asthma) can occur.

Development of a predictive equation for residual work capacity in the presence of chronic pulmonary disease

A significant factor causing decreased residual work capacity is the effect of normal aging.[10] Any equation using only a percentage of predicted value penalizes the older worker.[3] The amount of work required to accomplish a given task remains constant, yet physiologic work capacity deteriorates significantly as one grows older. Therefore, the older worker must work at a progressively higher percentage of his or her maximum work capacity.[8]

It has been demonstrated that if one selects a parameter for the ventilatory function of the lungs—the MVV—and a parameter for the gas transfer function of the lungs—the oxygen ventilation equivalent (Vo_2)—a linear relationship exists between these parameters and the maximum steady state aerobic capacity. Taking this one step further, my colleagues and I have added the parameter of age to a ventilatory function parameter (FEV_1) and to a gas transfer parameter (single breath D_{LCO}). We have demonstrated a remarkably good linear relationship between these parameters and symptom-limited Vo_2 max and power output max.[11] Unfortunately, the range in metabolic equivalents (METS) between the ability to sustain heavy work as described by Roemmich et al.[9] (7.5 METS) and the levels indicating total disability for any work stated in the Social Security Administration's handbook for physicians[12] (approximately 5.0 METS) is very narrow. The standard error of our equation is approximately 1.2 METS,[11] which creates a significantly large gray zone of imprecision concerning an individual's ability to perform a job of specific, mean metabolic, and power demands.

Power output is often expressed as kilopond-meters per minute, that is, the power required to raise 1 kg the distance of 1 m against the force of gravity in 1 minute. Further, although the relationship between aerobic capacity and power output is linear in a given individual and has a mean slope of approximately 100 kpm/min power output per 1 MET of oxygen consumption in a large group of individuals, the slope of this linear relationship varies strikingly among individuals, particularly among those with COPD.[11] The slope of this relationship can vary from 20 kpm/min power output per MET of oxygen consumption to 200+ kpm/min power output per MET of oxygen consumption. Therefore, in any given individual, the physician cannot accurately predict the maximum work capacity when knowing only maximum aerobic capacity.

History, physical examination, and laboratory investigations

The history and physical examination should describe in detail all pulmonary symptoms and signs exhibited by the patient, mentioning all relevant negatives. It should also detail current and prior exercise tolerance and rate of deterioration, if any, and describe any and all occupational or environmental exposures in detail, including intensity and duration of each exposure as well as the severity and duration of any symptoms noted at the time or immediately after such exposures. The physician should obtain the results, if possible, of previous relevant medical evaluations, such as preemployment physical and insurance examinations and physician and/or hospital records of previous physiologic testing. The examining physician should strive to determine the diagnosis of the pulmonary condition and any coexistent disease, especially heart disease, and the etiology of the pulmonary and coexistent diseases. The patient's current and prior smoking history should be described in detail as well as any other substance abuse of potential clinical relevance.

Also important are current and past exercise habits, past and present therapeutic management, and, finally, the patient's cooperation during examination and physiologic testing. Further, the examining physician should attempt to determine whether each of the patient's diseases are probably, possibly, or indeterminately related to his or her occupational or environmental exposures. Finally, a statement should be made on the prognosis of both the pulmonary and any coexisting diseases.

Before the examination and testing the patient should be receiving optimal tolerated therapy, be clinically as stable as possible, and have fully recovered from any intercurrent pulmonary or systemic illnesses. Patients with a highly unstable pulmonary disease, such as labile bronchial asthma, require a detailed description of the frequency and severity of attacks as well as a list and dosages of all medications and a description of any and all therapeutic complications. Patients with a rapidly deteriorating pulmonary condition such as bronchogenic cancer require a statement describing the rate of progression of the tumor and a description of any and all complications from the tumor and its therapy. An appropriate battery of laboratory investigations should be applied in order to determine as accurately as possible the diagnosis, appropriate therapy, necessary public health or industrial hygiene measures, and the presence or absence of common diseases in other systems that may affect work capacity, for example, ischemic heart disease or anemia. If industrial asthma is suspected, spirometry should be obtained before and after both work and exercise.

Rating of work impairment due to chronic pulmonary disease

Despite the previously described complexities, one can say with reasonable medical probability that an individual whose FEV_1 and single breath D_{LCO} are 80% percent or more of predicted value should be capable, from a pulmonary standpoint, of performing virtually any kind of work, even that requiring sustained, heavy exertion.[9] On the other hand, one can also say with reasonable medical probability that an individual whose FEV_1 or single breath D_{LCO} is less than 40% of predicted value has sufficient pulmonary impairment to make him or her incapable of performing all but the most sedentary of jobs.[7] These latter patients are frequently limited not only by metabolic job requirements, but by the metabolic and power requirements of getting to and from work.

The V_{O_2} max and power output max can be estimated from the following equations: V_{O_2} max in METS and/or power output in hundreds of kpm/min equals three times the fraction of predicted FEV_1 plus two times the fraction of the predicted single breath D_{LCO} minus age in years divided by 12.[11]

$$\text{METS and/or kpm/min} \times 100 = \frac{FEV_1 m}{FEV_1 p} \times 3 + \frac{D_{LCO}^m}{D_{LCO}^p} \times 2 - \frac{Age}{12}$$

Those individuals who have normal pulmonary function, that is, 80% or more of predicted value for FEV_1 and D_{LCO},[2] will generally achieve 8 METS or 800 kpm/min or more[11] and are probably fit for almost any job. Rare exceptions include persons with an extraordinarily physically demanding job or those suffering primarily from pulmonary vascular disease. Individuals with values of these two tests under 40% of predicted value will generally have a V_{O_2} max of less than 4.5 METS or a power output max of less than 450 kpm/min; they are probably unfit for any but the most sedentary of jobs.[7] Those patients whose estimated V_{O_2} max falls between 4.5 and 8.0 METS and/or those with estimated power output between 450 and 800 kpm/min need further evaluation, which should include (1) exercise testing—preferably on a treadmill while monitoring a 12-lead ECG, (2) arterial oxygen saturation, and (3) expired gases.[10] The patient is then exercised to his symptom-limited Vo_2 max and power output max; 40% of the symptom-limited Vo_2 max is then related to the mean metabolic or power output requirements of his specific job. If the average metabolic and power requirements of the job required more than 40% of the symptom-limited Vo_2 max and power output max, the patient would then be considered unfit from a pulmonary standpoint to continue in that job.[10]

Other indications for exercise testing include dyspnea out of proportion to the measured FEV_1 and single breath D_{LCO}, the suspicion of significant underlying heart or pulmonary vascular disease, the specific request of the claimant, respondent, administrative, or judicial authority, and the failure of the claimant to cooperate with the spirometric and diffusing capacity testing. Contraindications to exercise testing include, among others, recent myocardial infarction, severe heart disease, ominous arrhythmias, severe or uncontrolled hypertension, severe neuromuscular disease, or interfering severe orthopedic problems.

In addition to the diagnosis, etiology, and prognosis of the chronic pulmonary disease, the physician rating an individual's residual work capacity should state whether the patient can physiologically and medically return to his or her usual job and recommend restrictions, if any. If the patient is unable to return to his or her usual job, the physician should indicate jobs for which the patient could be retrained and any required follow-up, especially additional or repeated physiologic and other testing. Finally, the physician should recommend, if appropriate, how the patient's co-workers could prevent similar cases of chronic pulmonary disease.

• • •

This testing system is sensitive enough to include all individuals who are enough impaired so that they cannot comfortably perform their jobs, yet it is specific enough to exclude all those who are still able to perform their jobs comfortably despite a chronic pulmonary disease that has caused some permanent pulmonary functional impairment. Further, the majority of patients can be evaluated reliably, yet inexpensively, with widely available equipment. Relatively few patients will require further evaluation at a regional exercise testing facility.

REFERENCES

1. Richman, S.I.: Meanings of impairment and disability, Chest **78**:367, 1980.
2. Sharpe, I.K., and Tomashefski, J.F.: The physician's role in the evaluation of disability due to pulmonary disease. Clin. Respir. Dis. **17**:3, 1979.
3. Cotes, J.E.: Assessment of disablement due to impaired respiratory function, Bull. Physiopathol. Respir. **11**:210, 1975.

4. Musk, A.W., Bevan, C., Campbell, M.D., and Cotes, J.E.: Factors contributing to the clinical grade of breathlessness in coal workers with pneumoconiosis, Bull. Europ. Physiopathol. Respir. **15:**343, 1979.

5. Morgan, W.K.C.: Disability or disinclination? Chest **75:**712, 1979.

6. Lyons, J.P., Ryder, R., Campbell, H., and Gough, J.: Pulmonary disability in coal worker's pneumoconiosis, Brit. Med. J. **1:**713, 1972.

7. Epler, G.R., Ray, A.S., and Gaensler, E.A.: Determination of severe impairment (disability) in interstitial lung disease, Am. Rev. Respir. Dis. **121:**647, 1980.

8. Armstrong, B.W., Workman, J.N., and Hurt, H.H., Jr.: Clinicophysiologic evaluation of physical working capacity in persons with pulmonary disease, Am. Rev. Respir. Dis. **93:**90, 223, 1966.

9. Roemmich, W., Blumenfeld, H.L., and Moritz, H.: Evaluating remaining capacity to work in miner applicants with simple pneumoconiosis under 65 years of age under Title IV of public law 91-173, Ann. N.Y. Acad. Sci. **200:**608.

10. Astrand, P.O.: Quantification of exercise capability and evaluation of physical capacity in man, Prog. Cardiol. Dis. **19:**51, 1976.

11. Repsher, L.H., unpublished data.

12. Disability evaluation under social security: a handbook for physicians, DHEW pub. no. (SSA) 79-10089 23, Washington, DC, 1979, U.S. Department of Health, Education and Welfare.

Appendix A

CHECKLIST FOR READING CHEST FILMS

1. Verify right as opposed to left side as follows: observe stomach bubble and shape and position of left border and aorta; note identifying differences in ribs and parenchyma; note marker on film.
2. Was film taken at full inspiration, or is it a full or partial expiration film?
3. Soft tissues of neck and chest wall: air, foreign objects; calcifications; sinus tracts.
4. Bones and joints: old or recent fractures; degree of calcification; notching of upper and under margin of ribs; moth-eaten areas; cervical ribs; deformities.
5. Aorta: size; shape; calcification; tortuosity.
6. Trachea: position; patency; note normal narrowing at larynx and normal slight deviation to right at aorta.
7. Heart: size, shape; straight left border, calcified valves; prostheses; mediastinal air; cardiophrenic angles; double contour; enlarged atrium.
8. Hilums: pulmonary arteries—main and branches; enlarged nodes; calcium; egg-shells; relationship right versus left; left hilum normally slightly above right.
9. Costophrenic angles.
10. Hemidiaphragms: right hemidiaphragm normally slightly above left; scalloping; "adhesions"; calcific plaques.
11. Parenchyma: character of abnormal shadows, that is mottled; stringy, homogeneous, clear, or vague margins; calcific, spicular radiations; air bronchogram; silhouette sign; interstitial as opposed to alveolar infiltrates; vascularity or bronchovascular markings.
12. Obliques: posterior ribs can be identified as horizontal; anterior ribs run diagonally; abnormal shadows can be located as anterior or posterior by tendency to remain in relationship to one or the other in two different views.
13. Lateral view: substernal space; sternum; retrocardiac area (hiatal hernia); spine.

Appendix B

GLOSSARY OF TERMS IN RESPIRATORY PHYSIOLOGY

a arterial

A alveolar

Aa P_{O_2} difference $P_{A_{O_2}} - Pa_{O_2}$.

alveolar CO_2 tension (PA_{CO_2}) Usually equals arterial CO_2 tension, Pa_{CO_2}.

alveolar O_2 tension (PA_{O_2}) $= (P_B - 47) - PA_{CO_2} - PA_{N_2}$.

arterial O_2 tension (Pa_{O_2}) Depends on hemoglobin dissociation curve and lung function.

CO_2 output (V_{CO_2}) Depends on metabolic rate and ventilation.

compliance of lung ($\triangle V/\triangle P_{pl}$) $\triangle V$ = change in lung volume or depth of one breath; $\triangle P_{pl}$ = intrapleural pressure change with breathing.

D_L_{CO} Diffusing capacity using end-tidal P_{CO} for PA_{CO}.

diffusing capacity (D_L_{CO}) V_{CO}/PA_{CO}; also called transfer factor.

forced expiratory volume (FEV) Fast (1 sec) VC—liters of flow in first second (FEV_1).

maximum breathing capacity (MBC) or **maximum voluntary ventilation (MVV)** Total expired flow during 15 sec vigorous hyperventilation reported in L/min.

maximum midexpiratory flow (MMEF) Flow rate of midhalf of fast VC; reported in L/sec.

O_2 uptake (V_{O_2}) Depends on metabolic rate and blood flow.

resistance to gas flow ($\triangle P/V$) $\triangle P$ = alveolar-to-mouth gas pressure difference; V = total flow rate.

ventilation-perfusion ratio (V/Q) Usually refers to regional gas and blood flows.

vital capacity (VC) Maximum volume that can be expired after full inspiration.

Appendix C

RECOMMENDED TEXTS AND JOURNALS

TEXTS

Bates, D.V.: Respiratory function in disease: an introduction to the integrated study of the lung, ed. 2, Philadelphia, 1971, W.B. Saunders Co.

Baum, G.L., editor: Textbook of pulmonary diseases, ed. 2, Boston, 1974, Little, Brown & Co.

Ciba Foundation: Pulmonary structure and function: a symposium, Boston, 1962, Little, Brown & Co.

Comroe, J.H., Forster, R.E., DuBois, A.B., et al.: The lung: clinical physiology and pulmonary function tests, ed. 2, Chicago, 1962, Year Book Medical Publishers, Inc.

Cotes, J.E.: Lung function: assessment and application in medicine, ed. 2, Oxford, England, 1968, Blackwell Scientific Publications.

Crofton, J., and Douglas, A.: Respiratory diseases, Oxford, England, 1969, Blackwell Scientific Publications.

Deeley, T.J., editor: Carcinoma of the bronchus, New York, 1971, Appleton-Century-Crofts.

Filley, G.F.: Pulmonary insufficiency and respiratory failure, Philadelphia, 1967, Lea & Febiger.

Fraser, R.G., and Paré, J.A.P.: Diagnosis of diseases of the chest: an integrated study based on the abnormal roentgenogram, Philadelphia, 1970, W.B. Saunders Co.

Hinshaw, H.C.: Diseases of the chest, ed. 3, Philadelphia, 1969, W.B. Saunders Co.

King, E.J., and Fletcher, C.M., editors: Industrial pulmonary diseases, Boston, 1960, Little, Brown & Co.

Liebow, A.A., and Smith, D.E., editors: The lung, Baltimore, 1968, The Williams & Wilkins Co.

Medlar, E.M.: The behavior of pulmonary tuberculous lesions: a pathological study, Am. Rev. Tuberc. **71**(3), pt. 2, 1955.

Pepys, J.: Hypersensitivity diseases of the lungs due to fungi and organic dusts, Basel, Switzerland, 1969, S. Karger.

Petty, T.L.: Intensive and rehabilitative respiratory care: a practical approach to the management of acute and chronic respiratory failure, Philadelphia, 1971, Lea & Febiger.

Reid, L.: The pathology of emphysema, London, 1967, Lloyd-Luke (Medical Books) Ltd.

Spencer, H.: Pathology of the lung, excluding pulmonary tuberculosis, ed. 2, New York, 1968, Pergamon Press, Inc.

Sykes, M.K., Campbell, E.J.M., and McNicol, M.W.: Respiratory failure, Philadelphia, 1969, F.A. Davis Co.

Tsuboi, E.: Atlas of transbronchial biopsy: early diagnosis of peripheral pulmonary carcinomas, Stuttgart, Germany, 1971, Georg Thieme.

336

JOURNALS

American Review of Respiratory Disease
British Journal of Diseases of the Chest
Chest
Journal of Thoracic and Cardiovascular Surgery
Revue de la Tuberculose
Scandinavian Journal of Respiratory Diseases
Seminars in Respiratory Medicine
Thorax
Tubercle

Am. Thor. Soc., and Am. Coll. Chest. Phys.: Pulmonary terms and symbols, Chest **67**:583-593, 1975.

INDEX